HEMATOLOGY:
A PATHOPHYSIOLOGIC
APPROACH

MOSBY PHYSIOLOGY SERIES

HEMATOLOGY: A PATHOPHYSIOLOGIC APPROACH

MOSBY PHYSIOLOGY SERIES

S. David Hudnall, MD

Professor Emeritus
Pathology and Laboratory
Medicine
Yale University School of
Medicine
New Haven, Connecticut

2nd **EDITION**

ELSEVIER

Elsevier
1600 John F. Kennedy Blvd.
Ste 1800
Philadelphia, PA 19103-2899

HEMATOLOGY: A PATHOPHYSIOLOGIC APPROACH, SECOND EDITION   ISBN: 978-0-323- 59583-4

Notice

Previous Edition copyrighted 2012

Content Strategist: Marybeth Thiel
Content Development Specialist: Marybeth Thiel
Content Development Manager: Marybeth Thiel
Publishing Services Manager: Shereen Jameel
Project Manager: Haritha Dharmarajan
Design Direction: Ryan Cook

Printed in India

Last digit is the print number: 9 8 7 6 5 4 3 2 1

Working together to grow libraries in developing countries

www.elsevier.com • www.bookaid.org

In loving memory of my parents Stanley and Marjorie Hudnall

To my wife Amy and children Katie and Molly

Significant changes have been made in the second edition of the text *Hematology: A Pathophysiologic Approach*. Chapters have been extensively revised to reflect advances in our understanding of hematologic physiology and pathophysiology, with extra coverage of iron metabolism, the complement system, and the genetics of acute myeloid leukemia. To assist students, many new figures and tables have been included, along with color photomicrographs of normal and abnormal histology. To meet educational needs, each chapter is followed by a set of thought-provoking multiple-choice review questions and answers.

Hematology: A Pathophysiologic Approach is designed as an introductory hematology text for all students and trainees, including medical students, biomedical graduate students, pathology residents, and fellows in hematology/oncology and hematopathology. This book is based on my 26 years of experience practicing laboratory hematology and teaching hematology to medical students, residents, fellows, and graduate students at four medical schools in the United States. The idea of writing a textbook crystallized during my years as course director of an innovative 2-year, small-group, problem-based course in hematology at the University of Texas Medical Branch (UTMB) in Galveston. At that time, I was disappointed by the choice of hematology textbooks suitable for medical students. Over the years we tried several texts, and although some were quite good, both faculty and students expressed dissatisfaction with one thing or another. The possibility of writing a textbook suddenly became a reality when I was approached by Elsevier to write a hematologic physiology text for their Physiology Series—an opportunity that I gladly accepted.

It is important to state what this text is not. It is not a comprehensive textbook of clinical hematology. Clinical hematology is a vast, complex field that, to be thoroughly and expertly covered, requires many authors, many pages, and tracts of up-to-date references. To meet this demand, several excellent, large, and generously referenced textbooks written by multiple expert contributors are available. However, these textbooks are not appropriate as introductory texts. They are far too detailed, often presuming strong prior knowledge of basic anatomy and physiology of the hematologic system.

The text you are about to read is radically different. It is written by a single author and contains no references. Although some expert advice was sought, I have for the most part been able to draw on my own experience as a course designer and director and as a teacher of hematology to present a single unified overview of the field. Because reference materials are readily available on the Internet, I decided not to clutter the text with references that are seldom used by students. Instead, students interested in more depth of any topic can easily access the most recent literature online.

This is a book that first and foremost approaches hematology from a pathophysiologic perspective, with mechanistic explanations of normal and abnormal function. Hematopoiesis, blood physiology, immunology, neoplasia, transplantation, and hemostasis are presented as interrelated subjects. Because the practice of hematology is highly dependent on a relatively large number of diagnostic laboratory tests, fairly detailed descriptions of blood counting, histopathology, immunohistochemistry, flow cytometry, cytogenetics, and coagulation testing are provided. Numerous color photomicrographs of both normal and abnormal histology are also provided in full color.

Over many years of teaching hematology and designing and directing a hematology course, I have formulated a good idea of what students need to know about this complex subject. But with the primary goal of imparting an understanding of the subject by the student in mind, I have done my best to resist the temptation to assume that if I present the material, it will be understood. To this end, I have always encouraged students to question the material and contact me directly with their questions. Over the years, this has proven to be immensely valuable. Literally hundreds of insightful questions received from students have challenged me to provide more accurate, lucid explanations of difficult topics. In other cases, questions have led to my discovery that some facts we take for granted may be flawed, incomplete, or illogical. Based on this experience, I have tried to anticipate many of the issues that often lead to confusion and to provide a more explicit explanation than is usually offered. But because perfection is an elusive goal, I urge all readers of this text, whether expert or novice, to contact me with your questions, corrections, or concerns. With your help, the text can be continually improved.

I sincerely hope you enjoy the book.

S. David Hudnall, MD

PREFACE TO THE SECOND EDITION

Changes made to the second edition include many updates, additions, and corrections of the first edition. Updates include more extensive coverage of the diagnostics, genetics, and chemotherapy of myeloid neoplasms. Additions include more extensive coverage of the complement system, allergic hypersensitivity response, iron metabolism, and hemolysis, with new descriptions of netosis, familial Mediterranean fever, Job syndrome, cytokine storm, WHIM syndrome, and CHIP. Also, students are provided with study questions and answers for each chapter.

The second edition of this well-regarded single-authored text offers students at all levels an up-to-date comprehensive review of the field of hematologic pathophysiology.

S. David Hudnall, MD

ACKNOWLEDGMENTS

I would like to thank some special people who have played important roles in furthering my understanding of the science and practice of hematology and in bringing this book to life.

The list rightly begins with my late father-in-law, Abner H. Levkoff, MD, who unselfishly shared his interest in physiology, read the first drafts of the text, and provided me with incisive critiques and sage advice.

I am very grateful to my early mentors in immunology and hematology, Drs. Abul Abbas and Faramarz Naeim, for providing me with a strong foundation to build on.

Many thanks to my former colleagues at UTMB, Drs. Jack Alperin, David Bessman, Tarek Elghetany, and Frank Gardner, for their collective expertise regarding selected topics in hematology.

I would also like to thank my good friends and colleagues, Drs. Rolf Konig, Malcolm Brodwick, and Peter Rady, for their invaluable opinions about academic life, biomedical science, and the joys and challenges of teaching medical and graduate students.

And of course, thanks go to the hundreds of second-year medical students at UTMB, who took the course in hematology during my tenure as a course director, for all your wonderful questions—questions that always begged for more lucid answers and sometimes highlighted the incompleteness of our knowledge.

And finally, I would like to thank Marybeth Thiel, Haritha Dharmarajan, and other members of the editorial staff at Elsevier for their expert assistance in making the extensive changes to both text and figures in this new second edition of *Hematology: A Pathophysiologic Approach*. Without them, the book simply would not have seen the light of day.

CONTENTS

HEMATOLOGY:
A PATHOPHYSIOLOGIC APPROACH

MOSBY PHYSIOLOGY SERIES

Brief Overview of the Hematolymphoid System

Hematology is the medical science that deals with all things blood. Blood is a non-Newtonian fluid composed of liquid plasma and suspended blood cells. The volume of blood in the normal adult human is approximately 5 L, of which about 55% (v/v) is plasma and 45% cells.

Plasma is a slightly alkaline (pH, 7.4) saline solution (0.9% sodium chloride) containing about 8% proteins, lipids, amino acids, glucose, hormones, and metabolic waste products (including carbon dioxide, urea, bilirubin, uric acid, and lactic acid). The four most abundant plasma proteins are albumin, gamma globulins, transferrin, and fibrinogen, in that order. Albumin maintains blood volume by contributing to the colloid oncotic pressure and serving as a carrier protein for a large variety of hydrophobic molecules, including fat-soluble hormones, vitamins, unconjugated bilirubin, and fatty acids. The gamma globulin fraction of serum protein is largely composed of immunoglobulin (antibody) (IgG > IgA > IgM > IgD > IgE). **Transferrin** is the major iron transport protein, and fibrinogen is the most abundant coagulation factor. Although most plasma proteins are produced by the liver, **gamma globulins** are produced by B cell–derived plasma cells.

Serum, the residual fluid obtained from clotted blood, is essentially plasma depleted of fibrinogen and other coagulation proteins.

Peripheral blood obtained by venipuncture is usually drawn into glass tubes with or without anticoagulant (ethylenediaminetetraacetic acid [EDTA], citrate, or heparin). Blood drawn into tubes without anticoagulant forms a clot, leaving residual serum, the preferred substrate for most clinical laboratory tests. Blood drawn into tubes with anticoagulant does not clot and provides a source of whole blood for laboratory tests such as complete blood count, erythrocyte sedimentation rate, and Coombs test; plasma (after high-speed centrifugation to remove all cellular elements) for coagulation tests; and platelet-rich plasma (after low-speed centrifugation to remove **red blood cells [RBCs]** and leukocytes) for platelet function testing.

Blood volume is largely controlled by the kidneys in response to changes in renal arterial pressure. Specialized smooth muscle cells in the walls of the renal afferent arterioles called juxtaglomerular cells secrete the enzyme **renin** in response to decreased arterial pressure. Renin converts plasma angiotensinogen to **angiotensin** I, which is rapidly converted to angiotensin II by pulmonary endothelial cells. Angiotensin II increases arterial pressure by inducing systemic arteriolar vasoconstriction and inhibiting salt and water excretion by the kidneys.

Blood osmolarity is indirectly controlled by hypothalamic osmoreceptors that induce secretion of **antidiuretic hormone** (**ADH**, also known as vasopressin) from specialized neurons of the posterior hypothalamus in response to hyperosmolar (concentrated) extracellular fluid. ADH rapidly increases water reabsorption by the renal collecting ducts, thus increasing plasma volume and decreasing osmolarity. ADH secretion is also stimulated by decreased plasma volume, detected by atrial stretch receptors, and carotid, aortic, and pulmonary artery baroreceptors.

Blood cell formation (**hematopoiesis**) begins in the embryonic yolk sac and later migrates to the liver and spleen in a developing fetus. By birth, hematopoiesis has moved to the **bone marrow**, a fatty, highly vascular tissue found in the spaces within spongy bone in the interior of the central skeleton. The marrow contains rare hematopoietic stem cells, their numerous progeny, and supportive stromal cells.

Stromal cells include endothelial cells that line the vascular spaces, adventitial reticular cells that lay down the extracellular reticulin fiber scaffolding of the marrow, adipocytes (fat storage cells), macrophages that serve both as scavengers and as iron-rich nurse cells for developing erythroid precursors, osteoblasts (bone-forming cells), and osteoclasts (bone-resorbing cells).

Hematopoietic stem cells are pluripotential and are capable of proliferation and differentiation into erythroid, myelomonocytic, lymphoid, megakaryocytic, and stromal cell lineages. Proliferation, differentiation, and maturation of the various cell lineages occurs in response to small glycoproteins produced by a variety of cells and tissues termed **hematopoietic growth factors (cytokines)** that bind to cytokine receptor–bearing marrow cells. The hematopoietic cytokines include stem cell factor, interleukin (IL-3, IL-5, IL-7), **erythropoietin (EPO)**, **granulocyte colony-stimulating factor (G-CSF)**, **monocyte colony-stimulating factor (M-CSF)**, and **thrombopoietin (TPO)**.

The most abundant blood cells (~5 million/μL of blood) are the red RBCs or erythrocytes. RBCs contain the cytoplasmic oxygen-binding protein hemoglobin that is responsible for oxygen delivery from the lungs to other tissues. RBC production in the marrow is regulated by EPO, the renal synthesis of which is stimulated by low oxygen tension. The normal function of RBCs depends on the oxygen-carrying capacity of heme, an iron-containing tetrapyrrole contained within the hemoglobin molecule. Dietary iron is absorbed by the duodenum and transferred to the marrow by the iron-binding protein transferrin.

The second most abundant (~300,000/μL of blood) and smallest blood cells are the **platelets**. Platelets are produced by cytoplasmic budding of marrow megakaryocytes. Platelets express receptors for adhesion to regions of vascular damage and, after being activated, serve as the nidus for clot formation. Far less numerous but no less important are the **leukocytes**, or white blood cells (~5000/μL of blood). Unlike RBCs and platelets, most leukocytes spend only a small fraction of their lives in the blood, instead remaining in reserve within the marrow or spleen or rapidly entering other tissues to mature and perform their allotted functions.

Leukocytes are primed to respond to all variety of noxious materials, including infectious agents, foreign proteins (allergens), and cell debris. There are five leukocyte types, each with a particular function: **neutrophils**, **lymphocytes**, **monocytes**, **eosinophils**, and **basophils**, in that order of abundance in blood. One marrow leukocyte type, **mast cells**, do not normally circulate in the blood. Mast cells are found in perivascular tissues, where they help maintain vascular integrity by producing **heparin**.

Granulocytes, defined as blood leukocytes with prominent cytoplasmic granulation (neutrophils, eosinophils, and basophils), enter the blood from marrow fully mature and ready for action. Granulocytes rapidly enter inflamed tissues and contribute to the inflammatory response to infection, trauma, and allergic reactions by phagocytosis and granule release.

In contrast to granulocytes, most lymphocytes leave the marrow in an immature state. Immature **T cells** (precursor T lymphoblasts) released from the marrow rapidly migrate to the thymus, where they undergo selection and maturation into one of several T-cell subsets—CD4+ T-helper cells, CD4+ suppressor T cells, CD8+ cytotoxic T cells, CD4/CD8− gamma-delta T cells, and so on—before migrating to lymphoid tissues as mature antigen-specific T cells.

Natural killer (NK) cells are released from the marrow as fully functional cytotoxic lymphoid cells that recognize and kill abnormal cells, including virus-infected cells and tumor cells.

Unlike immature T cells, immature **B cells** that leave the marrow are antigen specific but naïve, not having yet encountered antigen in peripheral lymphoid tissues. Naïve B cells rapidly migrate from marrow to lymph nodes and spleen, where they first encounter antigen bound to dendritic cells, and with help from follicular T-helper cells, they undergo antigen-driven proliferation and affinity maturation in germinal centers. After germinal center maturation is complete, mature B cells differentiate into either antibody-secreting **plasma cells** or long-lived **memory B cells**.

Similar to lymphocytes, monocytes leave the marrow as immature cells and rapidly enter peripheral tissues, where they undergo cytokine-mediated maturation into a variety of highly specialized phagocytic **macrophages** and antigen-presenting **dendritic cells**.

Megakaryocytes are large cells with polyploid nuclei that normally reside only in the bone marrow. In response to the liver-derived cytokine TPO, megakaryocytes release small cytoplasmic fragments known as **platelets** into the circulation. Platelets maintain vascular integrity by binding to sites of vascular damage and, in conjunction with plasma coagulation factors, minimizing blood loss by forming blood clots.

Blood coagulation is usually triggered by adhesion of platelets to subendothelial **collagen** and **von Willebrand factor** and release of **tissue factor** from damaged endothelium. Tissue factor triggers a cascading series of enzymatic reactions (involving plasma coagulation factors produced mostly by the liver) that take place on the surface of adherent platelets and damaged endothelial cells, leading to **thrombin** activation, **fibrin** deposition, and clot formation. The mature clot is a platelet–fibrin meshwork that adheres to the site of vascular damage. After vascular repair, enzymatic digestion of the clot by the thrombin-activated fibrinolytic protease **plasmin** leads to clot resorption.

KEY WORDS AND CONCEPTS

- Angiotensin
- Antidiuretic hormone (ADH)
- Basophils
- B cells
- Blood coagulation
- Blood osmolarity
- Blood volume
- Bone marrow
- Collagen
- Cytokines
- Dendritic cells
- Eosinophils
- Erythropoietin (EPO)
- Fibrin
- Gamma globulins
- Granulocyte colony-stimulating factor (G-CSF)
- Granulocytes
- Hematopoiesis
- Hematopoietic growth factors
- Hematopoietic stem cells
- Heparin
- Leukocytes
- Lymphocytes
- Monocyte colony-stimulating factor (M-CSF)
- Macrophages
- Mast cells
- Megakaryocytes
- Memory B cells
- Monocytes
- Natural killer (NK) cells
- Neutrophils
- Plasma
- Plasma cells
- Plasmin
- Platelets
- Red blood cells (RBCs)
- Renin
- Serum
- Stromal cells
- T cells
- Thrombin
- Thrombopoietin (TPO)
- Tissue factor
- Transferrin
- von Willebrand factor

2

Hematopoiesis

KEY POINTS

- Hematopoiesis begins in the embryonal yolk sac and aorto-gonado-mesonephros (AGM), migrates to the fetal liver and spleen, and then moves to the bone marrow by birth.

- The nonhematopoietic marrow stroma provides a microenvironment conducive to growth and differentiation of hematopoietic cells.

- Hematopoietic marrow stem cells are small undifferentiated cells capable of both self-renewal and pluripotential differentiation.

- Growth and differentiating signals to hematopoietic cells are provided by both small protein cytokines released by stromal cells and by direct physical contact with marrow stroma.

- Pluripotential stem cells differentiate into common myeloid progenitors and common lymphoid progenitors under the influence of specific transcription factors, epigenetic factors, and cytokines.

- Myeloid stem cells differentiate into seven lineages: erythroid, neutrophilic, eosinophilic, basophilic,

- monocytic or dendritic, megakaryocytic, and mast cell or basophilic.

- Lymphoid stem cells differentiate into three lineages: B cell, T cell, and natural killer (NK) cell.

- Hematopoietic cells released from the marrow into the blood include erythrocytes, neutrophils, eosinophils, basophils, monocytes, platelets, immature B cells, immature T cells, and NK cells.

- Mast cells, megakaryocytes, and plasma cells do not normally circulate in the blood.

- Immature T and B cells rapidly migrate from the blood to extramedullary sites to complete the maturation process (T cell to the thymus, B cells to lymph nodes and spleen).

- Blood leukocytes are recruited to sites of inflammation by specific chemoattractant cytokines, known as chemokines, produced by a range of cell types.

- Blood leukocytes enter peripheral tissues by binding to activated endothelial cells and migrating through the vascular wall in a process termed *diapedesis*.

Pluripotential hematopoietic stem cells first develop from endothelial cells within the **embryonic yolk sac**, where they form erythroid blood islands. Embryonic red cells are large nucleated cells that contain **embryonic hemoglobin (hemoglobin Gower 1, hemoglobin Gower 2,** and **hemoglobin Portland**). Embryonic erythropoiesis in the yolk sac is followed by the appearance of nonerythroid progenitors in both the yolk sac and the **aorto-gonado-mesonephros (AGM) region** of the embryo. Progenitor cells from the yolk sac and AGM colonize the hepatic cords of the fetal liver and later the

red pulp of the spleen. Erythropoiesis predominates in the fetal liver and is associated with a switch from production of embryonic hemoglobin to fetal hemoglobin (**hemoglobin F**). The higher oxygen affinity of embryonic hemoglobin and hemoglobin F compared with adult **hemoglobin A** facilitates oxygen transport in the placenta from maternal blood to fetal blood.

Vascularization of intraosseous cartilage leads to formation of a well-vascularized cavity in the bones, known as the **bone marrow**. By week 20, hematopoietic cells from the fetal liver and spleen have migrated to the marrow. By birth, virtually all hematopoiesis takes place within the marrow, and hemoglobin F is steadily replaced by adult hemoglobin A and A$_2$. In young children, marrow production is found throughout the entire marrow space, including the long bones. In adults, marrow production is limited to the marrow space of the central axial skeleton, with the marrow space in peripheral bones of the extremities occupied primarily by fatty tissue.

The marrow contains many nonhematopoietic cells and a specialized extracellular matrix (ECM) that is collectively referred to as the **marrow stroma**. The stroma provides an environment conducive to stem cell growth and differentiation. Stromal cells include endothelial cells, adventitial cells, adipocytes, osteoblasts, osteoclasts, mast cells, and macrophages. The stromal ECM provides a physical site for binding of marrow stem cells. Stromal cells produce many of the growth factors required for marrow cell growth, including **stem cell factor (SCF)**, FMS-like tyrosine kinase 3 ligand (Flt-3 ligand), interleukin 6 (IL-6), interleukin 11 (IL-11), granulocyte colony-stimulating factor (G-CSF), and monocyte colony-stimulating factor (M-CSF). Growth factors produced by non-stromal cells include IL-1 (by monocytes and granulocytes); IL-3, IL-5, and granulocyte-monocyte colony stimulating factor (GM-CSF) (by T cells); erythropoietin (EPO) (by renal peritubular cells); and thrombopoietin (TPO) (by hepatocytes). These growth factors seldom act individually, instead acting synergistically to induce marrow cell growth and differentiation. Many growth factors bind to membrane receptors with inducible tyrosine kinase activity that trigger cell proliferation, activation, and differentiation. An example is **SCF receptor (CD117, c-kit)**, which is expressed by all hematopoietic stem cells. Many of these growth factors act not only to stimulate proliferation but also to inhibit programmed cell death (**apoptosis**).

Not all cytokines act on marrow cells to promote growth and differentiation. Instead, some cytokines inhibit hematopoiesis. Examples of **inhibitory cytokines** include IL-1, tumor necrosis factor (TNF), transforming growth factor beta (TGF-β), and interferon gamma (IFN-γ). These proinflammatory cytokines contribute to the marrow suppression seen in chronic inflammatory conditions.

Pathologic conditions caused by imbalances in hematopoietic cytokine production include anemia of renal failure caused by EPO deficiency, anemia of chronic disease (inflammation) caused by excess IL-1 and hepcidin, aplastic anemia caused by gamma interferon–mediated marrow suppression, and thrombocytopenia caused by TPO deficiency in chronic liver disease.

Hematopoietic stem cells undergo a process of stepwise differentiation from undifferentiated (multipotential) cells to fully differentiated (unipotential) cells. Multipotential stem cells can give rise to any marrow cell lineage. This process is largely controlled by differential binding of exogenous growth factors (secreted by numerous cell types, including marrow stromal cells, T cells, renal tubular cells, and hepatocytes) to growth factor receptors expressed by hematopoietic progenitor cells. Binding of growth factor ligands to cellular growth factor receptors leads to expression of nuclear transcription factors that activate lineage-specific gene expression. In addition to differentiation, growth factors (**cytokines**) acting at early stages of marrow cell differentiation induce cell proliferation. Thus, in general, progressive maturation is accompanied by a progressive increase in cell number.

Stem cells under the influence of growth factors SCF and TPO, and transcription factor ***Hox*** differentiate into common myeloid progenitors (CMPs), and stem cells under the influence of IL-7 and the transcription factor ***Ikaros*** differentiate into common lymphoid progenitors (CLPs). CMP respond to cytokines GM-CSF and G-CSF, GM-CSF, and M-CSF, SCF, or IL-5 by further differentiating into granulocytes, monocytes, mast cells, or eosinophils, respectively. Under the influence of cytokines IL-3 and TPO, CMP undergo differentiation into bilineal erythroid–megakaryocyte precursors that further differentiate into unilineal erythroid or megakaryocyte precursors induced by EPO or TPO, respectively. CLP respond to cytokines IL-2, IL-4, or IL-15 (among other factors), with further differentiation into T-cell, B-cell, or natural killer (NK) cell precursors, respectively (Figs. 2.1 and 2.2).

Hematopoietic stem cells are rare cells with the ability to self-renew and give rise to multilineage and unilineage progenitor cells. **Multilineage progenitor cells**, such as colony-forming unit–granulocytic-erythroid-monocytic-megakaryocytic cells (CFU-GEMM), can give rise to more than one type of lineage-committed precursor cell, whereas **unilineage progenitor cells**, such as colony-forming unit–erythroid (CFU-E) cells, give rise to only one type of precursor cell. Stem cells and progenitor cells are primitive undifferentiated

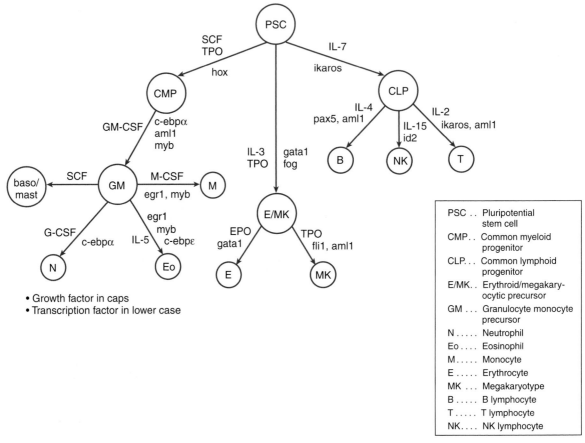

Fig. 2.1 Hematopoietic cytokines and transcription factors.

cells that display no identifiable morphologic features. Stem cells express specific cell surface proteins, including CD34, which mediates adhesion to marrow stroma; CD117 (c-kit), the SCF receptor that induces stem cell proliferation when bound by SCF (kit ligand, produced by endothelial cells); CD133, which induces development of cell membrane protrusions; and *c-mpl*, the TPO receptor that promotes stem cell growth.

In contrast to progenitor cells, **precursor cells** display lineage-specific morphologic and phenotypic features. For example, erythroid precursor cells contain hemoglobin-rich cytoplasm, myeloid precursor cells contain myeloperoxidase (MPO)–positive cytoplasmic granules, and megakaryocyte precursors display enlarged hyperlobated nuclei and cytoplasmic buds. Precursor cells also express lineage-specific molecules that can be exploited as phenotype markers when detected

with monoclonal antibodies by flow cytometry, immunohistochemistry, or cytochemistry. Examples include glycophorin A, CD71 (transferrin receptor), hemoglobin, and e-cadherin for erythroid precursors; CD13, CD33, MPO, and **alpha naphthyl acetate esterase (ANAE)** for myeloid precursors; CD41, CD61, and von Willebrand factor (VWF, factor VIII–related antigen) for megakaryocyte precursors; cytoplasmic CD3 (cCD3), CD7, and terminal deoxynucleotidyl transferase (TdT) for T cell precursors; CD19, paired box (PAX) protein 5 (PAX-5), cCD22, and TdT for B cell precursors; CD14, CD68, CD163, and **alpha naphthyl butyrate esterase (ANBE)** for monocyte precursors; and CD117 and mast cell tryptase for mast cell precursors (Table 2.1).

The normal bone marrow contains both stromal and hematopoietic elements (Fig. 2.3). Bone marrow cellularity can be determined by examination of a bone

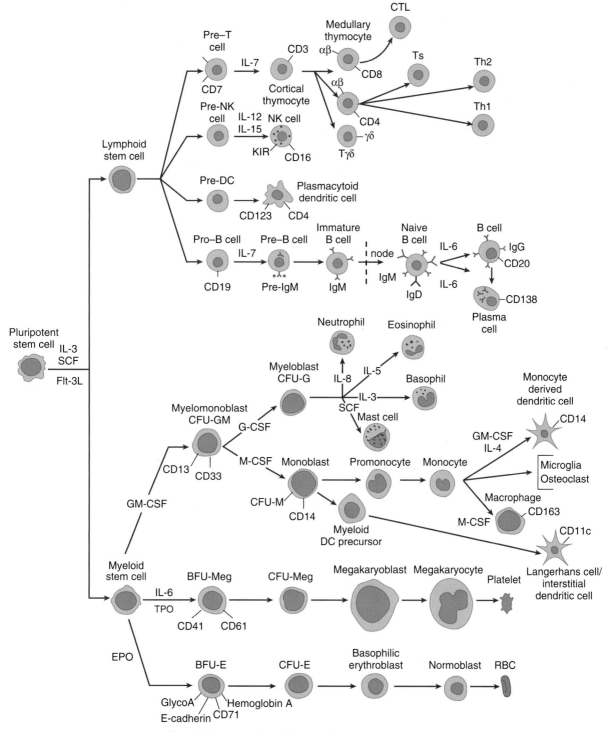

Fig. 2.2 Hematopoiesis. See text for abbreviations.

TABLE 2.1	Cell Types in Marrow Aspirates and Peripheral Blood Smears		
Cell Type	**Phenotype**	**Marrow (%)**	**Blood (%)**
Nucleated RBC	Glycophorin A, CD71, E-cadherin	23–32	0
Neutrophil	MPO, CD13, CD33, ANAE	45–52	40–60
Monocyte	CD14, CD163, ANBE	1–2	2–8
Eosinophil	Major basic protein	3	1–3
Basophil	Histamine	0–1	0–1
Megakaryocyte	CD41, CD61, VWF		0
Lymphocyte	CD3, CD7, CD4, CD8 (T cells)	14–16	20–40
	CD19, CD20, CD79a (B cells)		
	CD16, CD56 (NK cells)		
Plasmacytic	CD138, kappa, lambda	1–3	0

ANAE, Alpha naphthyl acetate esterase; *ANBE,* alpha naphthyl butyrate esterase; *MPO,* myeloperoxidase; *NK,* natural killer; *RBC,* red blood cell; *VWF,* von Willebrand factor.

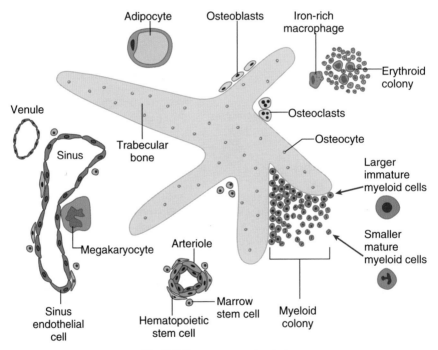

Fig. 2.3 Bone marrow structure.

marrow biopsy and aspirate. Bone marrow cellularity is calculated as the ratio of cellular marrow volume to fatty marrow volume. Normal iliac crest marrow cellularity in a newborn is 90%, with a steady reduction to 30% to 40% in older adults. The normal marrow is populated by myeloid and erythroid cells in approximately a 3:1 (myeloid predominant) ratio (Fig. 2.4).

Most myeloid cells are neutrophils, with scattered eosinophils, basophils, and mast cells (Fig. 2.5). In the normal marrow, most neutrophilic cells are mature (metamyelocytes, bands, and segmented neutrophils), with lesser numbers of myelocytes and promyelocytes. Myeloblasts (and stem cells) are rare cells in the normal marrow, accounting for no more than 3% of the

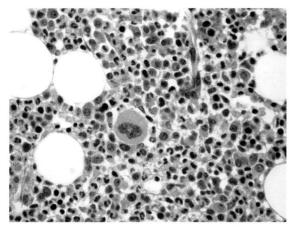

Fig. 2.4 Normal adult marrow biopsy (hematoxylin and eosin stained). Note the clear spaces that represent adipocytes removed by tissue processing and the large megakaryocyte at the left center. In this field, there is a predominance of myeloid cells with relatively few erythroid cells (small cells with dense basophilic nuclei).

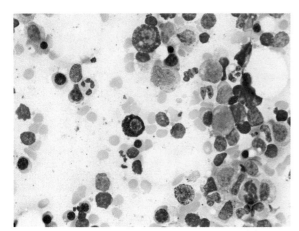

Fig. 2.5 Adult marrow aspirate smear with an eosinophil *(upper middle)*, mast cell *(center)*, and basophil *(lower middle)* (Wright-Giemsa stain).

marrow cell count. Lymphocytes account for 10% to 15% of the marrow cellularity in adults but in young children may account for up to 50%. Monocytes and promonocytes account for 2% to 3% of the marrow cellularity. Relatively few megakaryocytes (0.1%) are scattered throughout the normal marrow, often in proximity to vascular sinuses.

Under normal circumstances, only fully mature (enucleated) erythroid cells and myeloid cells are released into the bloodstream from the bone marrow (Fig. 2.6). Under stress conditions (e.g., infection, inflammation, blood loss, trauma), less mature cells are released into the blood. For example, acute bacterial infection leads to release of immature myeloid cells (band neutrophils, metamyelocytes, and myelocytes), and blood loss leads to release of reticulocytes and nucleated red cells. While mature erythrocytes remain in the bloodstream, myeloid cells (neutrophils, eosinophils, and basophils) and monocytes are recruited to inflamed tissues under the influence of a closely related group of chemoattractant cytokines known as **chemokines**. Chemokines are produced by a range of cell types, including endothelial cells, macrophages, T cells, fibroblasts, keratinocytes, and stromal cells.

Under normal conditions, neutrophils migrate from the blood to bronchial and intestinal submucosa, where they serve as first responders to infection. Blood neutrophils also rapidly migrate to localized sites of acute infection or injury. Intravascular neutrophils reside in two freely exchangeable pools: the circulating pool and the **marginal pool**. At any time, most intravascular neutrophils are not circulating, instead marginating along capillary and venular walls (the marginal pool) in the spleen and lungs. In response to infection or inflammation, cells within the marginal pool rapidly enter the

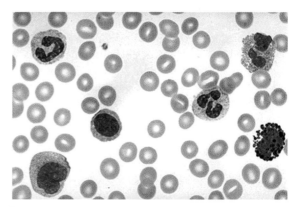

Fig. 2.6 Peripheral blood smear (Wright stained) with six leukocytes: band neutrophil *(upper left)*, eosinophil *(upper right)*, basophil *(lower right)*, monocyte *(lower left)*, lymphocyte *(middle left)*, and segmented neutrophil *(middle right)*. A single platelet is noted to the right of the band neutrophil. The remaining cells in the field are red blood cells.

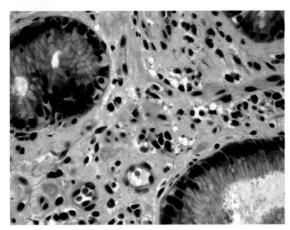

Fig. 2.7 Eosinophils and mast cells in the intestinal submucosa. Note the eosinophils with bright red cytoplasmic granules and the mast cells, small mononuclear cells with purple cytoplasm.

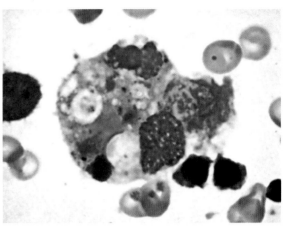

Fig. 2.8 Hemophagocytic histiocyte (macrophage) with abundant vacuolated cytoplasm and ingested cellular debris in hemophagocytic syndrome (bone marrow aspirate).

circulating pool. The total intravascular granulocyte pool (circulating and marginal) is supported by the marrow granulocyte reserve. This reserve, primarily composed of mature myeloid cells, is approximately 20 times larger than the blood granulocyte pool and capable of rapidly repleting the blood granulocyte pool in the face of infection or inflammation. The rapid migration of blood neutrophils into sites of inflammation is mediated by the chemokine IL-8 (CXCL-8) produced by activated macrophages.

Eosinophils and basophils in blood migrate to the submucosa of the aerodigestive tract (Fig. 2.7) and, like neutrophils, can migrate to other sites in response to inflammatory chemokines. Eosinophils are recruited to inflamed tissues by IL-5, eotaxin, and chemokine ligand 5 (CCL-5), and basophils are recruited by CCL-2 and CCL-5. Mast cells, unlike basophils, are not typically found in peripheral blood, instead homing to perivascular sites within a variety of connective tissues, including marrow stroma. Mast cells maintain vascular integrity by secretion of **heparin**, and like basophils, release the vasoactive factor **histamine** in response to allergens.

Many blood monocytes, like neutrophils, reside in the marginal pool and rapidly enter tissues to undergo further differentiation into several specialized cell types of the mononuclear phagocyte system, including histiocytes (macrophages), dendritic cells, osteoclasts, and microglial cells. Blood monocyte–derived macrophages are particularly numerous in organs such as the liver,

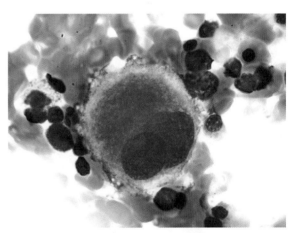

Fig. 2.9 A megakaryocyte is noted in the center of the field (marrow aspirate). Note the cytoplasmic blebs that will give rise to budding platelets.

spleen, lymph nodes, and lungs that capture and process antigen (Fig. 2.8). To replenish macrophages in inflamed tissues, blood monocytes are recruited to areas of inflammation by the chemokine CCL-2 (macrophage chemoattractant protein-1).

Megakaryocytes remain in the marrow in the vicinity of vascular sinuses, producing platelets by cytoplasmic budding and release directly into the bloodstream (Fig. 2.9).

In response to the chemokine IL-13 (CXCL-13), naïve immunoglobulin M (IgM) and/or IgD-positive B cells enter peripheral lymphoid tissues via high endothelial venules and home in on lymphoid follicles in lymph nodes and spleen to await antigen-driven germinal center maturation (Fig. 2.10). Naïve CD7+, CD3− T cells home to the thymic cortex to begin the complex process of T-cell maturation (Fig. 2.11). NK cells are released into the bloodstream as fully mature and functional cells, homing primarily to lymphoid tissues and submucosal sites. Circulating NK cells also enter sites of inflammation in response to the cytokine IL-12 released by activated macrophages.

TECHNICAL CONSIDERATIONS

Bone marrow biopsy and aspiration is most often obtained from the posterior iliac crest. The cylindrical core biopsy is fixed in formalin and decalcified to allow for thin sectioning of the bony tissue. Typically, the biopsy sections are stained with hematoxylin and eosin (Fig. 2.12). The aspirate, a liquid suspension of marrow cells, is smeared onto a glass slide or coverslip and stained with a Wright-Giemsa stain (Fig. 2.13). This stain renders nuclei and basophil or mast cell granules blue and hemoglobin and eosinophil granules red. The

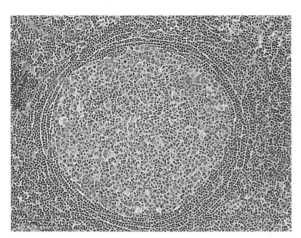

Fig. 2.10 Secondary lymphoid follicle with a large central germinal center composed of activated B cells surrounded by a cuff of small resting mantle zone B cells.

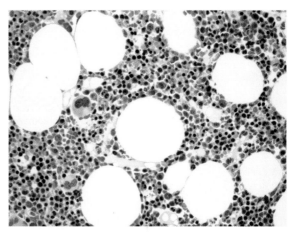

Fig. 2.12 Normal adult marrow biopsy (hematoxylin and eosin stained). Note the small, dark erythroid cells; the lighter stained myeloid cells; and the large, bilobated megakaryocyte.

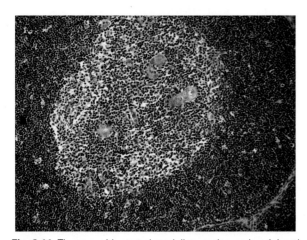

Fig. 2.11 Thymus with central medullary region and peripheral cortical zone. Note the pink epithelial whorls (Hassall corpuscles) in the medullary region.

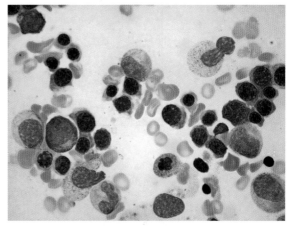

Fig. 2.13 Erythroid-predominant marrow aspirate (Wright-Giemsa stain).

marrow aspirate is particularly useful for enumerating individual marrow cell types and detecting cytologic abnormalities such as dysplasia. As a single cell suspension, the marrow aspirate is also amenable to flow cytometry (see next paragraph). The marrow biopsy is particularly useful for examining the in situ architectural features of the marrow, including detection of lymphoid aggregates, granulomas, and fibrosis. In some cases, clotted marrow particles devoid of bone may be fixed and embedded for sectioning. This specimen, the clot section, is often useful as a biopsy surrogate in cases for which biopsy sections are inadequate.

Flow cytometry is a technique that allows for antibody-mediated detection of specific cell types in cell suspensions. In this technique, aliquots of 10^6 cells in liquid suspension are incubated with fluorochrome-conjugated monoclonal antibodies, rinsed to remove unbound antibody, and passed through a flow cytometry instrument. As the stream of cells passes through the instrument, monochromatic laser light focused on the passing stream induces antibody-bound cells to fluoresce at specific wavelengths (Fig. 2.14A). The fluorescence is detected by a wavelength-selective detector and recorded for each cell. All cells, whether labeled or not,

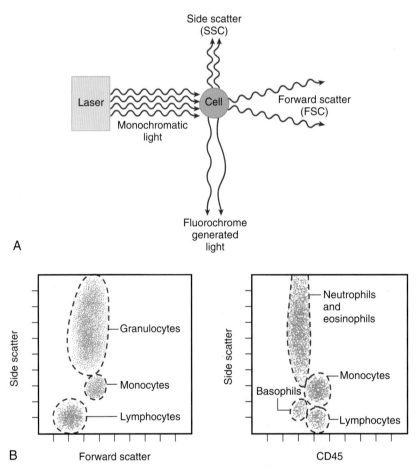

Fig. 2.14 A, Monochromatic laser light (ultraviolet) impacts each cell, generating several light signals. forward scatter (FSC) light is a measure of cell size. Side scatter (SSC) light is a measure of cell granularity. Fluorescent light emitted by fluorochrome-conjugated antibodies to cell-specific antigens is used to identify the cellular immunophenotype. Depending on the number of fluorochrome-conjugated antibodies used, many different antigens can be simultaneously detected on each cell. **B,** Flow cytometry histograms of peripheral blood leukocytes. An FSC-SSC plot yields distinct clusters of lymphocytes, monocytes, and granulocytes *(left)*. A CD45-SSC plot yields distinct clusters of lymphocytes, monocytes, granulocytes, and basophils *(right)*.

are identified by a light scatter detector that detects laser light deflected by each cell along the axis of the laser light beam. The intensity of the forward scatter (FSC) signal is directly proportional to cell size. For example, as shown in Figure 2.14B, lymphocytes are smaller cells than monocytes. Scattered light generated by each cell is also measured (at right angles to the incident laser light). The intensity of the side scatter (SSC) signal is directly proportional to the cytoplasmic *complexity* (i.e., cytoplasmic granularity). The FSC and SSC results for all cells are usually displayed as a dot plot histogram, with the two-dimensional signal intensity of each cell displayed as a single dot. Cells of similar type tend to form cell clusters. For example, lymphocytes, monocytes, and granulocytes nicely separate into distinct clusters when FSC and SSC results are plotted. Another commonly used technique for leukocyte display is to plot CD45 (common leukocyte antigen) expression against SSC (see Fig. 2.14B). Flow cytometry not only enumerates the relative percentages of each cell subset in a sample but also provides information regarding the relative fluorescence intensity of each cell, a measurement that is directly proportional to the antigen density expressed by each cell. Flow cytometry is applicable for samples that can be processed as single-cell suspensions. Examples include blood, bone marrow, body fluids, and lymphoid tissues. Generally, given the difficulty of disaggregation of the tumor cells into a single-cell suspension, most solid tumors cannot be processed for flow cytometry.

Immunohistochemistry is a technique that allows for detection of specific cell types by light microscopy after staining formalin-fixed, paraffin-embedded (or fresh frozen) tissue sections with antigen-specific antibodies. Tissue sections on glass slides are first incubated with a monoclonal antibody made in a mouse (or a polyclonal affinity-purified antibody made in a rabbit or goat), rinsed to remove unbound antibody, incubated with an enzyme-conjugated secondary anti-mouse (or anti-rabbit or anti-goat) antibody, rinsed to remove unbound secondary antibody, and incubated with an enzyme substrate that yields an insoluble colorfast product that deposits at the site of the reaction. After counterstaining the tissue with a nonspecific cellular dye such as hematoxylin (which stains nuclei blue), the slides are examined under a light microscope to detect the labeled cells of interest (Fig. 2.15). Immunohistochemistry is particularly suitable for solid tissue samples that cannot

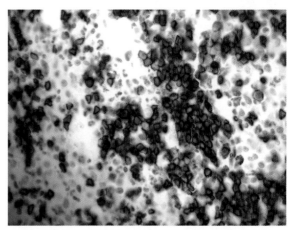

Fig. 2.15 Glycophorin A immunostain highlighting the large colonies of erythroid cells in the bone marrow *(brown staining of cell membranes)*. Myeloid cells are negative.

be disaggregated into a single cell suspension for flow cytometry or for those tissues in which the in situ distribution of the labeled cells is of particular interest. Marrow biopsy and clot sections can be incubated with a number of lineage-specific monoclonal antibodies for in situ detection of glycophorin A/CD71+ erythroid cells, MPO/CD33+ myeloid cells, CD41/CD61+ megakaryocytes, CD3/CD7+ T cells, CD20/CD79a+ B cells, CD56/CD57+ NK cells, CD14/CD68/CD163+ monocytes and macrophages, CD117/mast cell tryptase-positive mast cells, CD34/CD117+ myeloblasts, and CD34/TdT+ lymphoblasts.

Enzyme histochemistry is a colorimetric technique in which a fresh aliquot of cells in suspension is smeared (or pelleted) onto a glass slide, fixed, and incubated with an enzyme substrate that yields a colorfast product only within cells that express the desired enzyme. After counterstaining, the slide is examined with a microscope. A good example of enzyme histochemistry is the use of the dual esterase stain for simultaneous detection in marrow or blood of ANAE positive granulocytes (brown stain) and ANBE-positive monocytes (blue stain) (Fig. 2.16).

Fluorescence in situ hybridization is a technique that can be applied to freshly prepared smears (or pellets) of blood or marrow as well as sections of fixed tissue. The probes are small fluorescent-labeled single-stranded DNA oligonucleotides that bind to specific DNA sequences within cell nuclei. Whereas some probes are used to detect amplification or deletion of

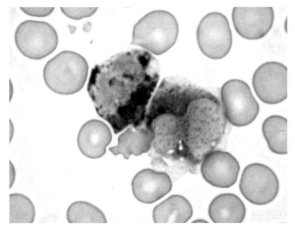

Fig. 2.16 Dual esterase stain with a chloroacetate esterase–positive myeloid cell *(red)* next to an alpha naphthyl butyrate esterase–positive monocyte *(brown)*.

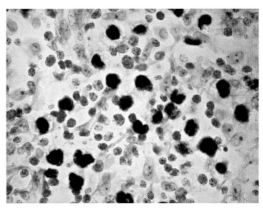

Fig. 2.18 Numerous large Epstein-Barr virus (EBV)–positive Reed-Sternberg cells (dark blue nuclear stain) detected with an EBV early RNA probe in a case of Hodgkin lymphoma (pink counterstain).

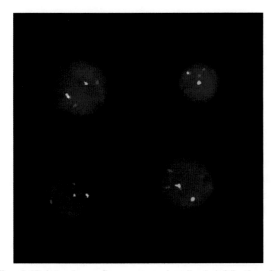

Fig. 2.17 Interphase fluorescence in situ hybridization for the detection of the t(9;22) translocation leading to a hybrid *BCR-ABL* gene characteristic of chronic myeloid leukemia. The *ABL* gene (on chromosome 9) probe generates two *orange* signals, and the *BCR* gene (on chromosome 22) probe generates two *green* signals. Note the presence of a *BCR-ABL* fusion gene in each cell.

disease-specific genes, other probes can be used to detect disease-specific gene translocations (Fig. 2.17).

Colorimetric in situ hybridization is a related technique that can be applied to sections of formalin-fixed, paraffin-embedded tissue, including bone marrow biopsy and clot sections. The probes are labeled, single-stranded oligonucleotide probes designed to specifically bind to nucleic acid target (RNA or DNA). Examples of probes used in hematopathology include the Epstein-Barr virus (EBV) early RNA probe for detection of EBV infection in lymphoma (Fig. 2.18) and immunoglobulin light chain probes for detection of kappa and lambda light chain mRNA in plasma cells.

For molecular studies, nucleic acids (DNA, RNA, or both) can be extracted from blood or tissues and subjected to **polymerase chain reaction (PCR)**–mediated amplification using primers to specific target sequences. The resulting (amplified) product can be detected by hybridization with labeled probes. The PCR product may also be sequenced in order to detect gene mutations, deletions, insertions, or translocations.

KEY WORDS AND CONCEPTS

- Alpha naphthyl acetate esterase (ANAE)
- Alpha naphthyl butyrate esterase (ANBE)
- Aorto-gonado-mesonephros (AGM) region
- Apoptosis
- Bone marrow
- Bone marrow biopsy and aspiration
- Chemokines
- Colorimetric in situ hybridization
- Cytokines
- Embryonic hemoglobin
- Embryonic yolk sac

- Enzyme histochemistry
- Flow cytometry
- Fluorescence in situ hybridization
- Hematopoietic stem cells
- Hemoglobin Gower 1
- Hemoglobin Gower 2
- Hemoglobin Portland
- Hemoglobin F
- Hemoglobin A
- Heparin
- Histamine
- *Hox*

- *Ikaros*
- Immunohistochemistry
- Inhibitory cytokines
- Marginal pool
- Marrow stroma
- Multilineage progenitor cells
- Polymerase chain reaction (PCR)
- Pluripotential hematopoietic stem cells
- Precursor cells
- Stem cell factor (SCF, kit ligand)
- SCF receptor (CD117, c-kit)
- Unilineage progenitor cells

REVIEW QUESTIONS

1. Embryonic and fetal hematopoiesis occurs in all sites below **except** the
   A. yolk sac.
   B. liver.
   C. kidneys.
   D. spleen.
   E. AGM.

2. Which of the following cytokines inhibit hematopoiesis?
   A. G-CSF
   B. IL-1
   C. TPO
   D. EPO
   E. IL-3

3. Which of the following cytokines specifically promote eosinophil growth and differentiation?
   A. SCF
   B. IL-4
   C. TPO
   D. EPO
   E. IL-5

4. Rapid migration of neutrophils from the marginal pool to sites of inflammation is mediated by which macrophage-derived chemokine?
   A. CCL-2
   B. IL-15
   C. CCL-5
   D. CCL-8
   E. Gamma interferon

Erythropoiesis and Oxygen Transport

KEY POINTS

- Red blood cell (RBCs) production is stimulated by erythropoietin (EPO), a secreted glycoprotein produced by renal peritubular cells in response to hypoxia.
- EPO binds to EPO receptor-bearing erythroid colony-forming unit cells in the marrow, inducing proliferation, maturation, and inhibition of apoptosis.
- EPO deficiency in renal disease is associated with a hypoproliferative anemia.
- EPO excess in patients with chronic hypoxia is associated with polycythemia.
- After enucleation, mature RBCs are released from the marrow into the circulation and with a half-life of 120 days.
- Reticulocytes are circulating anucleate RBCs newly released from the marrow that retain rough endoplasmic reticulum.

- In normal adults, reticulocytes account for approximately 1% of all circulating RBCs.
- Whereas anemia caused by marrow failure is characterized by an inappropriately low reticulocyte count, anemia caused by RBC destruction or loss is characterized by a high reticulocyte count.
- Anemia-induced hypoxia stimulates increased EPO from the kidneys with consequent erythroid hyperplasia in the marrow and increased reticulocytes in the blood.
- Hypoxia-induced lactic acidosis and increased 2,3-bisphosphoglycerate production lead to decreased hemoglobin oxygen affinity with enhanced release of oxygen to peripheral tissues.

The rate of erythropoiesis is primarily controlled by the positive growth effect of the glycoprotein hormone **erythropoietin (EPO)** on erythroid progenitors in the bone marrow. EPO is produced in fetuses primarily by hepatocytes, but after birth, it is primarily produced by peritubular fibroblasts in the renal cortex. EPO production is stimulated by tissue hypoxia. The key regulator of EPO synthesis is **hypoxia-inducible factor 1 (HIF-1)**, a transcription factor that binds to hypoxia response elements not only in the *EPO* gene but also in genes involved in glucose metabolism, including glucose transporters and glycolytic enzymes. Plasma EPO levels rapidly increase within 1 hour after initiation of hypoxia and peak within 1 to 2 days. Under normal circumstances,

increased EPO leads to a hypercellular marrow with erythroid predominance (erythroid hyperplasia).

Marrow stem cells under the influence of hematopoietic growth factors give rise to the earliest committed erythroid progenitors, **erythroid burst-forming unit (BFU-E)** cells and **erythroid colony-forming unit (CFU-E)** cells. BFU-E give rise to CFU-E. CFU-E express the highest density of cell surface EPO receptors and thus is highly sensitive to the positive influence of EPO. EPO binding to a dimerized pair of EPO receptor molecules induces a variety of cytoplasmic signal transduction pathways that ultimately lead to the prevention of apoptosis of CFU-E cells. Under normal conditions, relatively few CFU-E cells survive to form mature red blood cells (RBCs). In contrast, under hypoxic conditions, increased EPO enhances CFU-E survival, leading to an increased number of surviving CFU-E cells. Each CFU-E is capable of giving rise to 8 to 64 immature RBCs. EPO further contributes to erythropoiesis by directly stimulating proliferation and maturation of more differentiated proerythroblasts and normoblasts. After enucleation, mature RBCs are released into the circulation.

A burst in EPO-induced erythropoiesis is followed 3 to 4 days later by an increased number of **reticulocytes**, young RBCs with a high content of rough endoplasmic reticulum, in peripheral blood. Given the normal RBC half-life of 120 days, approximately 1% of RBCs are normally replaced each day with reticulocytes. Thus, under normal circumstances, reticulocytes account for approximately 1% of all RBCs in blood. In patients with anemia and a normal functional marrow reserve, hypoxia induces EPO production with consequent erythroid hyperplasia in the marrow; reticulocytosis in the blood; and eventual normalization of the RBC count, hemoglobin, and hematocrit.

OXYGEN TRANSPORT

The average resting adult human consumes about 250 mL of oxygen per minute to fuel aerobic metabolism. The oxygen-carrying capacity of RBCs in blood is 200 mL/L, and normal cardiac output is 5 L/min. Thus, the total circulating RBC mass can deliver 1 L of oxygen per minute to tissues. At rest, extraction of only 25% of the available blood oxygen by peripheral tissues provides the necessary delivery rate of 250 mL of oxygen per minute. In contrast, exercise requires greater consumption of oxygen, a need that can be met by a combination of increased cardiac output and increased blood oxygen extraction rate. If the need for additional oxygen is not met, hypoxia develops. Tissue hypoxia develops as a consequence of inadequate oxygen delivery in a variety of settings, including extreme physical activity, chronic anemia, decreased cardiac output, blood loss, or lung disease. **Hypoxia** leads to the rapid accumulation of lactic acid in tissues (**lactic acidosis**) because of the inability to efficiently operate the citric acid cycle. The lactic acidosis triggers an increased respiratory rate, leading to a compensatory respiratory alkalosis. Acidosis and increased production of RBC **2,3-bisphosphoglycerate (2,3-BPG)** lead to a shift to the right of the oxygen dissociation curve, that is, to decreased

hemoglobin oxygen affinity (see Fig. 4.16). Decreased oxygen affinity allows for more rapid release of oxygen from RBCs to hypoxic tissues. In acute (blood loss) anemia, vascular changes lead to shunting of blood to the gut, thus avoiding acute intestinal ischemia. On the other hand, in chronic anemia, blood is shunted to the skin and kidneys. Decreased oxygen in blood triggers renal peritubular cells to increase their production of EPO some 1000-fold. EPO binds to and stimulates the growth and maturation of EPO receptor-positive erythroid precursors in the marrow, ultimately leading to increased production of RBCs.

EPO deficiency, caused both by loss of EPO-producing renal peritubular epithelial cells and inhibition of EPO synthesis by uremia-associated metabolic factors, is responsible for the anemia seen in patients with chronic renal failure. **EPO excess** caused by chronic hypoxia from cyanotic heart disease, pulmonary insufficiency, or prolonged residence at high altitude leads to an increased number of RBCs (**polycythemia**). Secondary (reactive) polycythemia contrasts with primary polycythemia (**polycythemia vera**), a clonal neoplastic condition. The symptoms of polycythemia (headache, pruritus, plethora, paresthesia, and thrombosis) are caused by increased RBC mass, increased blood volume, and hyperviscosity.

Normal erythropoiesis depends on an adequate dietary supply of **iron**, folic acid, and cobalamin (active form of vitamin B_{12}). Iron is necessary for a variety of cellular functions, most prominently in hemoglobin synthesis in erythrocytes and myoglobin synthesis in myocytes of heart and skeletal muscle. Iron deficiency leads to an anemia because of the production of small (microcytic), hemoglobin-poor (hypochromic) RBCs with reduced half-lives. **Folic acid** and **cobalamin** are necessary for normal DNA synthesis, and their deficiency leads to impaired proliferation of rapidly growing tissues, most prominently in the bone marrow and gastrointestinal tract. In contrast to the small RBCs (microcytic) seen in iron deficiency, RBCs in folic acid and cobalamin deficiency are enlarged (macrocytic).

KEY WORDS AND CONCEPTS

- 2,3-Bisphosphoglycerate (2,3-BPG)
- Cobalamin
- EPO deficiency

- EPO excess
- Erythroid burst-forming unit (BFU-E)
- Erythroid colony-forming unit (CFU-E)
- Erythropoietin (EPO)
- Folic acid
- Hypoxia

- Hypoxia-inducible factor 1 (HIF-1)
- Iron
- Lactic acidosis
- Polycythemia
- Polycythemia vera
- Reticulocytes

REVIEW QUESTIONS

1. In response to hypoxia, EPO is produced by which cell type?
   A. Proerythroblasts
   B. Splenic macrophages
   C. Renal peritubular cells
   D. Pneumocytes
   E. Renal juxtaglomerular cells

2. In response to hypoxia, increased RBC 2,3-BPG leads to
   A. increased EPO-driven erythropoiesis.
   B. decreased hemoglobin oxygen affinity.
   C. increased respiratory rate.
   D. reticulocytosis.
   E. polycythemia.

3. Which of the conditions below is **not associated** with an elevated blood EPO level?
   A. Pulmonary insufficiency
   B. Cyanotic heart disease
   C. Life at high altitude
   D. EPO doping (athletic)
   E. Polycythemia vera

4. Which of the following conditions is partially responsible for the anemia in chronic kidney disease?
   A. Lactic acidosis
   B. Iron deficiency
   C. Uremia
   D. Increased 2,3-BPG
   E. Folate deficiency

Iron, Heme, and Hemoglobin

KEY POINTS

- Dietary iron is absorbed by duodenal enterocytes, transported in the blood bound to the iron carrier protein transferrin, and released to transferrin receptor-bearing hepatocytes and macrophages.

- Hereditary hemochromatosis is an iron-overload condition often caused by high iron (Fe) protein (HFE) mutations that lead to excess iron absorption by the duodenum.

- Heme synthesis in erythroid precursors occurs in mitochondria by incorporation of ferrous iron into protoporphyrin IX by the enzyme ferrochelatase.

- Defective heme synthesis can lead to toxic accumulation of porphyrin intermediates (porphyria) or to ineffective erythropoiesis (sideroblastic anemia).

- Each molecule of hemoglobin produced by erythroid cells is composed of a complex of four globin chains (two alpha and two non-alpha) and four ferric heme molecules, each of which can reversibly bind one molecule of oxygen (O_2).

- The oxygen affinity of hemoglobin is dependent on temperature, pH, and level of 2,3-bisphosphoglycerate (2,3-BPG).

- In the presence of high temperature (fever), low pH (acidosis), and high 2,3-BCG, hemoglobin oxygen affinity is reduced, allowing for more rapid oxygen delivery to peripheral tissues.

- Whereas hemoglobin variants with high oxygen affinity present with polycythemia, hemoglobin variants with low oxygen affinity present with cyanosis.

- Senescent or damaged red blood cells are removed from blood by splenic macrophages and digested within lysosomes.

- Lysosomal digestion of hemoglobin yields iron, bilirubin, and amino acids.

- Albumin-bound bilirubin in blood is absorbed by hepatocytes, conjugated to glucuronic acid to increase solubility, and excreted into bile and urine.

- Iron deficiency caused by inadequate dietary intake or to chronic bleeding often leads to reduced erythropoiesis and a microcytic hypochromic anemia caused by inadequate hemoglobin production (iron-deficiency anemia).

- Chronic inflammation- (or infection-) mediated release of hepcidin from hepatocytes coupled with inadequate erythropoietin production by the kidneys leads to reduced erythropoiesis and impaired iron delivery to erythroid precursors in the bone marrow (anemia of chronic disease).

IRON UPTAKE IN THE DUODENUM

The human body contains about 3 to 4 g of **iron**, of which 70% to 80% is complexed to protoporphyrin IX to form **heme**, the oxygen-binding prosthetic group of hemoglobin and **myoglobin**. Although iron plays a role in many enzymatic reactions, most nonheme iron is stored in the marrow (80%) and liver (20%) as **ferritin** and **hemosiderin**. A small amount (1/1000th) of total body iron circulates in blood plasma, complexed to the iron transport protein **transferrin**. Free iron (esp. ferrous iron) is toxic, with formation of reactive oxygen species (ROS). To minimize damage, a small amount of intracellular ferrous iron necessary for immediate needs is bound to **iron chaperone protein (ICP)**, forming the **labile iron pool (LIP)**. Surplus iron, on the other hand, is stored in ferric form as ferritin and hemosiderin. Iron is stored primarily in hepatocytes and macrophages in the spleen and marrow. There is no physiologic mechanism for controlled release of excess iron. A small amount of iron is lost through daily shedding of intestinal epithelial cells and keratinocytes as well as intermittent menstrual blood loss. Chronic iron loss leading to iron-deficiency anemia may be seen in gastrointestinal (GI) bleeding, menorrhagia, and hemolytic anemia.

Iron in food is present as heme iron and non-heme (ionic) iron. **Nonheme (ionic) iron** is present in fruits and vegetables, while **heme iron** is present in meats. Ionic non-heme iron is primarily ferric (Fe3+), while heme iron is ferrous (Fe2+). Acid digestion of food in the stomach releases non-heme iron and heme. In the duodenum (Fig. 4.1), ferric iron (Fe3+) is converted to ferrous iron (Fe2+) by **duodenal cytochrome B** and **vitamin C ferrireductase** and absorbed at the luminal surface of villus enterocytes through the **divalent metal transporter (DMT1)**. Heme bound to **heme carrier protein (HCP)** is absorbed by villus enterocytes and transported to endosomes for acid and **heme oxygenase (HO)** mediated release of ferrous iron. Ferrous iron, bound to ICP, is transported to the basolateral surface of the enterocyte and released to the blood through the iron transporter **ferroportin** where it is rapidly re-oxidized to ferric iron by membrane-bound **hephaestin (HAE)** or **extracellular ceruloplasmin**, and bound to the iron transporter transferrin for release to the bloodstream.

Duodenal **crypt cells** differentiate into absorptive **villus epithelium** within 2 to 3 days. In crypt cells, the level of plasma iron, as detected by the TFR1–HFE complex (transferrin receptor–high iron [Fe] protein), programs the level of expression of iron transport proteins DMT1 and ferroportin in villus cells. Low plasma iron detected by crypt cells leads to increased expression of DMT1 and ferroportin by villus cells and increased duodenal iron uptake. In contrast, high plasma iron detected by crypt cells leads to decreased expression of DMT-1 and ferroportin by villus cells and decreased duodenal iron uptake.

IRON STORAGE AND REGULATION: HEPATOCYTES

Hepatocytes play two roles in iron metabolism, as a site of iron storage and as a regulator of iron uptake

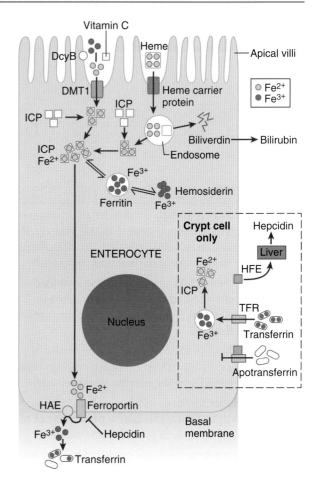

Fig. 4.1 The Iron Cycle in the Duodenum.
1, Iron is absorbed by duodenal enterocytes—elemental iron from vegetables and heme iron from meats. Elemental iron is absorbed by divalent metal transporter (DMT1) after reduction of ferric to ferrous form by duodenal cytochrome B (DcytB).
2, Ferrous iron migrates through the cell bound to iron chaperone protein (ICP) and enters the labile iron pool (LIP) or stored in the ferric form as ferritin.
3, Heme is absorbed by heme carrier protein (HCP) and digested in endosomes with release of ferrous iron to LIP or ferritin.
4, Ferrous iron exits the cell through the ferroportin (FP) transporter, oxidized to ferric iron by hephaestin (HAE), and enters the bloodstream bound to transferrin.
5, On duodenal crypt cells, the iron sensor protein (HFE) competes with transferrin (TF) for binding to transferrin receptor (TFR1). When serum iron is reduced, HFE binds to and inhibits iron uptake by TFR1. Conversely, when serum iron is elevated, HFE is released from TFR1, and iron uptake is increased.

and release (Fig. 4.2). Transferrin-bound iron in plasma binds to **TFR1** and enters hepatocytes by receptor-mediated endocytosis. Within acidic endosomes, TF-TFR complexes are disassembled, ferric iron (Fe3+) and converted to ferrous iron (Fe2+) by **ferric reductase (STEAP3)**. Ferrous iron exits the endosome through the divalent metal transporter (DMT1), binds ICP, and enters the LIP to meet immediate needs. Surplus iron (ferric) is stored as ferritin and hemosiderin. Ferritin is composed of an outer

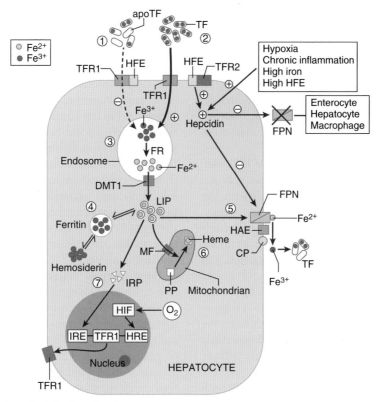

Fig. 4.2 The Iron Cycle in Hepatocytes.

1, If transferrin-bound iron is low (iron deficiency), HFE forms a complex with transferrin receptor (TFR1), leading to a reduction in the rate of iron uptake.

2, If transferrin-bound iron is high (iron overload), HFE is released from TFR1, leading to increased iron uptake, and is bound instead to TFR2. The HFE–TFR2 complex signals increased production of hepcidin. Hepcidin binds to and blocks ferroportin, preventing release of intracellular iron to the bloodstream.

3, Absorbed transferrin is delivered to acidic endosomes, where the iron is converted from ferric to ferrous iron by ferric reductase (FR). Ferrous iron exits the endosome through the transporter protein DMT1 and enters the cytoplasm bound to iron carrier protein (ICP). In aggregate, the ICP–iron constitutes the labile iron pool (LIP).

4, Surplus ferrous iron in the LIP can be stored in ferritin or hemosiderin as ferric iron. This iron can be reused after conversion back to ferrous iron.

5, Ferrous iron passes through the hepatocyte iron transporter ferroportin (FP), converted to ferric iron by membrane bound hephaestin (HAE) or serum ceruloplasmin (CP), and released bound to transferrin.

i6, Ferrous iron from the labile iron pool (LIP) enters mitochondria by passing through the mitoferrin transporter and bound to protoporphyrin IX (PP) by the enzyme ferrochelatase to form heme. In hepatocytes, heme is used primarily as an oxidizing co-factor for cytochrome P450 (CYP450), which is important in hepatic clearance of a number of compounds, including steroids, fatty acids, and toxins.

7, Hepatocyte iron content is monitored and controlled by intracellular iron-sensing proteins (IRPs) and iron-responsive DNA elements (IREs). Iron binds to IRE that flank the *TFR1* gene.

shell of apoferritin protein enclosing a dense core of crystalline ferrihydrite. Hemosiderin, formed by lysosomal degradation of the apoferritin shell, is composed almost entirely of ferric iron.

The transferrin iron saturation of plasma is monitored by the TFR1–HFE complex on hepatocytes. HFE, the plasma iron sensor, competes with transferrin for binding to TFR1. With normal to low transferrin iron saturation, HFE (high iron (Fe) protein) binds to TFR1, reducing iron uptake. With high transferrin iron saturation, transferrin outcompetes HFE for TFR1 binding, leading to increased iron uptake. The released HFE binds instead to **TFR2**, triggering hepcidin production. **Hepcidin** blocks iron transport by irreversible inactivation of ferroportin expressed by villus enterocytes, hepatocytes, and macrophages.

In a setting of chronic inflammation or infection, release of the liver hormone hepcidin blocks systemic iron uptake and release by inactivating ferroportin, the major iron exporter. Plasma iron (transferrin) saturation is monitored by the hepatocyte TFR1–HFE complex. As a counterbalance to hepcidin, the hormone HFE (high Fe) produced by GI tract, macrophages, and granulocytes blocks transferrin receptor and blocks hepcidin production in the liver. When iron saturation is high, HFE translocates from TFR1 to TFR-2, triggering hepcidin release. Inactivating HFE mutations are the most common cause of **hereditary hemochromatosis (HH)**. Less common HH-related mutations include those of **TFR-2** and HAMP (hepcidin).

The level of intracellular iron is regulated at both transcriptional and translational levels. Iron binds to **iron-responsive proteins**, which bind to **iron-responsive elements** in iron-related genes. Hypoxia increases expression of **hypoxia-inducible factor**, which binds to **hypoxia-responsive elements** in iron-related genes. High iron triggers increased ferritin and ferroportin and decreased TFR1 and DMT1. Low iron triggers decreased ferritin and increased TFR1 and DMT1. Low oxygen (hypoxia) triggers increased TFR1.

IRON STORAGE AND RECYCLING: MACROPHAGES

Splenic macrophages are responsible for the removal of senescent and damaged red blood cells (RBCs) from the blood circulation (Fig. 4.3). Given their critical role in oxygen transport, RBCs are naturally subject to irreparable and progressive free radical damage. Because of increased rigidity, senescent RBCs are trapped in the splenic cords and by virtue of **phosphatidylserine (PS)** expression are recognized and engulfed by **PS receptor**–bearing macrophages. In normal RBCs, the enzyme **flippase** restricts PS expression to the inner leaflet of the RBC plasma membrane, unrecognized by macrophages. In contrast, the enzyme **scramblase** leads to expression of PS on the RBC outer leaflet and recognized by the macrophage PS receptor. Ingested RBCs are confined to membrane-bound phagosomes that fuse with lysosomes to form **phagolysosomes**. In the acidic environment of the phagolysosome, hemoglobin is degraded to ferric iron, heme, and globin. The iron is stored as ferritin and hemosiderin. Heme is converted to **biliverdin**, and globin is converted to amino acids. Biliverdin is reduced to bilirubin, transported to the liver for conjugation to glucuronic acid (to increase solubility), and excreted in bile, urine, and feces. In hemolytic anemia, free heme and hemoglobin bind to carrier proteins **hemopexin (HPX)** and **haptoglobin (HPG)**, respectively, and absorbed by HPX/HPG receptor-bearing macrophages.

Bone marrow macrophages (nurse cells) provide iron to developing erythroid precursors for production of hemoglobin. Ferritin released from iron-laden macrophages is directly transferred to small groups of developing erythroid cells (erythroid islands) by the process of **pinocytosis**. Erythroid precursors in marrow also acquire iron by binding of plasma transferrin to RBC transferrin receptors (Fig. 4.4).

Cellular iron that is not immediately used for heme synthesis or enzymatic reactions or as low-molecular-weight chelates is primarily stored in the cytoplasm as ferritin. Ferritin is composed of a core of crystalline **ferrihydrite** (ferric iron) enclosed within an **apoferritin** protein shell. Under normal circumstances, nearly all ferritin is found in the cytoplasmic compartment of cells. A very small amount of ferritin is present in the blood. In most circumstances, the serum ferritin level in blood correlates closely with the level of intracellular ferritin, thus providing a useful measure of total body iron stores. However, as an **acute-phase reactant**, serum ferritin is elevated in chronic inflammatory states and thus may not accurately reflect low storage iron in patients with both iron deficiency and chronic inflammation. In the marrow, most storage iron is present in macrophages as both ferritin

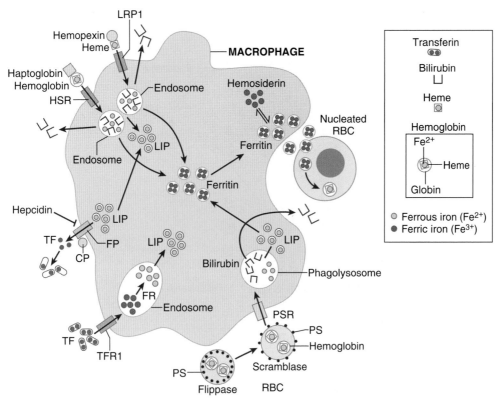

Fig. 4.3 The iron cycle in macrophages. *CP,* ceruloplasmin; *HSR,* hemoglobin scavenger receptor; *LIP,* labile iron pool; *LRP1,* lipoprotein receptor protein 1; *PS,* phosphatidylserine; *PSR,* phosphatidyl serine receptor; *RBC,* red blood cell; *TF,* transferrin; *TFR1,* transferrin receptor 1.

and hemosiderin, an aggregated, iron-rich ferritin degradation product with very low apoferritin content. Approximately 20% to 50% of normal marrow erythroid precursors are **sideroblasts,** nucleated erythroid cells that contain a few small, ferritin-rich lysosomes called **siderosomes.** Storage iron distribution in macrophages and sideroblasts can be visualized by staining of marrow smears or biopsy sections with Prussian Blue, a dye that stains aggregates of ferritin and hemosiderin (Fig. 4.5). Even without Prussian blue staining, golden-brown refractile aggregates of hemosiderin can often be seen by light microscopy (Fig. 4.6).

IRON-DEFICIENCY ANEMIA

The **anemia of iron deficiency** may occur as a result of an iron-deficient diet, inadequate intestinal iron absorption, chronic blood loss (menorrhagia or GI), or intravascular hemolysis with hemoglobin loss in the urine (hemoglobinuria). Iron deficiency in infants and children is most often caused by an iron-poor diet. Cow's milk, dairy products, and nonsupplemented infant formulas do not provide the necessary iron content. Iron deficiency in pregnant or lactating women is often caused by inadequate dietary compensation for the increased iron requirements of fetal growth and milk production. Inadequate duodenal iron uptake is seen in patients with intestinal malabsorption (as in celiac disease) and after gastrectomy (caused by achlorhydria with inadequate release of iron from organic matter). Menorrhagia in premenopausal women is the most common cause of iron deficiency. GI blood loss is the most common cause of iron deficiency in men and postmenopausal women.

Lack of iron in erythroid cells reduces the rate of hemoglobin synthesis by interfering with the rate-limiting **ferrochelatase** step of heme synthesis. In the absence

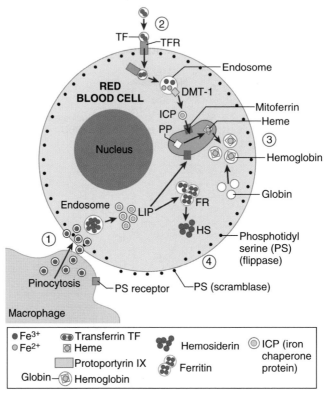

Fig. 4.4 The iron cycle in erythroid cells. *FR,* ferritin; *HS,* hemosiderin; *LIP,* labile iron pool; *TF,* transferrin; *TFR1,* transferrin receptor.

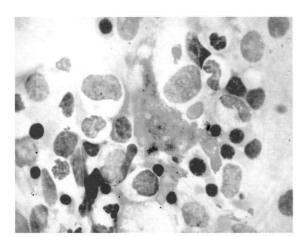

Fig. 4.5 Iron-laden bone marrow macrophage (Prussian blue stain, marrow aspirate). The large cell in the center of the field is a macrophage-rich cell with cytoplasmic storage iron (ferritin and hemosiderin). Surrounding this macrophage are erythroid precursors (with bright pink-red nuclei) that obtain the iron required for heme synthesis directly from the macrophage.

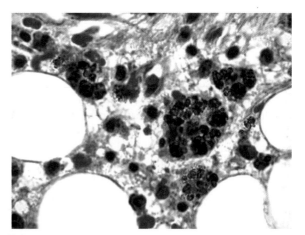

Fig. 4.6 Marrow biopsy with increased hemosiderin (brown granular material) within macrophages (Wright stain). This asymptomatic phenomenon, often seen in marrows of patients with a history of multiple blood transfusions, is termed *hemosiderosis* and should be distinguished from primary hemochromatosis, a serious medical condition.

of iron, **zinc protoporphyrin (ZP)** is produced. Measurement of serum ZP is a convenient laboratory marker for detection of iron deficiency or **lead poisoning**. In iron deficiency, the reduction in hemoglobin synthesis leads to production of small (microcytic), pale (hypochromic) RBC. The mildly reduced lifespan of hemoglobin-deficient RBCs, uncompensated by a normal rate of production, leads to anemia, a condition marked by reductions in RBC count, hemoglobin concentration, and hematocrit (percentage of RBC volume per blood volume). In response to hypoxia, erythropoietin (EPO) production by the kidneys increases. However, because RBC production is hampered by the defect in heme synthesis, the marrow response is ineffective. **Ineffective erythropoiesis** is characterized by an inappropriately low reticulocyte count in peripheral blood (**reticulocytopenia**).

Clinical findings in patients with chronic iron deficiency may include pallor, fatigue, irritability, headache, glossitis, stomatitis, angular cheilitis, koilonychia, paresthesia, and restless leg syndrome. The diagnosis of iron-deficiency anemia can be confirmed by **complete blood count (CBC)** and serum iron measurements. CBC findings include anemia (low RBC, hemoglobin, and hematocrit), microcytosis (low mean corpuscular volume), hypochromia (low mean corpuscular hemoglobin concentration), anisocytosis (high RBC distribution width), and decreased reticulocyte count. Although iron deficiency itself is not typically associated with neutropenia or thrombocytopenia, patients with iron deficiency caused by blood loss (bleeding) often present with thrombocytosis (increased platelet count). The peripheral smear reveals small hypochromic RBCs, often accompanied by pencil-shaped **elliptocytes** (Fig. 4.7), and reduced numbers of **polychromatophilic** RBCs (**reticulocytes**). Serum iron studies typically reveal decreased serum iron, increased total iron-binding capacity (largely caused by transferrin), decreased percent iron (transferrin) saturation, and decreased serum ferritin. Of these tests, serum ferritin is generally considered to be the most useful because it most accurately reflects total body iron stores with the caveat that as a positive acute-phase reactant, ferritin levels may be increased in patients with inflammatory disorders, thereby limiting its use as a marker of iron deficiency in this setting. Bone marrow examination reveals a normocellular marrow with absent stainable iron. Iron supplementation leads to a rapid

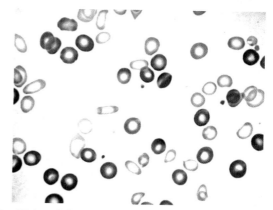

Fig. 4.7 Iron-deficiency anemia after transfusion (blood smear). About half of the red blood cells (RBC) in this field are hypochromic and microcytic, many with elongated elliptical shapes (elliptocytes). These findings are characteristic of iron-deficiency anemia. The other RBCs in this field are normochromic and normocytic, consistent with donor cells from a recent blood transfusion. A few small blue platelets are also present in this field.

regenerative erythroid hyperplasia in the marrow and a peripheral blood reticulocytosis followed by eventual replacement of hypochromic microcytic RBCs with normochromic, normocytic RBCs in the peripheral blood.

HEMOCHROMATOSIS

Hemochromatosis is a family of conditions associated with excessive accumulation of iron in parenchymal tissue. Classical HH is an autosomal recessive disorder seen most often in northern Europeans caused by mutations of the *HFE* gene. Only 1% of those with homozygous HFE mutations are symptomatic. HFE defects render the transferrin receptor–HFE complex expressed by duodenal crypt cells unresponsive to high levels of interstitial fluid transferrin iron, preventing downregulation of DMT-1 and ferroportin by apical enterocytes, leading to inappropriately high iron absorption by the duodenum. Secondary (acquired) hemochromatosis (aka hemosiderosis) is seen in patients with a history of multiple RBC transfusions. The reduced half-life of transfused RBCs leads to increased RBC turnover and excess iron. In either form of hemochromatosis, iron accumulates in multiple tissues (skin, bone marrow, liver, gallbladder, pancreas, and myocardium), leading ultimately to oxidative tissue damage largely mediated

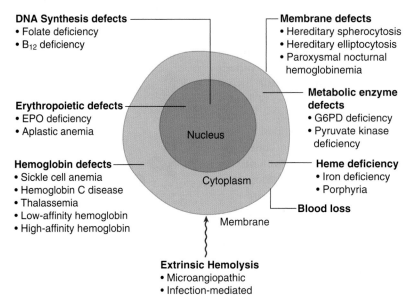

DNA Synthesis defects
• Folate deficiency
• B$_{12}$ deficiency

Membrane defects
• Hereditary spherocytosis
• Hereditary elliptocytosis
• Paroxysmal nocturnal hemoglobinemia

Erythropoietic defects
• EPO deficiency
• Aplastic anemia

Metabolic enzyme defects
• G6PD deficiency
• Pyruvate kinase deficiency

Nucleus

Hemoglobin defects
• Sickle cell anemia
• Hemoglobin C disease
• Thalassemia
• Low-affinity hemoglobin
• High-affinity hemoglobin

Cytoplasm

Heme deficiency
• Iron deficiency
• Porphyria

Blood loss

Membrane

Extrinsic Hemolysis
• Microangiopathic
• Infection-mediated

Fig. 4.8 Causes of anemia. *EPO,* Erythropoietin; *G6PD,* glucose-6-phosphate dehydrogenase.

by the highly reactive hydroxyl radical. Patients with hemochromatosis are at increased risk of infection, veno-occlusive disease, and liver disease.

Anemia may result from a variety of intrinsic RBC defects, as well as extrinsic causes (Fig. 4.8). Based on physiologic mechanisms, the anemias can be broadly classified into those caused by blood loss, decreased RBC production, or increased RBC destruction (Table 4.1). More simply, anemia can also be classified into two broad groups based on the presence or absence of a compensatory reticulocyte response. Types of anemia marked by deficient erythropoiesis (and thus a low reticulocyte count) include those caused by nutrient deficiencies and heme biosynthetic defects. Types of anemia marked by increased reticulocytes (**reticulocytosis**) include those caused by chronic blood loss and hemolysis. Under normal conditions, given the 120-day lifespan of RBCs, about 1% to 2% of RBCs must be replaced each day. The replacements are primarily reticulocytes, relatively large RBCs newly released from the marrow that retain a loose (polychromatophilic) with the Wright stain (Fig. 4.9). Staining reticulocytes with RNA-binding dyes such as new methylene blue or the fluorochrome thiazole orange provides for improved accuracy in enumerating reticulocytes (Fig. 4.10).

HEME

Heme, the oxygen-carrying prosthetic group of hemoglobin, is an iron-containing tetrapyrrole that functions in electron exchange (Fig. 4.11). Heme is incorporated as a prosthetic group into many proteins, including hemoglobin, myoglobin, **cytochrome P450**, catalase, and peroxidase. Most heme synthesis (85%) takes place in erythroid cells, where it is incorporated into hemoglobin; most of the remainder is produced in the liver (as cytochrome P450) and skeletal muscle (as myoglobin). Steps in heme synthesis take place in both cytoplasm and mitochondria (Fig. 4.12). The first step of heme synthesis is formation of **delta aminolevulinic acid** (ALA) from **glycine** and **succinyl coenzyme A** by the enzyme ALA **synthase**. Deficiency of the ALA synthase cofactor **pyridoxine (vitamin B6)** leads to decreased heme synthesis and accumulation of mitochondrial iron (sideroblastic anemia). The last (and rate-limiting) step in heme synthesis is the binding of ferrous iron (Fe^{2+}) to protoporphyrin IX by the mitochondrial enzyme ferrochelatase.

PORPHYRIA

Enzyme defects in heme biosynthesis lead to a group of disorders known collectively as **porphyria**. Most types

TABLE 4.1 Major Causes of Anemia

Decreased Production (Low Reticulocyte Count)	Increased Destruction or Loss (High Reticulocyte Count)
Nutritional Deficiency Iron deficiency: hemoglobin production defect Folic acid deficiency: DNA production defect Cobalamin deficiency: DNA production defect	**Blood Loss** Menorrhagia Gastrointestinal bleeding Trauma
Bone Marrow Failure Fanconi anemia: autosomal recessive DNA repair defect Aplastic anemia: autoimmune or toxin mediated	**Hemolytic Anemia (Intrinsic)** Hemoglobinopathy Thalassemia (reduced alpha- or beta-globin synthesis)
Red Blood Cell Aplasia Diamond-Blackfan anemia: autosomal dominant Anemia of renal disease: EPO deficiency Parvovirus B19 infection	Production of mutant globin protein (hemoglobins S, C, D, E, and so on) Cell membrane defects (spectrin, ankyrin)—membrane instability Hereditary spherocytosis Hereditary elliptocytosis Enzyme deficiency: oxidative damage to cellular proteins G6PD deficiency
Sideroblastic Anemia (Defective Heme Synthesis) Lead poisoning Ethanol toxicity Myelodysplasia	Pyruvate kinase deficiency Paroxysmal nocturnal hemoglobinuria—glycosylphosphatidylinositol anchoring defect (*PIG-A* mutation) leading to loss of CD55 and CD57 and hypersensitivity to complement-mediated lysis
Myelophthisis (Marrow Infiltration with Loss of Normal Hematopoietic Tissue) Granulomatous disease Metastatic cancer Leukemia	**Hemolytic Anemia (Extrinsic)** Autoimmune hemolytic anemia: immune-mediated hemolysis Microangiopathic hemolytic anemia: mechanical damage to red blood cells by microvascular thrombi, cardiac valve defects, thermal injury Hypersplenism: congestive and infiltrative diseases of the spleen
Chronic Inflammation Anemia of chronic disease: hepcidin-mediated iron utilization defect	Drug induced Nonimmune (dapsone, sulfasalazine) Immune mediated (penicillin, cephalosporin, methyldopa, levodopa, quinidine)

EPO, Erythropoietin; *G6PD,* glucose-6-phosphate dehydrogenase.

of porphyria are inherited autosomal dominant disorders. Excess heme precursors produced by hepatocytes, erythroid precursors, or both accumulate in various tissues, leading to a wide variety of symptoms, including cutaneous photosensitivity, abdominal pain, neuropathy, behavioral disturbances, hemolytic anemia, and liver disease. Heme deficiency also plays a role in the neurologic dysfunction. **Acute intermittent porphyria (AIP)** is caused by mutations of the **porphobilinogen deaminase** gene. Only about 10% of patients who carry this mutation present with clinical disease, with attacks often precipitated by drugs. During an attack, patients with AIP present with severe abdominal (neurovisceral) pain, motor paralysis, neuropsychiatric symptoms, or a combination of these. During an attack, clear, freshly voided urine slowly darkens when exposed to light as porphyrinogen is oxidized to porphyrin. In chronic **porphyria cutanea tarda (PCT)**, porphyrin deposition

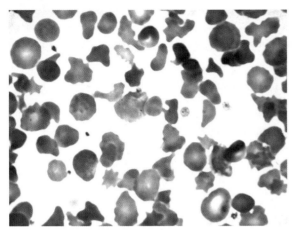

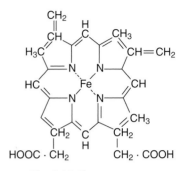

Fig. 4.11 Heme structure.

Fig. 4.9 Increased polychromatophilic (blue-tinged) red blood cells (RBCs) (4%) and fragmented RBCs (schistocytes) indicative of severe hemolytic anemia. The grayish blue polychromatophilic cells represent young RBCs (reticulocytes) that retain abundant cytoplasmic RNA. The light blue polychromasia is caused by binding of both the methylene blue dye present in the Wright stain to the RNA and the eosin (red) dye to the hemoglobin. The tiny faintly blue bodies in the background are platelets.

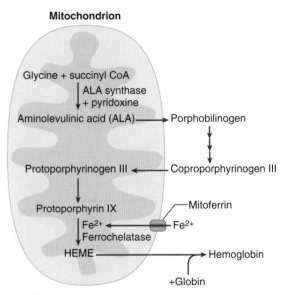

Fig. 4.12 Heme biosynthesis. *CoA*, Coenzyme A.

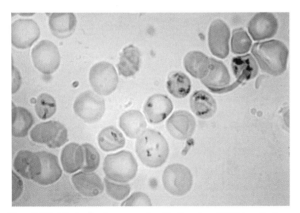

Fig. 4.10 Markedly increased reticulocytes (24%) noted on this blood smear stained with the alcoholic RNA-binding dye new methylene blue. The blue reticulum is an artifact caused by alcohol-mediated aggregation of the numerous mitochondria and ribosomes in the young red blood cells. In many laboratories, the reticulocyte count is now performed on an automated instrument using fluorescent RNA-binding dyes.

in the epidermis induce bullous formation and hyperpigmentation after sun exposure. Patients with PCT may also develop cirrhosis caused by porphyrin deposition in the liver. **Erythropoietic protoporphyria**, caused by mutations of the ferrochelatase gene, is characterized by severe cutaneous photosensitivity and chronic liver disease in later life. Some patients with erythropoietic protoporphyria also present with mild microcytic anemia and increased ring sideroblasts in the marrow, a process termed *sideroblastic anemia*.

SIDEROBLASTIC ANEMIA

Sideroblastic anemia is caused by a variety of inherited and acquired intramitochondrial defects in heme synthesis that lead to mitochondrial accumulation of iron within bone marrow erythroid precursors and abnormal erythroid maturation (**dyserythropoiesis**). Iron staining of the marrow in sideroblastic anemia reveals numerous **ring sideroblasts**, nucleated RBCs with a

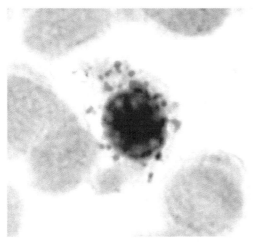

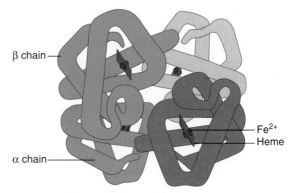

Fig. 4.14 Hemoglobin A structure.

Fig. 4.13 Ringed sideroblast (Prussian blue stain, marrow aspirate). The nucleated red blood cell contains numerous small, Prussian blue-positive, iron-laden mitochondria that form a ring around the nucleus. This is an abnormal finding. Normal sideroblasts contain only a few (one or two) particles of iron.

perinuclear ring-shaped distribution of iron-laden mitochondria (Fig. 4.13). Ring sideroblasts fail to properly develop and undergo apoptotic death within the marrow. The hypercellular erythroid predominant marrow is caused by EPO-driven dyserythropoiesis. The most common form of acquired sideroblastic anemia is classified as a clonal myelodysplasia (**MDS with ring sideroblasts**), associated with mutation of the *SF3B1* gene. Other causes of acquired sideroblastic anemia include drug therapy (e.g., cytotoxic agents, isoniazid, chloramphenicol), radiation therapy, alcohol abuse, and lead poisoning. Lead poisoning leads to sideroblastic anemia by directly inhibiting multiple steps of heme synthesis.

HEMOGLOBIN

Hemoglobin, an oxygen-binding molecule produced only by erythroid cells, is composed of two alpha chains and two non-alpha chains (beta, gamma, or delta), each of which binds one heme molecule (Fig. 4.14). Because each heme molecule can reversibly bind one molecule of oxygen, each hemoglobin molecule can bind four molecules of oxygen (O_2). The three hemoglobin variants normally seen in healthy adults are hemoglobin A ($\alpha_2\beta_2$) hemoglobin A_2 ($\alpha_2\delta_2$), and hemoglobin F ($\alpha_2\gamma_2$). Some globin gene mutations lead to imbalanced production of otherwise normal alpha or beta chains, with

damaging accumulation of excess unpaired globin chains, leading to **thalassemia** (see Chapter 4). Other globin gene mutations lead to synthesis of dysfunctional alpha or beta globin chains, conditions broadly classified as **hemoglobinopathy**. These structural mutations yield hemoglobin with poor solubility, altered oxygen affinity (high or low), and instability, all of which (except for high-affinity hemoglobin) lead to anemia.

Aged and damaged RBCs engulfed by splenic and hepatic macrophages are digested within lysosomes to yield lipids, peptides, and heme. Aged (senescent) RBCs that express high levels of PS in the outer leaflet of the plasma membrane are recognized and bound by PS receptor-positive macrophages (see Figs. 4.3, 4.4, and 7.1). Normally, PS is maintained within the inner leaflet of the plasma membrane through the action of the adenosine triphosphate–dependent enzyme flippase. During **apoptosis**, flippase is inactivated, and the enzyme scramblase leads to redistribution of PS to the outer leaflet, where it is recognized by the PS receptor on macrophages. Hemoglobin is degraded within macrophages to yield amino acids from globin, iron and biliverdin from heme, and **carbon monoxide**. Iron is recycled back to immature erythroid cells in the marrow for heme synthesis. Carbon monoxide bound to hemoglobin as **carboxyhemoglobin** is eventually expelled in the breath. Biliverdin (green pigment) is reduced to unconjugated (fat soluble) **bilirubin** (yellow pigment), transported to the liver bound to albumin (indirect bilirubin), and conjugated to glucuronic acid to form the more soluble form **bilirubin diglucuronide**. Conjugated bilirubin (termed direct bilirubin) is then excreted in the bile, where it is converted to **urobilinogen** and **stercobilin** (brown pigment) by colonic bacteria. Some urobilinogen is reabsorbed, converted to **urobilin**, and excreted in the urine, along with a small amount of bilirubin. Excess bilirubin deposited in skin and mucosa yields a yellowish discoloration termed **jaundice (icterus)**. Jaundice is often seen in patients with chronic liver disease.

There is no normal physiologic mechanism for release of excess iron, with minimal iron loss occurring by GI mucosa cell loss, skin cell desquamation of skin cells, and menstruation in women. Thus, iron balance is maintained primarily by the rate of intestinal absorption. The rate of intestinal absorption is controlled by **intestinal crypt epithelial cells** that monitor the transferrin iron content of the interstitial fluid via the membrane-bound TFR–HFE complex. HFE is a human class I leukocyte antigen (HLA) class I protein that associates in the plasma membrane with the transferrin receptor. In iron-deficient states, the low level of iron detected in the interstitial fluid by intestinal crypt cells triggers increased villus enterocyte expression of DMT-1 and ferroportin, leading to increased intestinal iron absorption. Also, because low serum iron leads to a reduction in hepcidin production by the liver, reduced hepcidin likely contributes to increased iron uptake by ferroportin.

Anemia of chronic disease is a mild to moderate anemia associated with chronic inflammation and chronic infection. This form of anemia is due to a combination of decreased RBC survival and inadequate erythropoiesis. Inflammatory cytokine-mediated activation of splenic and hepatic macrophages and increased binding of antibody and complement to RBCs leads to increased hemolysis. EPO production in anemia of chronic disease is blunted by inhibition of EPO synthesis by the inflammatory cytokines **interleukin-1** and **tumor necrosis factor α**. Complicating the EPO production defect is **EPO resistance**, which is caused by functional iron deficiency, preventing RBCs from producing adequate hemoglobin. The inflammatory cytokine interleukin-6 induces hepatic synthesis of the iron-regulating hormone hepcidin. Hepcidin binding to the cell membrane iron transporter protein ferroportin leads to ferroportin degradation, blocking the release of iron by macrophages and intestinal cells and preventing the transfer of iron to RBC precursors in the marrow. Although typically normochromic and normocytic, the anemia may be hypochromic, microcytic, or both hypochromic and microcytic in some cases. Serum iron and iron-binding capacity are decreased, and serum ferritin

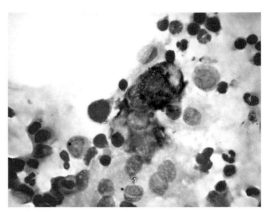

Fig. 4.15 Increased macrophage iron (Prussian blue stain, marrow aspirate) and decreased sideroblasts (iron-positive nucleated blood red cells) as seen in anemia of chronic disease.

is increased. The decrease in iron-binding capacity is caused by reduced production of apotransferrin by the liver. In contrast to blood levels of positive acute-phase reactants such as C-reactive protein, fibrinogen, and ferritin that rise in response to inflammation, blood levels of the negative acute-phase reactant transferrin drop in response to inflammation. Examination of the marrow in anemia of chronic disease reveals numerous iron-laden macrophages and markedly decreased sideroblasts (nucleated RBCs with small particles of stainable iron) (Fig. 4.15).

HEMOGLOBIN OXYGEN AFFINITY

The oxygen affinity of hemoglobin depends primarily on three factors—temperature, pH, and concentration of RBC **2,3-bisphosphoglycerate (2,3-BPG)** (also known as 2,3-diphosphoglycerate [2,3-DPG]). Oxygen affinity declines with increasing temperature, decreasing pH, and increasing 2,3-BPG concentration. Oxygen affinity is usually expressed in terms of the p50—the oxygen tension (partial pressure) at which hemoglobin is half-saturated (Fig. 4.16). It is important to keep in mind that the oxygen affinity and the p50 are inversely related; that is, a decrease in oxygen affinity translates to an increase in the p50. Increased metabolic activity requires an increased supply of oxygen. As body temperature rises, the oxygen affinity of hemoglobin drops, allowing for more rapid delivery of oxygen to metabolically active tissues. Similarly, a decrease in pH (acidosis) usually signifies hypoxia, a condition for which more

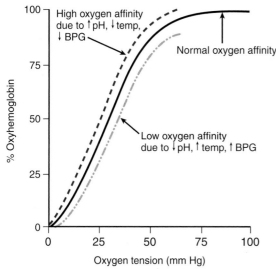

Fig. 4.16 Hemoglobin oxygen affinity. *BPG,* Bisphosphoglycerate; *temp,* temperature.

rapid delivery of oxygen to tissues is highly advantageous. Thus, as with high temperature, a decreasing pH triggers a decrease in hemoglobin oxygen affinity and more efficient delivery of oxygen to hypoxic tissues. Acidosis and hypoxia are both associated with increases in RBC 2,3-BPG concentration. 2,3-BPG stabilizes the structure of deoxyhemoglobin A by loosely and reversibly binding to the beta globin subunits of deoxyhemoglobin A, thereby reducing oxygen affinity.

Some mutant hemoglobins are characterized by altered oxygen affinity. Patients with **high-affinity hemoglobin** present with increased RBC mass (**polycythemia**). The reduced delivery of high-affinity hemoglobin–bound oxygen to tissues triggers the kidney to release high levels of EPO, consequently stimulating increased erythropoiesis. **Low-affinity hemoglobins,** on the other hand, are associated with **cyanosis** and mild anemia. Cyanosis is caused by the rapid, inappropriate release of low-affinity hemoglobin–bound oxygen to tissues, with enhanced conversion of *bright red* oxyhemoglobin to *dark red* (cyanotic) deoxyhemoglobin. The mild anemia is caused by resetting of the EPO set point to a lower hematocrit.

KEY WORDS AND CONCEPTS

- 2,3-Bisphosphoglycerate (2,3-BPG)
- Acute intermittent porphyria (AIP)
- Acute-phase reactant
- Aminolevulinic acid (ALA) synthase
- Anemia of chronic disease
- Anemia of iron deficiency
- Apoferritin
- Apoptosis
- Bilirubin
- Bilirubin diglucuronide
- Biliverdin
- Bone marrow macrophages
- Carbon monoxide
- Carboxyhemoglobin
- Complete blood count (CBC)
- Ceruloplasmin
- Cytochrome p450
- Delta aminolevulinic acid
- Divalent metal transporter 1 (DMT-1)
- Duodenal cytochrome B
- Dyserythropoiesis
- Elliptocyte
- EPO resistance
- Erythropoietic protoporphyria
- Extracellular ceruloplasmin
- Ferrihydrite
- Ferritin
- Ferrochelatase
- Ferroportin
- Flippase
- Glycine
- Haptoglobin (HPG)
- Heme
- Heme carrier protein (HCP)
- Heme iron
- Heme oxygenase (HO)
- Hemochromatosis
- Hemoglobin
- Hemopexin (HPX)
- Hemoglobinopathy
- Hemosiderin

- Hepcidin
- Hephaestin (HAE)
- Hereditary hemochromatosis (HH)
- HFE (high iron protein)
- High-affinity hemoglobin
- Hypoxia-inducible factor (HIF1)
- Hypoxia-responsive elements (HRE)
- Ineffective erythropoiesis
- Interleukin-1
- Intestinal crypt epithelial cells
- Iron
- Iron chaperone protein (ICP)
- Iron-responsive elements
- Iron-responsive proteins
- Jaundice (icterus)
- Labile iron pool (LIP)
- Lead poisoning
- Low-affinity hemoglobin
- Myoglobin
- Nonheme (ionic) iron
- Oxygen affinity
- Phagolysosomes
- Phosphatidylserine (PS)
- Pinocytosis
- Polychromatophilic
- Polycythemia

- Porphobilinogen deaminase
- Porphyria
- Porphyria cutanea tarda (PCT)
- Protoporphyrin IX
- PS receptor
- Pyridoxine (vitamin B_6)
- MDS with ring sideroblasts
- Reticulocytopenia
- Reticulocytosis
- Ring sideroblast
- Scramblase
- Sideroblastic anemia
- Sideroblast
- Siderosome
- Stercobilin
- Succinyl coenzyme A
- Thalassemia
- Transferrin (TRF)
- Transferrin receptor (TFR1, TFR2)
- Tumor necrosis factor alpha
- Urobilin
- Villus epithelium
- Vitamin C ferrireductase
- Urobilinogen
- Zinc protoporphyrin (ZP)

REVIEW QUESTIONS

1. Which of the following is blocked by hepcidin?
   A. Ferroportin
   B. DMT-1
   C. HCP
   D. Transferrin receptor
   E. Hephaestin
2. Intestinal crypt cells modulate intestinal iron uptake by interaction of transferrin receptor with
   A. DMT-1.
   B. HFE.
   C. ferritin.
   D. HCP.
   E. hephaestin.

3. Heme synthesis is dependent on which vitamin?
   A. Vitamin C
   B. Vitamin B_{12}
   C. Vitamin B6
   D. Folic acid
   E. Vitamin A
4. Porphyria is caused by defects of
   A. heme synthesis.
   B. globin chain production.
   C. iron uptake.
   D. hemoglobin oxygen affinity.
   E. Erythropoiesis.

5

Hemoglobinopathy

KEY POINTS

- Normal adult hemoglobins include hemoglobins A (97%), A_2 (2%–3%), and F (<1%).

- Trace quantities of nonfunctional hemoglobins (methemoglobin, carboxyhemoglobin, sulfhemoglobin, and nitrosohemoglobin) are present in normal blood.

- Specific inherited point mutations of the beta-globin gene lead to abnormal unstable hemoglobin and resultant hemolytic anemia (e.g., hemoglobins S, C, and E).

- The hemolysis seen with hemoglobins S and C is caused by intraerythrocytic precipitation of the unstable abnormal hemoglobin with increased red blood cell (RBC) rigidity.

- Thalassemias are anemias caused by defects in globin gene synthesis leading to unbalanced production of globin chains and formation of unstable globin chain homo-tetramers.

- In alpha thalassemia reduced alpha chains leads to excess beta chains and formation of unstable beta-chain tetramers. In beta thalassemia reduced beta chains leads to excess alpha chains and formation of increased hemoglobin A2, hemoglobin F, and unstable alpha chain tetramers.

- Some hemoglobin variants with poor solubility (often due to alpha gene mutation) lead to formation of red cells with intracellular aggregates of unstable hemoglobin (Heinz bodies).

Normal hemoglobin types differ in the identity of the non-alpha globin chains—that is, beta chains in hemoglobin A, gamma chains in hemoglobin F, and delta chains in hemoglobin A_2. The proportions of normal hemoglobin variants in red blood cells (RBCs) vary with age. Synthesis of embryonic hemoglobins Gower and Portland is rapidly followed during the first trimester of pregnancy by synthesis of hemoglobin F. At birth, the predominant hemoglobin is **hemoglobin F (fetal hemoglobin)**. Composed of two alpha and two gamma-globin chains, hemoglobin F is especially well-suited to meet the needs of fetuses by binding more avidly to oxygen than adult hemoglobin A, thus facilitating oxygen transfer from maternal blood to fetal blood in the placenta. The synthesis of hemoglobin A begins in fetal life, but at birth, it accounts for less than 45% of total hemoglobin. After birth, gamma-chain synthesis rapidly declines, and hemoglobin F levels fall such that by 1 year of age, the proportion of hemoglobin variants reaches adult levels: greater than 95% hemoglobin A, 1% to 3% hemoglobin A_2, and 0% to 2% hemoglobin F. **Hemoglobin A** is composed of two alpha- and two beta-globin chains, and **hemoglobin A_2** is composed of two alpha- and two delta-globin chains. Hemoglobins A and A_2 bind to oxygen less avidly than hemoglobin F and thus deliver oxygen to tissues at a higher oxygen tension. Poorly controlled diabetes mellitus is characterized by increased amounts of **hemoglobin A_{1c}**, a hemoglobin A variant formed by irreversible nonenzymatic glycation of the beta-globin chain.

NONFUNCTIONAL HEMOGLOBIN VARIANTS

Trace amounts of nonfunctional hemoglobin are present in normal blood. These include methemoglobin, carboxyhemoglobin, nitrosohemoglobin, and sulfhemoglobin. **Methemoglobin**, or oxidized hemoglobin, is formed from hemoglobin by oxidation of heme iron from the ferrous to the ferric form. In nearly all cases, methemoglobinemia is caused by hemoglobin oxidation induced by drugs or toxins. Although methemoglobin itself does not bind oxygen reversibly, the interaction of methemoglobin with normal hemoglobin in the blood of patients with methemoglobinemia leads to increased oxygen affinity and consequent tissue hypoxia. **Carboxyhemoglobin** results from the binding of carbon monoxide to heme iron. Because carbon monoxide binds to hemoglobin 200 times more strongly than oxygen, exposure to very small amounts of carbon monoxide leads to a large amount of carboxyhemoglobin. Tissue hypoxia is caused not only by the inability of carboxyhemoglobin to carry oxygen but also by the increased oxygen affinity of hybrid oxygen–carbon monoxide tetramers. Nitric oxide binds reversibly to hemoglobin to form **nitrosohemoglobin**. However, the physiologic and clinical significance of this interaction are unclear at this time. **Sulfhemoglobin** is formed by heme sulfation, most often by sulfur-containing drugs, leading to reduced oxygen affinity. Low hemoglobin oxygen affinity leads to more rapid oxygen delivery to tissues with reduced erythropoietin production and mild anemia.

BETA-GLOBIN MUTATIONS

Nearly all common inherited disorders of hemoglobin are caused by beta-globin gene mutations that lead to single amino acid substitutions in the beta-globin molecule. These disorders, known collectively as the beta hemoglobinopathies, are autosomal recessive conditions, with the symptomatic homozygous state often referred to as "*disease*" and the asymptomatic heterozygous form referred to as "*trait*." Having said this, homozygous hemoglobin S (beta hemoglobin genotype SS) is best known as **sickle cell anemia** (rather than sickle cell disease), and heterozygous hemoglobin S (beta-hemoglobin genotype AS) is known as **sickle cell trait**. In sickle cell anemia, hemoglobin S is the predominant hemoglobin, and no hemoglobin A is present. In sickle cell trait, hemoglobin A is the predominant hemoglobin, and hemoglobin S accounts for 35% to 45% of total hemoglobin. Other common inherited beta-chain defects include **hemoglobins C, D, and E**. In every case,

only the homozygous or mixed heterozygous condition (e.g., hemoglobin SC) is associated with anemia. **Hemoglobin E** is perhaps the most common hemoglobin variant worldwide, with the highest prevalence in Southeast Asia. **Hemoglobin E disease** is an asymptomatic condition associated with mild microcytosis. **Hemoglobin D trait** is an entirely asymptomatic condition, with the highest prevalence seen in people of northwest Indian descent.

Hemoglobins S and C are poorly soluble hemoglobin variants that form intraerythrocytic crystalline precipitates in the deoxygenated state. Whereas precipitated hemoglobin S forms rigid tactoids that induce RBC sickling (Fig. 5.1), precipitated hemoglobin C forms discrete rhomboid structures that less significantly alter the shape of RBCs (Fig. 5.2). In the case of sickle cell disease, the increased rigidity of sickle cells impedes their flow through small capillaries and splenic red pulp, leading to hemolysis, thrombosis, ischemia, and ultimately, end-organ failure. Sudden episodes of severe bone pain caused by ischemia in patients with sickle cell anemia are termed **sickle cell crises**. The multiple bouts of thrombosis and infarction of the spleen in patients with sickle cell disease ultimately lead to splenic atrophy and increased susceptibility to pneumococcal (*Streptococcus pneumoniae)* sepsis caused by the loss of splenic function. **Howell-Jolly bodies** are discrete basophilic intraerythrocytic inclusions of DNA commonly seen on peripheral smears of patients with asplenia caused by splenectomy or splenic atrophy (Fig. 5.3).

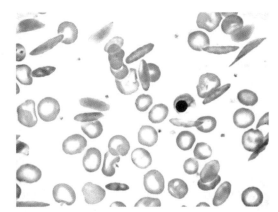

Fig. 5.1 Sickle cell anemia (peripheral blood smear). Numerous sickle-shaped red blood cells (RBCs), along with a nucleated RBC (nucleus partially extruded) and increased polychromasia (indicative of hemolysis with some compensation).

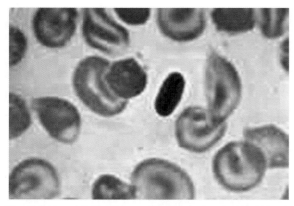

Fig. 5.2 Hemoglobin C crystal (dense rhomboid object in center) and numerous target cells (peripheral smear).

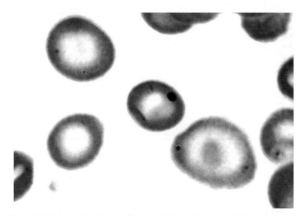

Fig. 5.3 Howell-Jolly bodies (peripheral smear). The discrete dark blue, round particle in the central blood red cell is the best example in this field. This structure stains blue because it consists of retained DNA. Howell-Jolly bodies are often found in patients with a nonfunctional (or absent) spleen. Also seen in this field is a target cell.

The highest prevalence of the hemoglobin S allele is found in tropical Africa, ranging from 20% to 40%. In African Americans, the frequency is about 8%. Hemoglobin S is also found in the Middle East, Greece, and India.

Hemoglobin C disease, seen most often in people of West African descent, is a microcytic hypochromic anemia with splenomegaly and numerous target cells on peripheral smears.

Hemoglobin SC disease is a mild sickling disorder caused by the coinheritance of a hemoglobin S allele and a hemoglobin C allele. Numerous target cells and relatively few plump sickle cells are seen on peripheral smears.

THALASSEMIA

The **thalassemias** are another common group of hemoglobin defects caused by autosomal codominant mutations or deletions in the alpha- or beta-globin gene region that lead to reduced synthesis of normal alpha or beta-globin chains (Table 5.1). These defects lead to variable degrees of anemia caused both by ineffective erythropoiesis (caused by increased RBC destruction in the marrow) and production of microcytic hypochromic RBCs with shortened lifespans.

A tandem pair of alpha-globin genes is inherited from each parent, yielding four alpha-globin genes per diploid genome. In **alpha thalassemia**, one or more alpha-globin genes are deleted. Reduced alpha-globin synthesis leads to an imbalance in alpha and non-alpha (beta, gamma, delta)-globin synthesis, leading to reduced hemoglobin synthesis and production of microcytic hypochromic RBCs. Decreased production and the shortened half-lives of alpha thalassemic RBCs (with consequent anemia) are caused by formation of unstable homotetramers of excess non-alpha globin chains, leading to RBC destruction in the bone marrow (ineffective erythropoiesis) and spleen (extravascular hemolysis). Inheritance of four deleted alpha-globin genes (genotype $--/--$) prevents production of all normal hemoglobins (hemoglobins F, A, and A_2). In this situation, the major hemoglobin that forms in the fetus is **hemoglobin Barts**, a nonfunctional gamma chain homotetramer ($\gamma4$). Oxygen delivery to fetal tissues is markedly reduced, leading to a severe hypoxic condition incompatible with extrauterine life known as **hydrops fetalis**. Inheritance of three deleted alpha-globin genes ($--/+-$) leads to a moderate to severe hypochromic microcytic anemia known as **hemoglobin H disease**. In this condition, up to 25% hemoglobin Barts is present during infancy, and up to 30% hemoglobin H, the beta-chain homotetramer ($\beta4$), is present after 1 year of age. Hemoglobin Barts and hemoglobin H are both high-affinity hemoglobin variants, avidly binding oxygen and releasing it only at a very low oxygen tension. As such, they do not function properly in tissue oxygenation. These variant hemoglobins are easily detected by hemoglobin fractionation as differentially charged hemoglobin species.

In contrast to the insoluble alpha-chain tetramers formed in beta thalassemia, the gamma- and beta-chain tetramers (hemoglobins Barts and H) formed in alpha

TABLE 5.1 **Thalassemia Syndromes**

Clinical Variant	Genotype	Complete blood Count	Hemoglobin Variants	Clinical Severity
Alpha Thalassemia				
Silent carrier	$-\alpha/\alpha\alpha$	Normal: mild microcytosis	Normal	Asymptomatic
Trait	$-\alpha/-\alpha$ $--/\alpha\alpha$	Microcytosis: minimal anemia	Normal	Asymptomatic: mild anemia
Hemoglobin H disease	$--/-\alpha$	Severe microcytic hypochromic anemia	Hemoglobin H ($\beta4$)	Moderately severe anemia
Hydrops fetalis	$--/--$	Severe microcytic hypochromic anemia	Hemoglobin Barts ($\gamma4$)	Severe anemia
Beta Thalassemia				
Thalassemia minor	β^0/β β^+/β β^+/β^+	Microcytosis, target cells	↑ Hemoglobin A_2 Slight ↑ hemoglobin F	Asymptomatic
Thalassemia major	β^0/β^0 β^0/β^+ β^+/β^+	Severe microcytic anemia, targets, schistocytes, nucleated RBCs	↑↑ Hemoglobin F ↓↓ Hemoglobin A	Severe anemia
HPFH[a]	$\delta\beta^0/\delta\beta^0$ $\delta\beta^0/\delta\beta$	Microcytosis: normal	↑↑ Hemoglobin F Hemoglobin A_2	Asymptomatic
Delta–beta thalassemia	$\delta\beta^0/\delta\beta^0$ $\delta\beta^+/\delta\beta^+$ $\delta\beta^0/\delta\beta$ $\delta\beta^+/\delta\beta$	Microcytic hypochromic anemia, target cells	↑↑ Hemoglobin F ↑ Hemoglobin Lepore	Mild to moderate anemia

[a]Other forms of hereditary persistence of fetal hemoglobin (HPFH) not listed here are nondeletional, with point mutations upstream of the delta-globin locus.
RBC, Red blood cell.

thalassemia are relatively soluble and form damaging intracellular precipitates only within aged RBCs. Hemoglobin H precipitates can be identified in older RBCs on peripheral blood smears only after staining with a redox dye, such as brilliant cresyl violet. Thus, in contrast to beta thalassemia, there is little destruction of developing RBCs within the bone marrow in alpha thalassemia. Instead, the major causes of the anemia in alpha thalassemia are production of microcytic hypochromic RBCs and extravascular (intrasplenic) hemolysis of aged RBCs.

Inheritance of two deleted alpha-globin genes ($--/++$ or $+-/+-$) leads to the asymptomatic condition **alpha thalassemia trait**, characterized by production of hypochromic microcytic RBCs and target cells. Inheritance of a single deleted alpha gene ($+-/++$) leads to the asymptomatic condition **alpha thalassemia silent carrier** with no hematologic abnormalities.

In **beta thalassemia**, reduced beta-chain synthesis leads to decreased hemoglobin A production, and compensatory increased production of gamma- and delta-globin leads to increased levels of hemoglobins A_2 and F, respectively. Excess alpha chains form insoluble **alpha-chain tetramers** ($\alpha4$) and poorly deformable RBCs that are either destroyed in the bone marrow (**ineffective erythropoiesis**) or removed by the spleen (**extravascular hemolysis**). The alpha-chain aggregates are not usually seen on routine blood smears but may be detected after exposure of smears to reducing agents. There are three clinical conditions—beta thalassemia major (homozygous), thalassemia intermedia, and beta thalassemia minor (heterozygous). **Thalassemia major** (homozygous β^0/β^0) is marked by severe microcytic hypochromic anemia with **anisopoikilocytosis** (significant variation in both size and shape) (Fig. 5.4). In this condition, no beta chain is produced at either allele (β^0 signifying a nonfunctional gene), and nearly all the hemoglobin is hemoglobin F with a small fraction of hemoglobin A_2. Patients with thalassemia major have severe transfusion-dependent anemia. Inadequate transfusion support leads to childhood growth retardation,

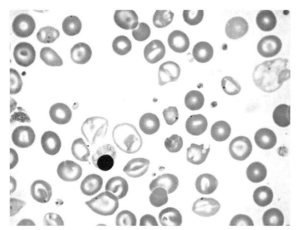

Fig. 5.4 Thalassemia major (peripheral smear). Hypochromic microcytic red blood cells (RBCs) with anisopoikilocytosis, Howell-Jolly bodies, and basophilic stippling. Also present is a nucleated RBC.

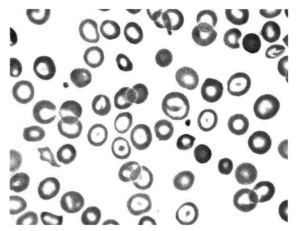

Fig. 5.5 Thalassemia minor (peripheral smear). Slight anisopoikilocytosis and numerous target cells.

skeletal abnormalities, hepatosplenomegaly, hyperpigmentation, and high risk of infection. With transfusion therapy alone, by the second decade, many patients develop endocrine and cardiac abnormalities caused by deposition of excess iron (siderosis) in endocrine organs and the heart, complications that can largely be avoided by iron chelation therapy.

In contrast to thalassemia major, patients with **thalassemia intermedia** present with mild anemia that seldom requires transfusion therapy. In many cases, patients with homozygous β^+ thalassemia (β^+/β^+), beta-chain production is moderately reduced (β^+ signifying a hypofunctional gene). Thus, patients with this condition produce less hemoglobin A, with increased amounts of hemoglobins F and A_2. **Thalassemia minor** (the heterozygous condition) is marked by microcytosis, hypochromia, elevated RBC count (a compensatory mechanism), and numerous target cells (caused by the reduction in RBC hemoglobin content) (Fig. 5.5).

Coinheritance of a beta hemoglobinopathy such as sickle cell trait with thalassemia sometimes occurs. **Sickle-alpha thalassemia**, sickle trait inherited with alpha thalassemia trait, results in a mild microcytic anemia, with an increased proportion of hemoglobin A and a reduced amount of hemoglobin S ($<35\%$). **Sickle-beta thalassemia**, sickle trait inherited with beta thalassemia trait, results in a microcytic anemia with reduced hemoglobin A and increased hemoglobin S.

Delta–beta thalassemia is a condition in which synthesis of both delta and beta chains are reduced. The delta and beta genes are located near each other on chromosome 11. Thus, some deletions in this region affect synthesis of both globin chains. Delta–beta thalassemia is broadly divided into those in which both genes are deleted ($\delta\beta^0$) and those in which the genes are only partially deleted ($\delta\beta^+$). In homozygous $\delta\beta^0$ thalassemia, the only hemoglobin produced is hemoglobin F; in the heterozygous condition, hemoglobin F is only moderately increased (5%–20%), and most of the remaining hemoglobin is hemoglobin A. In homozygous $\delta\beta^+$ thalassemia, most (80%) of the hemoglobin is hemoglobin F, with the remaining hemoglobin (20%) being hemoglobin Lepore. **Hemoglobin Lepore** is composed of two hybrid delta–beta chains (delta–beta fusion gene product) paired with two normal alpha chains. In heterozygous $\delta\beta^+$ thalassemia, hemoglobin Lepore accounts for only about 8% of total hemoglobin, most of the remaining hemoglobin being hemoglobin A.

Hereditary persistence of fetal hemoglobin (HPFH) is a clinically silent condition closely related to delta–beta thalassemia. In **homozygous $\delta\beta^0$ HPFH**, a condition caused by deletions of the delta–beta region on chromosome 11, hemoglobin F accounts for 100% of all hemoglobin, a feature shared with homozygous $\delta\beta^0$ thalassemia. Although $\delta\beta^0$ thalassemia is accompanied by microcytic hypochromic anemia with target cells, the blood count and peripheral smear in HPFH are normal. In the heterozygous state, these two related disorders

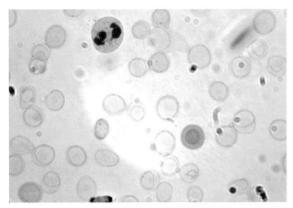

Fig. 5.6 Acid elution for detection of F cells (Kleihauer-Betke test). Most red blood cells (RBCs) in this field have been rendered devoid of hemoglobin by acid treatment (pale, ghostlike cells), a feature consistent with (adult) hemoglobin A–positive cells. Hemoglobin F, unlike all other hemoglobins, resists acid elution. One RBC (1:50, 2%) in this field has retained its hemoglobin, a feature consistent with a hemoglobin F cell (F cell). Note the single neutrophil in the upper field. Because normal adult blood contains less than 0.01% F cells, this field contains a significant increase in F cells. The Kleihauer-Betke technique allows for calculation of the percentage of fetal cells in maternal blood for purposes of gauging the degree of fetomaternal hemorrhage in prevention of hemolytic disease of the newborn. The test may also be useful in distinguishing beta thalassemia trait from hereditary persistence of fetal hemoglobin (HPFH). In beta thalassemia trait, the distribution of hemoglobin F in individual RBCs is quite heterogeneous; in HPFH, it is relatively uniform.

can be distinguished by the level of hemoglobin F: 20% to 30% in $\delta\beta^0$ HPFH compared with 5% to 20% in $\delta\beta^0$ thalassemia.

These two related conditions can also be distinguished by performing an **acid elution test** on a peripheral blood smear. In this assay, acid treatment of RBCs elutes out hemoglobin A, leaving acid-resistant hemoglobin F. After being stained, the presence and distribution of bright red hemoglobin F-positive RBCs (F cells) and pale hemoglobin A–positive cells is easily determined (Fig. 5.6). Although a homogenous distribution of F cells is seen in $\delta\beta^0$ HPFH, a heterogeneous distribution of positive and negative cells is seen in $\delta\beta^0$ thalassemia.

Nondeletional HPFH is a heterogeneous group of clinically silent disorders characterized by mildly to moderately increased hemoglobin F (5%–25%) caused by point mutations upstream of the gamma-globin locus. Recall that gamma chains associate with alpha chains to form hemoglobin F. Patients who coinherit both mild HPFH and beta thalassemia often express a milder illness, presumably because of the protective effects offered by high hemoglobin F levels.

UNSTABLE HEMOGLOBIN VARIANTS

Inheritance of **unstable hemoglobin**, usually caused by an alpha-globin mutation, may lead to a (usually) mild form of hemolytic anemia with high reticulocyte count. The unstable hemoglobin denatures and precipitates within the RBCs, forming inclusions called **Heinz bodies**. By reducing RBC deformability, Heinz bodies lead to accelerated removal of the abnormal RBCs by macrophages in the splenic cords (extravascular hemolysis). Heinz bodies can be visualized in RBCs after staining peripheral smears with the reducing dye brilliant cresyl blue (Fig. 5.7). Unstable hemoglobins can also be detected by their poor solubility in isopropanol using the **isopropanol solubility test**.

Hemoglobin fractions are detected by a variety of techniques, including agar gel electrophoresis, isoelectric focusing, and chromatography of peripheral blood hemolysates. All these techniques are based on separation of hemoglobin types by charge density. In **alkaline gel electrophoresis** (pH, 8.6), all forms of hemoglobin are negatively charged and move toward the anode at varying rates depending on amino acid composition. For example, hemoglobin S forms a distinct, slow-moving band in comparison with hemoglobin A. In **acid gel electrophoresis** (pH, 6.2), most forms of hemoglobin are positively charged and move toward the

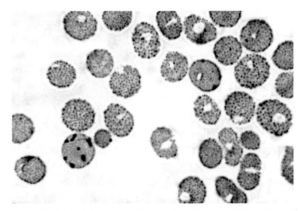

Fig. 5.7 Heinz body preparation with multiple aggregates of precipitated hemoglobin (Heinz bodies) in peripheral blood.

cathode at varying rates. Each agar electrophoresis technique has limitations in distinguishing among some hemoglobin variants.

Isoelectric focusing provides better separation of hemoglobin variants than agar electrophoresis. This gel method uses a set of small proteins (ampholytes) with a range of isoelectric points that are incorporated into an agarose gel. When a current is applied, the ampholytes form a pH gradient across the gel (pH, 6–8). Each hemoglobin molecule then migrates to the point (isoelectric point) in the gel at which the pH of its charge becomes neutral. For example, hemoglobins A, C, and S are readily distinguished given their respective isoelectric points of 6.95, 7.40, and 7.25. A limitation of isoelectric focusing is that some hemoglobin variants have nearly identical isoelectric points (e.g., hemoglobins C and A_2) and thus cannot be separated by this technique. In this case, the technique of **high-performance liquid chromatography** (**HPLC**) has proved useful (Fig. 5.8). In HPLC, the hemolysate is injected into the end of a thin tube filled with a stationary matrix through which a solution is passed under pressure. The chemical properties of the matrix and solution are such that the hemoglobin molecules pass through the tube at different rates depending on both molecular size and charge.

KEY WORDS AND CONCEPTS

- Acid elution test
- Acid gel electrophoresis
- Alkaline gel electrophoresis
- Alpha-chain tetramers
- Alpha thalassemia
- Alpha thalassemia silent carrier
- Alpha thalassemia trait
- Anisopoikilocytosis
- Beta thalassemia
- Carboxyhemoglobin
- Delta–beta thalassemia
- Extravascular hemolysis
- Heinz bodies
- Hemoglobin A
- Hemoglobin A_{1c}
- Hemoglobin A_2
- Hemoglobin Barts
- Hemoglobin C
- Hemoglobin D
- Hemoglobin D trait
- Hemoglobin E
- Hemoglobin E disease
- Hemoglobin F (fetal hemoglobin)
- Hemoglobin H disease
- Hemoglobin Lepore
- Hemoglobin SC disease
- Hereditary persistence of fetal hemoglobin (HPFH)
- High-performance liquid chromatography (HPLC)
- Homozygous $\delta\beta^0$ HPFH
- Howell-Jolly bodies
- Hydrops fetalis
- Ineffective erythropoiesis

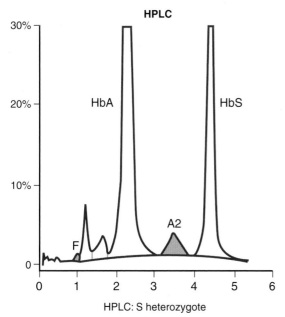

Fig. 5.8 Hemoglobin high-performance liquid chromatography (HPLC) (sickle trait). Notable hemoglobins *(from left to right)* are hemoglobin F *(tiny peak)*, glycosylated hemoglobins *(two small, unlabeled peaks)*, hemoglobin A *(major peak)*, hemoglobin A_2 *(small peak)*, and hemoglobin S *(major peak)*. The nearly equal amounts of hemoglobins A and S (A > S) and the slightly increased hemoglobin A_2 are highly characteristic of sickle cell trait (hemoglobin AS).

- Isoelectric focusing
- Isopropanol solubility test
- Methemoglobin
- Nitrosohemoglobin
- Non-deletional HPFH
- Sickle cell anemia
- Sickle cell crises
- Sickle cell trait

- Sickle-alpha thalassemia
- Sickle-beta thalassemia
- Sulfhemoglobin
- Thalassemia intermedia
- Thalassemia major
- Thalassemia minor
- Thalassemias
- Unstable hemoglobin

REVIEW QUESTIONS

1. Hydrops fetalis, a condition incompatible with extra-uterine life, is caused by complete absence of
   A. alpha-globin chains.
   B. beta-globin chains.
   C. gamma-globin chains.
   D. delta-globin chains.
2. Which of the nonfunctional hemoglobin variants below contain heme bound to ferric iron?
   A. Sulfhemoglobin
   B. Hemoglobin Barts
   C. Carboxyhemoglobin
   D. Methemoglobin

3. Which feature below is **not** characteristic of sickle cell anemia?
   A. Thrombosis
   B. Splenic infarction
   C. Bleeding
   D. Bone pain
4. Which of the following is **not** increased in beta thalassemia?
   A. Hemoglobin F
   B. Hemoglobin Barts
   C. Hemoglobin A_2
   D. Alpha-chain homotetramers

6

Red Blood Cell Metabolism and Enzyme Defects

KEY POINTS

- Red blood cell (RBC) energy is supplied entirely by anerobic glycolysis.

- Three auxiliary metabolic pathways branch from the glycolytic pathway: the hexose monophosphate (HMP) shunt, the 2,3-bisphosphoglycerate (2,3-BPG) pathway, and the methemoglobin reductase pathway.

- The HMP shunt produces glutathione, a reducing agent that protects RBCs from oxidative damage.

- Bisphosphoglycerate produced by the 2,3-BPG pathway leads to decreased hemoglobin oxygen affinity and more rapid release of oxygen to hypoxic tissues.

- Nicotinamide adenine dinucleotide plus hydrogen (NADH)–dependent methemoglobin reductase converts nonfunctional methemoglobin to functional hemoglobin by reduction of ferric iron (Fe^{3+}) to ferrous (Fe^{2+}) iron.

- Inherited defects in metabolic enzymes glucose-6-phosphate dehydrogenase (G6PD) and pyruvate kinase lead to hemolytic anemia caused by either oxidative damage to hemoglobin (G6PD deficiency) or loss of RBC membrane integrity (PK deficiency).

- Methemoglobinemia, a cyanotic nonhemolytic condition, is most often seen as an acquired condition associated with exposure to oxidant drugs.

After enucleation, red blood cell (RBC) metabolism is maintained by mitochondria, a short supply of residual mRNA, and preformed enzymes. Glucose, which enters RBCs in an insulin-independent fashion, is catabolized via the anaerobic **Embden-Meyerhof-Parnas glycolytic pathway**. Because the aerobic citric acid cycle does not function in the RBCs, both end products of glycolysis (pyruvate and lactate) are released into the blood. **Glycolysis** yields a net energy gain of two molecules of adenosine triphosphate (ATP) per molecule of glucose. This energy is primarily used by the RBCs to maintain osmotic equilibrium and membrane integrity. Glycolysis also yields reducing power (from nicotinamide adenine dinucleotide plus hydrogen [NADH] and nicotinamide adenine dinucleotide phosphate [NADPH]) that can be used to reverse oxidant damage sustained by RBCs.

Three important auxiliary metabolic pathways branch from the glycolytic pathway: the **hexose monophosphate**

(HMP) shunt, the **2,3-bisphosphoglycerate (2,3-BPG)** pathway, and the methemoglobin reductase pathway (Fig. 6.1).

The **HMP shunt**, by converting NADP to its reduced form, NADPH, replenishes the supply of **glutathione**, a sulfhydryl-containing tripeptide that serves as a protective reducing agent in RBCs by inactivation of hydrogen peroxide and reduction of oxidized proteins, including hemoglobin. The first reaction in the HMP shunt, the conversion of glucose-6-phosphate to 6-phosphogluconolactone, is catalyzed by the enzyme **glucose-6-phosphate dehydrogenase (G6PD)**.

Under conditions of hypoxia or acidosis, oxygen delivery to tissues is enhanced by a reduction in hemoglobin oxygen affinity due to reversible binding of **2,3-BPG** to hemoglobin. The conversion of 1,3-BPG to 2,3-BPG leads to reduced hemoglobin oxygen affinity at the expense of one molecule of ATP. Increased 2,3-BPG

41

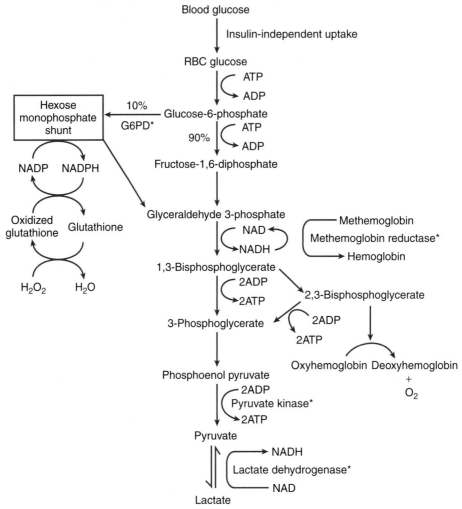

Fig. 6.1 Erythrocyte metabolism. Red blood cells need energy to maintain heme iron in reduced Fe^{2+} form, to maintain reduced sulfhydryl groups in proteins, to preserve the osmotic gradient with ion pumps, and to prevent oxidation of membrane lipids. *Asterisks* mark enzymes for which deficiency is associated with hemolytic anemia. *ADP,* Adenosine diphosphate; *ATP,* adenosine triphosphate; *G6PD,* glucose-6-phosphate dehydrogenase; *NAD,* nicotinamide adenine dinucleotide; *NADH,* nicotinamide adenine dinucleotide plus hydrogen; *NADPH,* nicotinamide adenine dinucleotide phosphate; *RBC,* red blood cell.

deoxyhemoglobin with greater affinity than oxyhemoglobin, leading to more rapid oxygen delivery to hypoxic tissues.

Methemoglobin, a nonfunctional hemoglobin variant formed by oxidation of heme iron from the ferrous to the ferric state, is normally reconverted to hemoglobin by NADH-dependent methemoglobin reductase—a complex of flavine adenine dinucleotide (FAD) and cytochrome *b5*. The source of the NADH (reduced NAD)

is the glycolytic conversion of glyceraldehyde 3-phosphate to 1,3-bisphosphoglycerate.

RED BLOOD CELL ENZYME DEFECTS

Several chronic hemolytic anemias result from inherited deficiency of RBC enzymes. By far, the most common inherited RBC metabolic disorder is deficiency of the HMP enzyme, G6PD. The gene for G6PD is located on the X chromosome; thus, **G6PD deficiency** is a sex-linked disorder primarily affecting males. G6PD deficiency is sometimes seen in female carriers in whom a large proportion of the RBCs derive from nucleated precursors expressing the mutated X chromosome. This disorder presents with episodic acute hemolysis triggered by a variety of oxidant stresses, including infection, exposure to oxidant drugs, and ingestion of fava beans. The disease is most often seen in men and boys of African and southern European descent. Infection-associated hemolysis may be triggered by hydrogen peroxide produced by activated leukocytes. Fava beans contain substances that destroy reduced glutathione. Deficiency of G6PD prevents the conversion of oxidized glutathione to reduced glutathione, a reducing agent that converts (nonfunctional) oxidized hemoglobin (methemoglobin) to hemoglobin. In patients with G6PD deficiency, (homozygous or heterozygous) damaged hemoglobin rapidly accumulates to form insoluble precipitates within RBCs called **Heinz bodies**. Heinz body–positive RBCs are poorly deformable, become trapped within the splenic cords, and are destroyed in a process termed *extravascular hemolysis*. **Bite cells**, RBCs with bitelike defects secondary to removal of Heinz bodies by splenic macrophages, may be seen on peripheral smears. In contrast, Heinz bodies are not visible on peripheral smears but can be identified after incubation with certain oxidant dyes, such as crystal violet (see Fig. 5.7). Laboratory features of hemolysis include increased indirect (unconjugated) bilirubin, decreased haptoglobin (hemoglobin carrier protein), and increased serum **lactate dehydrogenase (LDH)**, a ubiquitous cytoplasmic enzyme released by damaged and dying cells. Unlike most cells, erythrocytes depend entirely on glycolysis for energy production. Inherited deficiencies of glycolytic pathway enzymes lead to chronic hemolytic anemia caused by the inability to maintain energy (ATP)-dependent cell membrane integrity. Although quite rare, the most common anemia of this type results from **pyruvate kinase (PK) deficiency**. PK catalyzes the conversion of phosphoenol-pyruvate to pyruvic acid, yielding a molecule of ATP. Thus, PK-deficient RBCs are ATP deficient and unable to maintain cell membrane integrity. PK deficiency is an autosomal recessive disorder. Homozygous deficiency leads to a chronic nonspherocytic hemolytic anemia associated with jaundice, splenomegaly, and gallstones.

The splenomegaly results from the massive sequestration and destruction of the abnormal RBCs within the red pulp. The darkly pigmented gallstones are composed of insoluble calcium salts of unconjugated bilirubin derived from the chronic hemolysis. In contrast to the acute episodic hemolysis seen with G6PD deficiency, chronic hemolysis is seen in PK deficiency. Also, unlike G6PD deficiency, methemoglobinemia and Heinz body formation are not typical of PK deficiency.

Methemoglobin, a brown, nonfunctional hemoglobin variant with heme iron in the oxidized (ferric) state, is normally reduced to hemoglobin by **methemoglobin reductase** (a complex of FAD and cytochrome $b5$). **Methemoglobinemia** is a cyanotic (nonhemolytic) condition with a variety of causes, including methemoglobin reductase deficiency, **hemoglobin M** (a hemoglobin variant in which heme iron cannot be maintained in a reduced state), and exposure to drugs with oxidizing properties (sulfonamides, nitrites, nitroglycerin, and lidocaine).

Lactate dehydrogenase converts lactic acid to pyruvic acid with reduction of NAD to NADH, an antioxidant important in repair of cellular damage caused by reactive oxygen species (ROS). Given the high level of exposure to ROS in RBCs, the loss of LDH in RBCs leads to unrepaired oxidant injury and hemolytic anemia.

KEY WORDS AND CONCEPTS

- 2,3-Bisphosphoglycerate (2,3-BPG)
- Bite cells
- Embden-Meyerhof-Parnas glycolytic pathway
- G6PD deficiency
- Glucose-6-phosphate dehydrogenase (G6PD)
- Glutathione
- Glycolysis
- Hexose monophosphate (HMP) shunt
- Heinz bodies
- Hemoglobin M
- Lactate dehydrogenase
- Methemoglobinemia
- Methemoglobin reductase
- Pyruvate kinase (PK) deficiency

REVIEW QUESTIONS

1. The product of the HMP shunt in RBCs is
   A. 2,3-BPG.
   B. lactic acid.
   C. glutathione.
   D. glucose 6 phosphate.

2. Which of the following findings is **not** typically seen in G6PD deficiency?
   A. Methemoglobinemia
   B. Heinz bodies
   C. Bite cells
   D. Splenic atrophy

3. The primary defect in pyruvate kinase (PK) deficiency is
   A. unstable hemoglobin.
   B. nonfunctional hemoglobin.
   C. ATP deficiency.
   D. heme synthesis.

4. Laboratory findings in chronic hemolysis include all **except**
   A. increased serum ferritin.
   B. increased unconjugated bilirubin.
   C. increased LDH.
   D. decreased haptoglobin.

7

Hemolytic Anemia

KEY POINTS

- Hemolytic anemia can be caused by intrinsic red blood cell (RBC) defects (hemoglobin defects, enzyme defects, or membrane defects) or extrinsic causes (autoimmune, vascular defects, toxins, or heat).

- Intravascular hemolysis results from direct destruction of circulating s by extreme heat, toxins, infectious agents, complement, or shear forces.

- Extravascular hemolysis results from phagocytosis of intact (but abnormal) RBCs by macrophages of the spleen and liver.

- Free hemoglobin released into the blood is rapidly bound by the serum protein haptoglobin and delivered to hepatic and splenic macrophages for degradation to peptides (from globin), iron, and bilirubin (from heme).

- Free heme released into the blood is rapidly bound to the serum protein hemopexin and delivered to splenic and hepatic macrophages for degradation to iron and bilirubin.

- Unconjugated (hydrophobic) bilirubin is converted by hepatocytes to conjugated (hydrophilic) bilirubin (**bilirubin diglucuronide**) and is excreted in the bile and urine.

- The most common inherited forms of hemolytic anemia (hereditary spherocytosis and hereditary elliptocytosis) result from intrinsic RBC membrane defects.

Hemolysis, defined as shortened red blood cell (RBC) survival, may result from any number of abnormalities, whether intrinsic or extrinsic to the RBCs. Intrinsic abnormalities include membrane defects, abnormal hemoglobin, and enzyme defects. Extrinsic abnormalities include microangiopathy and anti-RBC antibody. *Hemolysis* is sometimes defined as intravascular or extravascular. Intravascular hemolysis occurs within the bloodstream with release of hemoglobin and phospholipids, and extravascular hemolysis occurs in the marrow, spleen, or liver (Fig. 7.1).

Intravascular hemolysis is caused by destruction of circulating RBCs by extreme heat, toxins, infectious agents, complement lysis, or shear forces induced by damaged capillaries or mechanical heart valves. The loss of plasma membrane integrity destabilizes the RBC osmotic gradient, leading to a rapid influx of sodium and water, cell swelling, and physical disintegration. In intravascular hemolysis, circulating **haptoglobin**-bound hemoglobin and haptoglobin-bound heme are absorbed by hepatosplenic macrophages, where heme is converted to **biliverdin** by **heme oxidase**, reduced to **bilirubin** by **bilirubin reductase**, and bound to **albumin** for transport to hepatocytes for conjugation to diglucuronide form, and excetion in bile. Heme iron is transferred to plasma apotransferrin for transport to tissues, most prominently to the bone marrow.

As a thrombogenic material, free RBC membrane phospholipid can initiate **disseminated intravascular coagulation (DIC)**. Free hemoglobin can be deposited in the kidneys and lead to renal tubular damage. Laboratory abnormalities indicative of intravascular hemolysis include increased serum lactate dehydrogenase (LDH) released from RBC cytoplasm, decreased serum haptoglobin (rapidly removed from the circulation upon binding to heme), and increased serum bilirubin. When bilirubin is measured in the laboratory, a distinction is made between soluble (direct) and insoluble (indirect)

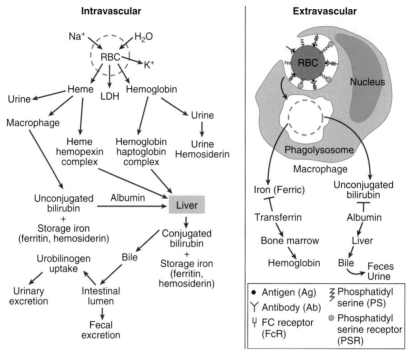

Fig. 7.1 Hemolysis. *LDH,* Lactate dehydrogenase; *RBC,* red blood cell.

forms of bilirubin. Hemolysis, whether intravascular or extravascular, is associated with an increase in **unconjugated (indirect) bilirubin**. Indirect bilirubin is converted to direct bilirubin by the liver and normally excreted in the bile. In the small bowel, gut bacteria reduce bilirubin to **urobilinogen**. A small amount of urobilinogen is absorbed by the small bowel and excreted in the urine.

Extravascular hemolysis results from phagocytosis of circulating damaged or senescent RBCs by macrophages in the spleen, liver, and marrow. Under normal circumstances, aged RBCs progressively lose the ability to prevent and repair **oxidative damage** to the cell membrane, cytoskeleton, and hemoglobin. A certain degree of extravascular hemolysis is normal, related to the physiological removal of senescent RBCs from the circulation, primarily by splenic macrophages.

The susceptibility of aged RBCs to removal results from changes in cell membrane composition, with consequent decreased deformability and physical entrapment within the splenic red pulp, and phagocytosis by splenic macrophages. Aged or senescent RBCs are recognized by splenic macrophages by several mechanisms. Expression of phosphatidyl serine (PS) is normally

confined to the inner leaflet of the RBC plasma membrane, maintained as such by the enzyme **flippase**. Expression of the enzyme **scramblase** by aged RBCs leads to expression of PS on the RBC surface and removal from the circulation by PS receptor-bearing splenic macrophages. Loss of terminal **sialic acid** residues on aged RBC surface glycoproteins exposes **galactosyl** residues that bind to macrophage galactosyl receptors. **CD47** loss from old RBCs prevents **SIRP1-alpha**–mediated "don't eat me" signaling of macrophages. Aggregates of damaged **Band 3** cytoskeletal protein are recognized by natural antibodies, inducing immunoglobulin (Fc) receptor–mediated phagocytosis.

Engulfed RBCs are degraded within macrophage phagolysosomes. Heme is degraded by heme oxidase to biliverdin, reduced to bilirubin, enters the blood bound to albumin, conjugated in the liver to bilirubin diglucuronide, and excreted in the bile. Several pathologic conditions are characterized by an abnormal degree of extravascular hemolysis, leading to anemia. Although extravascular hemolysis often accompanies intravascular hemolysis—for example, damaged RBCs that escape intravascular lysis are phagocytosed and destroyed by splenic and liver macrophages—this term is more commonly applied to situations in which little to no intravascular hemolysis occurs. Examples of such situations include **hypersplenism** and **autoimmune hemolytic anemia (AIHA)**.

Laboratory abnormalities in hemolytic anemia of any cause may include normochromic normocytic anemia, elevated reticulocyte count, increased serum LDH, hyperbilirubinemia, decreased serum haptoglobin, increased plasma hemoglobin, hemoglobinuria, and hemosiderinuria. In severe cases, the anemia may be macrocytic because of the compensatory release from the marrow of larger immature RBCs (reticulocytes). In contrast to other forms of macrocytic anemia, the heterogeneity in RBC size caused by admixed erythrocytes and reticulocytes may yield an increased **RBC distribution width (RDW)** on the complete blood count.

Hemolytic anemia can be broadly classified into two etiologic types, **extrinsic hemolytic anemia** resulting from extracorpuscular factors and **intrinsic hemolytic anemia** resulting from RBC defects.

EXTRINSIC HEMOLYTIC ANEMIA

The most common types of extrinsic hemolytic anemia are microangiopathic, autoimmune, drug induced, infection mediated, and alloimmune (hemolytic disease of the newborn).

Microangiopathic hemolytic anemia results from traumatic RBC fragmentation during passage through abnormal arterioles laden with fibrin-platelet thrombi. The arteriolar thrombi are secondary to a coagulopathy induced by a variety of underlying conditions, including disseminated adenocarcinoma, (pre)eclampsia, malignant hypertension, DIC, **thrombotic thrombocytopenic purpura**, hemolytic uremic syndrome, and immune-mediated vasculitis. Abnormalities noted on peripheral smear include fragmented RBCs (**schistocytes**) (Fig. 7.2); increased polychromatophilic RBCs (reticulocytes); and in severe cases, nucleated RBCs (Fig. 7.3). Evidence of consumptive thrombotic coagulopathy (or DIC) may include prolonged prothrombin time and activated partial thromboplastin time, increased fibrin split products, increased D-dimer, decreased fibrinogen, and thrombocytopenia.

Autoimmune hemolytic anemia results from hemolysis of antibody- or complement-bound RBCs. The autoantibodies are directed against widely expressed RBC

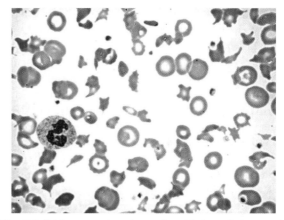

Fig. 7.2 Schistocytes in microangiopathic hemolytic anemia (peripheral smear).

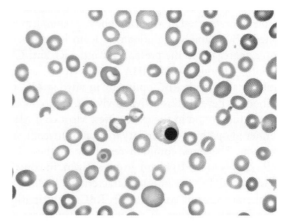

Fig. 7.3 Nucleated red blood cell (peripheral smear).

antigens, so-called public antigens, the most common being Rhesus (Rh) antigens. Extravascular hemolysis of antibody- or complement-bound (opsonized) RBCs occurs after Fc- or complement receptor–mediated phagocytosis by splenic and hepatic macrophages. Although the spleen is the primary site of phagocytosis, RBCs coated with high levels of immunoglobulin G (IgG) and C3b also undergo Kupffer cell–mediated phagocytosis in the liver. Opsonized RBCs, especially those coated with IgM, a pentavalent immunoglobulin isotype with strong complement-binding properties, may also undergo intravascular complement-mediated hemolysis. AIHA is subclassified as either warm or cold on the basis of the optimal temperature at which the antibody binds to RBCs in vitro (37° or <37°C, respectively). In general, the warm form results from IgG antibodies and the cold form results from IgM antibodies. **Warm AIHA**, the most common form of AIHA, may be primary (idiopathic) or secondary to lymphoma, autoimmune disease (systemic lupus erythematosus or ulcerative colitis), drugs, or infections. The most characteristic finding on peripheral smear in warm AIHA is increased **spherocytes** (Fig. 7.4). In AIHA, spherocytes form as a result of binding of antibody-bound (opsonized) RBCs to **Fc receptor**–bearing splenic macrophages, with progressive loss of cell membrane. The selective loss of cell membrane (with normal cell volume) induces a change in RBC shape from biconcave discs to spherocytes. Spherocytes and **elliptocytes** are easily detected on peripheral blood smears, and the diagnosis can be confirmed by an increase in RBC **osmotic fragility**. Confirmation of AIHA can be made by the **direct antiglobulin test (Coombs test)**, a simple laboratory test in which antibody- or complement-coated RBCs rapidly agglutinate to form large macroscopic aggregates in the presence of anti-IgG, anti-C3b, or both. Although **cold AIHA** is defined by an IgM antibody that binds RBC optimally in vitro at 4°C, the antibody is nevertheless active in vivo at 25° to 30°C, a temperature found in the extremities. Most cold AIHA is either idiopathic or secondary to viral or mycoplasma infection. The most common reactivity of these IgM antibodies is to the I/i blood group antigen. In contrast to warm AIHA, the most characteristic finding on peripheral smear of cold AIHA is **RBC agglutination**, with variable presence of spherocytes. Treatment for these conditions include corticosteroids and splenectomy and in refractory cases, anti-CD20 antibody

(which depletes B cells) or cytotoxic drugs. Steroids and splenectomy are often more effective for warm than for cold AIHA. Patients with cold AIHA are also advised to avoid cold exposure that may accelerate hemolysis.

Hemolytic disease of the newborn is an alloimmune hemolytic anemia caused by transplacental passage of IgG **anti-Rh (blood group) antibody** from the mother to the fetus. The disease is seen in Rh-negative mothers who carry anti-Rh antibody from previous exposure to Rh antigen, either from previous pregnancies with Rh-positive fetuses or by transfusion of Rh-positive blood. See Chapter 18 for further details.

Drug-induced hemolytic anemia occurs by one of three mechanisms. In one case, exemplified by penicillin, drug-coated RBCs are subject to splenic destruction mediated by **drug-specific antibody**. In the second case, exemplified by quinidine, the drug bound to an RBC membrane protein creates a neoantigen, which provokes production of a **neoantigen-specific antibody** that when bound to RBCs in the presence of complement induces hemolysis. In the third case, exemplified by alpha methyldopa, the drug induces (by an unknown mechanism) the formation of an **autoantibody** (often with anti-Rh specificity) with reactivity to autologous RBCs. Hemolytic anemia is caused by splenic macrophage-mediated phagocytosis of the autoantibody-coated RBCs.

Infection-mediated hemolytic anemia may result from direct intraerythrocytic invasion by the mosquito-borne protozoan *Plasmodium* spp. (Fig. 7.5) or the tick-borne protozoan *Babesia microti* (Fig. 7.6) or by release of hemolytic toxins by *Clostridium perfringens* and hemolytic autoantibody formation by *Mycoplasma pneumoniae*. Other causes of extrinsic hemolytic anemia include thermal burns; lead poisoning; and envenomation by an insect, spider, or snake bite.

INTRINSIC HEMOLYTIC ANEMIA

Hemolytic anemia caused by intrinsic RBC defects may be broadly classified into those caused by metabolic defects, hemoglobin defects, and membrane defects. The two most common membrane defects associated with hemolytic anemia are hereditary spherocytosis and hereditary elliptocytosis.

Hereditary spherocytosis is usually seen as an autosomal dominant hemolytic anemia in people of northern European ancestry. It results from defects of one of several cytoskeletal proteins, including **ankyrin**, **spectrin**,

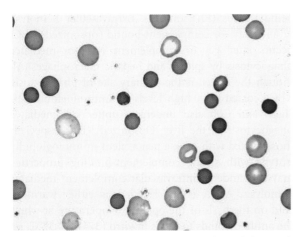

Fig. 7.4 Spherocytes in severe autoimmune hemolytic anemia (AIHA) (peripheral smear).

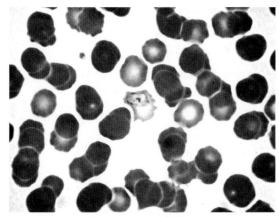

Fig. 7.5 Malaria parasite (peripheral smear). In the center of the field is a red blood cell with a *Plasmodium falciparum* ring form with associated brown pigment (degraded hemoglobin).

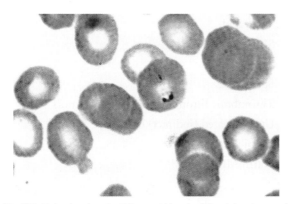

Fig. 7.6 *Babesia microti* within a red blood cell (peripheral smear). In contrast to malaria, there is no associated pigment.

and Band 3. These defects lead to progressive loss of membrane lipid, which in turn leads to decreased RBC surface-to-volume ratio and transformation of the normally flexible biconcave discs to rigid spherocytes (see Fig. 7.4). The rigid spherocytes become trapped in splenic sinuses and destroyed by splenic macrophages (extravascular hemolysis). Spherocytes are easily detected on peripheral smears as small, round RBCs without central pallor. The decreased surface-to-volume ratio often leads to an increased **mean corpuscular hemoglobin concentration**. Spherocytes alone are not diagnostic of hereditary spherocytosis because they are also commonly encountered in AIHA. In clinically suspected cases, diagnosis of hereditary spherocytosis can be confirmed by laboratory demonstration of increased **osmotic fragility** of RBCs in hypotonic salt solutions. In symptomatic cases, splenectomy often leads to improvement.

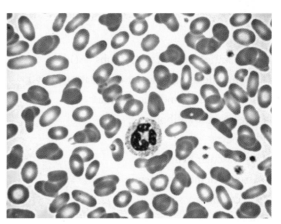

Fig. 7.7 Elliptocytosis (peripheral smear).

Hereditary elliptocytosis is usually seen as an autosomal dominant disorder affecting primarily people of African descent. It results from defects in the RBC membrane proteins spectrin, **protein 4.1**, or **glycophorin C**. Unlike hereditary spherocytosis, hereditary elliptocytosis is usually asymptomatic. Elliptocytes are easily detected on peripheral smears as oblong RBCs (Fig. 7.7). Elliptocytes may be seen in a variety of other conditions, including iron-deficiency and megaloblastic anemia. In these conditions, the percentage of elliptocytes seldom reaches 50%, but nearly all RBCs in hereditary elliptocytosis are elliptocytes. **Hereditary pyropoikilocytosis (HPP)** is a rare form of hereditary elliptocytosis caused by increased expression of a spectrin gene mutation. In HPP, peripheral smears reveal numerous bizarrely shaped and fragmented RBCs (**poikilocytes** and schistocytes).

KEY WORDS AND CONCEPTS

- Albumin
- Ankyrin
- Anti-Rh (blood group) antibody
- Autoantibody
- Autoimmune hemolytic anemia (AIHA)
- Band 3
- Bilirubin
- Bilirubin diglucuronide
- Bilirubin reductase
- Biliverdin
- Biliverdin reductase

- CD47
- Cold AIHA
- Direct antiglobulin test (Coombs test)
- Disseminated intravascular coagulation (DIC)
- Drug-induced hemolytic anemia
- Drug-specific antibody
- Elliptocyte
- Extravascular hemolysis
- Extrinsic hemolytic anemia
- Fc receptor
- Flippase
- Galactosyl
- Galactosyl residues
- Haptoglobin
- Heme oxidase
- Hemolytic disease of the newborn
- Hemopexin
- Hereditary elliptocytosis
- Hereditary pyropoikilocytosis (HPP)
- Hereditary spherocytosis
- Hypersplenism
- Infection-mediated hemolytic anemia
- Intravascular hemolysis
- Intrinsic hemolytic anemia
- Mean corpuscular hemoglobin concentration
- Microangiopathic hemolytic anemia
- *Mycoplasma pneumoniae*
- Neoantigen-specific antibody
- Osmotic fragility
- *Plasmodium* spp.
- Poikilocyte
- Protein 4.1
- Red blood cell agglutination
- Red blood cell distribution width (RDW)
- Schistocyte
- Scramblase
- Sialic acid
- SIRP1 alpha
- Spectrin
- Spherocyte
- Thrombotic thrombocytopenic purpura
- Unconjugated (indirect) bilirubin
- Urobilinogen
- Warm AIHA

REVIEW QUESTIONS

1. Intravascular hemolysis is accompanied by all the following **except**
   A. binding of free hemoglobin to haptoglobin.
   B. binding of free heme to hemopexin.
   C. binding of free iron to hemosiderin.
   D. release of RBC membrane phospholipid.

2. Which statement regarding heme is **false**?
   A. During intravascular hemolysis, free heme is delivered to liver as a heme–hemopexin complex.
   B. Heme is composed of protoporphyrin IX and ferric iron.
   C. Heme is degraded to yield iron and bilirubin.
   D. Heme is an "Impossible Burger" ingredient.

3. Which statement about autoimmune hemolytic anemia (AIHA) is **false**?
   A. Cold-acting IgM autoantibodies are directed to Ii blood group antigens.
   B. Spherocytes are commonly seen on peripheral smears in warm AIHA.
   C. Warm-acting IgG autoantibodies are directed to ABO blood group antigens.
   D. Antibody coated RBCs are destroyed by macrophages in the spleen and liver.

4. Which of the following statements about heme catabolism is **false**?
   A. Heme oxidase converts heme protoporphyrin to biliverdin.
   B. Bilirubin is converted to bilirubin diglucuronide.
   C. Bilirubin diglucuronide is excreted in bile and urine.
   D. Biliverdin oxidase converts biliverdin to bilirubin.

Aplastic Anemia and Related Disorders

KEY POINTS

- Aplastic anemia is broadly defined as pancytopenia (low hemoglobin, leukocyte count, and platelet count) with a hypocellular bone marrow.

- Some inherited forms of aplastic anemia present in early childhood and may be associated with increased risk for development of malignancy.

- Idiopathic aplastic anemia is an autoimmune condition most often seen in adults that may respond to immunosuppressive drugs.

- Pure red blood cell (RBC) aplasia, marked by loss of marrow RBC precursors only, is often caused by parvovirus infection in adults and in children is presumably caused by infection by an unrecognized virus.

- Some forms of aplastic anemia are seen in association with nonhematopoietic organ dysfunction (kidney, liver, thyroid, adrenal, pituitary, and parathyroid).

Pancytopenia associated with marrow aplasia is known as aplastic anemia. The diagnosis of severe aplastic anemia rests on the findings of pancytopenia; hypocellular marrow (Fig. 8.1); and two of the following: low reticulocyte count (<1%), neutropenia (<500/μL), or thrombocytopenia (<20,000/μL). Although most cases are seen in adolescents and young adults (ages 15–25 years), cases are also seen in older adults. The marrow failure results from a marked reduction in the number of hematopoietic progenitor cells (granulocyte–macrophage colony-forming unit and erythroid burst-forming unit cells).

Idiopathic aplastic anemia is an autoimmune condition in which autoreactive T cells suppress hematopoiesis by direct cytotoxicity and production of interferon-γ. Idiopathic aplastic anemia often responds to treatment with immunosuppressive drugs. Aplastic anemia may also be caused by chronic exposure to toxic organic chemicals (benzene, the insecticide lindane, the wood preservative pentachlorophenol, and toluene), drugs (chloramphenicol, ticlopidine, and alkylating agents), and viral infections (Epstein-Barr virus [EBV]). Some cases of aplastic anemia are seen in association with pregnancy, connective tissue disorders (rheumatoid arthritis), and thymoma. No cytogenetic abnormalities are seen in aplastic anemia. Clonal cytogenetic defects indicate the presence of an underlying neoplastic myeloid disorder (myelodysplastic syndrome [MDS], or acute myelogenous leukemia [AML]).

Paroxysmal nocturnal hemoglobinuria (PNH) is a rare intrinsic hemolytic disorder caused by acquired mutations in the *Pig-1* gene. *Pig-1* is a phosphatidylinositol glycosyltransferase that is essential in synthesis of the glycosylphosphatidylinositol (GPI)–linked family of cell membrane proteins. Although many GPI-anchored proteins (in all marrow cells) are deficient in PNH, hemolysis specifically results from deficiency of CD59, the membrane inhibitor of reactive lysis, a GPI-anchored membrane protein that blocks complement-mediated red blood cell (RBC) lysis by preventing incorporation of the lytic terminal complement component C9 into the C5b-8 membrane attack complex. In addition to intermittent bouts of intravascular hemolysis and hemoglobinuria, patients with PNH suffer from recurrent bouts of venous thrombosis most likely caused by complement-mediated activation of

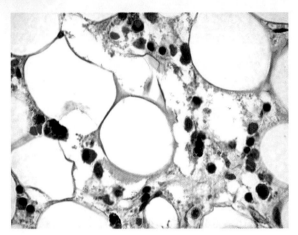

Fig. 8.1 Aplastic anemia (marrow biopsy). Note the extreme hypocellularity with a few scattered, small lymphocytes and plasma cells. Also note the hemosiderosis (brown granular material in histiocytes) that likely reflects the history of multiple transfusions to maintain the hematocrit.

GPI-deficient platelets. Neuromuscular symptoms of dysphagia, abdominal pain, and lethargy have been attributed to **nitric oxide deficiency** mediated by binding of nitric oxide to free plasma hemoglobin to form **nitrosohemoglobin**. Because marrow cells carrying the PNH defect do not exhibit malignant potential, it is unclear how these cells overgrow the normal marrow. Because PNH is often seen in association with aplastic anemia, it is thought that under these circumstances PNH cells may accumulate as a result of some unexplained survival advantage over normal marrow cells. The diagnosis of PNH can be established either by demonstration of increased sensitivity of PNH red cells to complement-mediated, sucrose-enhanced hemolysis (sucrose lysis test) or acid-enhanced hemolysis (Ham test) or by demonstration of decreased expression of GPI proteins such as CD14, CD16, CD24, CD55, and CD59 on blood cells by flow cytometry. More recently, a flow cytometry test using a recombinant fluorescent-labeled form of bacterial aerolysin (FLAER) has gained popularity for detection of the PNH defect. FLAER binds specifically to GPI-anchored proteins, and demonstration of FLAER-negative blood leukocytes by flow cytometry is characteristic of PNH.

Some forms of aplastic anemia are inherited conditions that present in childhood. The most common hereditary aplastic anemia, **Fanconi anemia**, is an autosomal recessive condition caused by mutations in genes of the **FA pathway**. Proteins of the FA pathway repair damage to DNA during DNA replication. Patients typically present in the latter half of the first decade of life with anemia, thrombocytopenia, and mucocutaneous bleeding in association with skeletal anomalies, including short stature and abnormal thumbs. Allogeneic stem cell transplantation is curative. Otherwise, death resulting from marrow failure, myeloid neoplasia, or other cancers usually occurs by 20 years of age. Recently, less severe forms of Fanconi anemia have been recognized in young adults.

Isolated acquired aplasia of erythroid cells is known as **pure red cell aplasia (PRCA)**. PRCA is characterized by normochromic normocytic anemia, a markedly reduced reticulocyte count, and markedly decreased to absent erythroid cells in the marrow. In adults, acquired PRCA develops in parvovirus B19 infection, MDS, thymoma, or rarely as a drug reaction. Drugs implicated in PRCA include diphenylhydantoin, sulfa drugs, azathioprine, and ribavirin.

The DNA virus **parvovirus B19** directly infects erythroid precursors, leading to intramedullary erythroid cell death (Fig. 8.2). Under normal circumstances, parvovirus infection in adults is transient and seldom leads to clinically significant anemia. In immunosuppressed people incapable of producing neutralizing humoral antibody, persistent parvovirus infection leads to chronic PRCA. Acute parvovirus infection in young patients with a chronic hemolytic anemia such as sickle

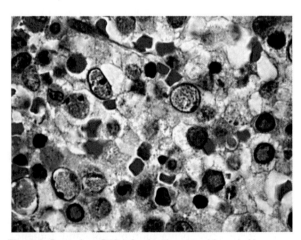

Fig. 8.2 Parvovirus B19 infection (marrow biopsy). Numerous erythroid precursors with pink granular intranuclear viral inclusions are shown. Note the thin rim of nuclear chromatin displaced by the viral inclusion.

cell disease or hereditary spherocytosis can trigger a **transient aplastic crisis** by interfering with compensatory erythroid hyperplasia. **Transient erythroblastopenia of childhood** is a self-limited form of PRCA seen in previously healthy children, presumably secondary to infection with an unrecognized virus. The marrow is normocellular with markedly decreased numbers of erythroid precursors.

Diamond-Blackfan anemia (DBA), also known as **constitutional PRCA**, results from defects in erythroid precursors that prevent them from responding to growth signals. In up to 40% of cases, DBA is associated with congenital defects (craniofacial, neck, or thumb). Patients with DBA are at increased risk for development of AML, carcinoma, and MDS. The anemia is normochromic and macrocytic. The reticulocyte count is decreased, and EPO levels are increased. DBA results from sporadic abnormalities at chromosome 19q13 involving the *RPS19* gene that encodes for a protein involved in ribosome assembly.

Other forms of aplastic marrow failure include Shwachman-Diamond-Oski syndrome, dyskeratosis congenita, amegakaryocytic thrombocytopenia, severe congenital neutropenia, and cyclic neutropenia. **Shwachman-Diamond-Oski syndrome** is an autosomal recessive condition marked by short stature, skeletal defects, exocrine pancreatic insufficiency, and cytopenia caused by marrow failure. Patients with this syndrome are at increased risk for MDS and AML. **Dyskeratosis congenita** is an X-linked or autosomal recessive disorder marked by a triad of lacy reticulated pigmentation of the upper body, leukoplakia, and nail dystrophy. Patients with this disorder develop aplastic anemia, with an increased risk for development of MDS and carcinoma. This disorder is caused by mutations that encode subunits of *TERC* (telomerase RNA component) gene, thus interfering with proper telomere maintenance and accelerated senescence of highly proliferative tissues such as the bone marrow. **Amegakaryocytic thrombocytopenia** is an autosomal recessive condition marked by thrombocytopenia and petechial rash in the first year of life, sometimes associated with neurologic and cardiac defects. Aplastic anemia often develops. The disease results from the inheritance of inactivating mutations in *c-MPL*, the **thrombopoietin (TPO)** receptor gene. This defect renders the megakaryocytes unresponsive to the growth-promoting properties of TPO. **Severe congenital neutropenia (Kostmann syndrome)** is an autosomal

recessive (sometimes autosomal dominant) condition marked by congenital neutropenia and recurrent life-threatening infections. The condition results from maturation arrest and increased apoptosis of early myeloid precursors (promyelocytes and myelocytes) that carry mutations in *ELA-2* (neutrophil elastase), an enzyme normally present in primary granules. The primary treatment is the granulocyte growth factor granulocyte colony-stimulating factor (G-CSF). Kostmann syndrome should be differentiated from other forms of neutropenia that are seen in young children, including **viral-induced neutropenia**, chronic benign neutropenia of infancy and childhood, and cyclic neutropenia. Viral infection is the most common cause of neutropenia in early childhood. The most common viral infections associated with neutropenia in children are varicella, measles, rubella, hepatitis A and B, Epstein-Barr virus EBV, influenza, parvovirus, and cytomegalovirus. Recovery from virus-induced neutropenia usually follows resolution of active infection. **Chronic benign neutropenia of infancy and childhood** usually presents within the first 14 months of life. At birth, blood neutrophil counts are normal, but they decline to very low levels with no increase in infection risk. Examination of the bone marrow reveals an increase in immature granulocytes, a result indicative of an appropriate compensatory marrow response. Because **antineutrophil antibodies** are commonly detected and treatment with steroids is often effective, the disorder is presumably immune in nature. **Cyclic neutropenia** is a rare autosomal dominant condition that presents most often in the first year of life. The disorder is marked in most cases by 21-day cycles of neutropenia associated with recurrent fever, pharyngitis, and stomatitis. Like severe congenital neutropenia, cyclic neutropenia is associated with mutations of the **elastase gene ELA2**. To prevent development of severe chronic dental caries, gingivitis, or stomatitis, patients are treated with G-CSF.

ANEMIA SECONDARY TO NONHEMATOPOIETIC DISEASE

Anemia of chronic renal failure is a hypoproliferative normochromic normocytic anemia caused primarily by **EPO deficiency** and exacerbated by RBC damage induced by uremic metabolites. Deficient in the hexose monophosphate shunt enzyme transketolase and the sodium–potassium pump enzyme adenosine triphosphatase (ATPase), uremic RBCs are defective in reversing oxidant damage and maintaining transmembrane cation gradients. These enzyme defects lead to the formation of rigid, burr-shaped RBCs (echinocytes and burr cells) with shortened lifespans. Given the hypoproliferative nature of this process, the reticulocyte count is inappropriately low. EPO administration is usually highly effective in treatment.

The cause of **anemia of liver disease** is multifactorial. To the extent that the liver disease is associated with chronic inflammation, reduced erythropoiesis caused by hepcidin excess may play a role. In cirrhosis, congestive splenomegaly caused by portal hypertension may lead to excessive splenic pooling (**hypersplenism**) and enhanced splenic clearance of RBCs. Liver defects in lipid metabolism lead to alterations in RBC membrane lipid composition and reduced RBC survival. Abnormalities in the lipid content of the RBCs can lead to RBC shape changes, including macrocytes, target cells, and **acanthocytes** (misshapen RBCs with irregular cytoplasmic spikes). **Spur cell anemia** is a specific form of hemolytic anemia seen in the context of chronic liver disease.

Anemia of endocrine disease is a mild normocytic normochromic anemia described in hypothyroidism, adrenal insufficiency, pituitary insufficiency, hyperparathyroidism, and androgen deficiency. Thyroid hormone deficiency impairs hypoxia-induced EPO synthesis and blunts the stimulatory effect of EPO on marrow erythroid precursors. Anemia in **hypothyroidism** may result from a combination of increased plasma volume, decreased RBC survival, and ineffective erythropoiesis. Anemia in **adrenal insufficiency** may be at least partly caused by glucocorticoid deficiency. Glucocorticoids enhance the stimulatory effects of EPO on erythroid proliferation. Androgens enhance erythropoiesis by stimulating EPO secretion and supporting the growth of marrow stromal cells. In contrast, estrogens have been shown to suppress erythropoiesis. The anemia seen in **hypopituitarism** indirectly results from a combined deficiency of the anterior pituitary hormones that lead to deficiencies of thyroid hormones, adrenal hormones (corticosteroids), and androgens. Posterior pituitary hormone deficiency (vasopressin or oxytocin) is not associated with anemia. The marrow in hypopituitarism is hypocellular and may be associated with pancytopenia.

KEY WORDS AND CONCEPTS

- Acanthocyte
- Adrenal insufficiency
- Amegakaryocytic thrombocytopenia
- Anemia of chronic renal failure
- Anemia of endocrine disease
- Anemia of liver disease
- Antineutrophil antibodies
- c-MPL mutation
- Chronic benign neutropenia of infancy and childhood
- Constitutional pure red cell anemia (PRCA)
- Cyclic neutropenia
- Diamond-Blackfan anemia (DBA)
- Dyskeratosis congenita
- ELA-2
- EPO deficiency
- Fanconi anemia
- FA pathway
- Hypersplenism
- Hypopituitarism
- Hypothyroidism
- Idiopathic aplastic anemia
- Nitric oxide deficiency
- Nitrosohemoglobin
- Paroxysmal nocturnal hemoglobinuria (PNH)
- Parvovirus B19
- *Pig-1*
- Pure blood red cell aplasia (PRCA)
- *RPS19* gene
- Severe congenital neutropenia (Kostmann syndrome)
- Shwachman-Diamond-Oski syndrome
- Spur cell anemia
- *TERC*
- Thrombopoietin (TPO)
- Transient aplastic crisis
- Transient erythroblastopenia of childhood
- Viral-induced neutropenia

REVIEW QUESTIONS

1. All of the following are potential causes of aplastic anemia **except**
   A. bacterial infection.
   B. autoimmune disease.
   C. organic chemicals.
   D. drugs.

2. All of the following statements about PNH are true **except**
   A. complement-mediated hemolysis is caused by deficiency of CD59 (the membrane inhibitor of reactive lysis).
   B. venous thrombosis likely caused by activation of GPI-deficient platelets.
   C. increased sulfhemoglobin leads to neuromuscular symptoms.
   D. it is often seen in the context of aplastic anemia.

3. Uremia contributes to anemia of chronic renal failure by what mechanism?
   A. Hepcidin-mediated ferroportin deficiency
   B. Oxidant injury of RBCs caused by glutathione deficiency
   C. Formation of glomerular microthrombi
   D. Complement-mediated hemolysis

4. Which of the following defects **does not** lead to aplastic anemia in infancy and childhood?
   A. Defective ribosome assembly in Diamond-Blackfan anemia
   B. Parvovirus infection in PRCA
   C. Elastase gene deficiency in severe congenital neutropenia
   D. EPO deficiency in amegakaryocytic thrombocytopenia

9

Megaloblastic Anemia

KEY POINTS

- Megaloblastic anemia is a type of macrocytic anemia resulting from inhibition of normal DNA synthesis caused in most cases by dietary deficiency of folic acid or cobalamin.

- Folic acid is present in most fruits and vegetables; cobalamin is present in meats and dairy products.

- Folic acid deficiency results from an inadequate diet, malabsorption, increased requirements, and drugs.

- Cobalamin deficiency most often results from pernicious anemia, an autoimmune disease characterized by gastric atrophy with consequent intrinsic factor (IF) deficiency.

- If is required for cobalamin absorption, the cobalamin–IF complex binds to IF receptor–bearing mucosal cells in the terminal ileum.

- Deficiency of folate or cobalamin leads to misincorporation of deoxyuridine triphosphate (dUTP)—instead of deoxythymidine triphosphate (dTTP)—into DNA.

- Unsuccessful attempts at DNA repair to replace dUTP with dTTP lead to DNA damage and mitotic arrest.

- Megaloblastic anemia is marked by production of enlarged (megaloblastic) red blood cell precursors, many of which undergo apoptosis in the marrow (ineffective erythropoiesis).

The **megaloblastic anemias** are a group of disorders caused by defects in DNA synthesis. Anemia develops as a result of the production of enlarged erythroid precursors that are destroyed within the marrow (ineffective erythropoiesis) as a result of their inability to undergo normal DNA replication and cell division. Specifically, in those cases caused by deficiency of folic acid or cobalamin, the inability to synthesize deoxythymidine monophosphate (dTMP) from deoxyuridine monophosphate (dUMP) leads to a deficiency of deoxythymidine triphosphate (dTTP). In the absence of dTTP, DNA polymerase incorporates deoxyuridine triphosphate (dUTP) into DNA. Incorporation of dUTP into DNA can lead to errors in base pairing that likely interfere with DNA replication. Furthermore, futile attempts on the part of the DNA repair apparatus to replace dUTP with dTTP lead to DNA damage and markedly reduced DNA synthesis. Despite the mitotic arrest, the cells continue to produce protein and

undergo cytoplasmic maturation, with production of greatly enlarged cells with **nuclear–cytoplasmic dyssynchrony**, that is, cells with immature nuclei and mature cytoplasm (Figs. 9.1 and 9.2). Large erythroid precursors with immature nuclei and giant band neutrophils are present in the marrow. Macrocytic red blood cells and hypersegmented neutrophils are seen in peripheral blood (Fig. 9.3). Other rapidly growing tissues are affected, most notably in the gastrointestinal tract. In most cases, megaloblastic anemia is caused by deficiency of folic acid or cobalamin. Folic acid and cobalamin are both involved in the conversion of dUMP to dTMP, a critical step in DNA synthesis (Fig. 9.4).

Folic acid is found in a variety of fruits and vegetables and is absorbed by the proximal jejunum. Causes of folate deficiency include a fruit- and vegetable-poor diet, malabsorption, increased requirements caused by cell proliferation (pregnancy, infancy, chronic hemolytic anemia, malignancy, or psoriasis), and drugs (alcohol or

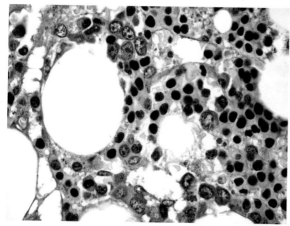

Fig. 9.1 Megaloblastic anemia (marrow biopsy). Erythroid predominant marrow with clusters of enlarged immature erythroid precursors *(upper and lower middle)* is shown.

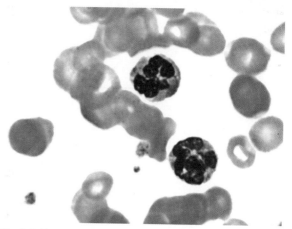

Fig. 9.3 Hypersegmented neutrophils (more than five lobes) in megaloblastic anemia (peripheral smear).

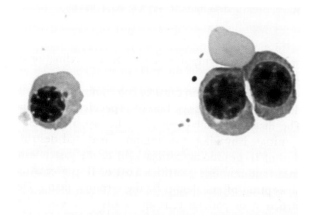

Fig. 9.2 Megaloblastic RBC precursors (marrow aspirate). Enlarged cells with nuclear–cytoplasmic dyssynchrony are shown.

methotrexate). Alcohol directly inhibits intestinal absorption, and methotrexate blocks **dihydrofolate reductase**, the enzyme that catalyzes conversion of dihydrofolate to tetrahydrofolate. Body stores of folic acid are limited, enough to maintain normal levels for only a few months.

Cobalamin is a macromolecule composed of a cobalt-containing tetrapyrrole linked to a nucleotide that is produced by certain bacteria and found in meats and dairy products. Cobalamin released from ingested food after gastric digestion binds to an R protein and enters the duodenum (Fig. 9.5). In the duodenum, the

cobalamin is released from R protein and bound to **intrinsic factor** (**IF**) produced by gastric parietal cells. The cobalamin–IF complex, resistant to proteolytic digestion, passes to the terminal ileum, where it is absorbed by IF receptor-bearing mucosal cells. After uptake, cobalamin is bound to the transport protein **transcobalamin** II and is released into the bloodstream, where it is rapidly taken up by the liver, the marrow, and other tissues. Recirculating cobalamin is bound primarily to transcobalamin I. Cobalamin acts as a cofactor in the coupled conversions of homocysteine to methionine and methyltetrahydrofolate to tetrahydrofolate. Tetrahydrofolate is necessary for the conversion of dUMP to dTMP. dTMP is converted to dTTP and used in DNA synthesis. Thus, both folate deficiency and cobalamin deficiency lead to dTTP deficiency and impaired DNA synthesis. The neurologic damage associated with cobalamin deficiency results from methionine deficiency and a toxic excess of methyl-malonyl coenzyme A.

Megaloblastic anemia caused by cobalamin deficiency can be reversed by cobalamin or folate, whereas megaloblastic anemia caused by folate deficiency can only be reversed by folate. Thus, in cobalamin deficiency, the megaloblastic anemia actually results from a defect in folate metabolism. However, the neurologic abnormalities in cobalamin deficiency cannot be reversed with folate.

The brain, spinal cord, and peripheral nerves are all affected in cobalamin deficiency. The earliest neurologic manifestation of cobalamin deficiency is paresthesia of

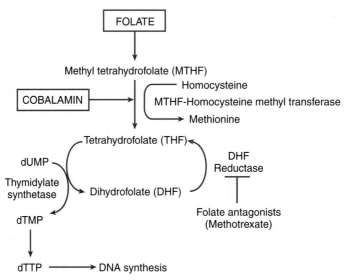

Fig. 9.4 Folate and cobalamin function. Deficiency of folate or cobalamin leads to defective DNA synthesis. DHF, Dihydrofolate; dTTP, deoxythymidine triphosphate; dUMP, deoxyuridine monophosphate; dUTP, deoxyuridine triphosphate.

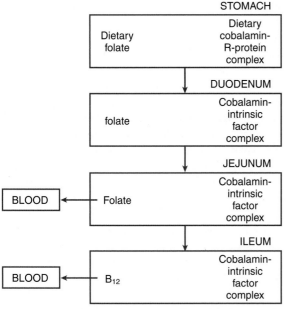

Fig. 9.5 Folate and cobalamin absorption.

nervous system symptoms result from demyelination of white matter.

The most common cause of cobalamin deficiency is the autoimmune disease known as **pernicious anemia**. The disease, usually seen after the age of 40 years, is initiated by idiopathic immune-mediated destruction of IF-producing parietal cells of the gastric mucosa (autoimmune gastritis). Loss of IF prevents the absorption of cobalamin by the terminal ileum. Destruction of parietal cells also leads to achlorhydria (reduced gastric acid production). Although vitamin B_{12} supplementation corrects the megaloblastic anemia, the more advanced neurologic symptoms are generally irreversible.

KEY WORDS AND CONCEPTS

- Cobalamin
- Combined system disease
- Dihydrofolate reductase
- Folic acid
- Intrinsic factor (IF)
- Megaloblastic anemias
- Nuclear–cytoplasmic dyssynchrony
- Pernicious anemia
- Transcobalamin

the fingers and toes. If untreated, the disease progresses to spastic ataxia caused by demyelination of the dorsal and lateral columns of the spinal cord, a process termed **combined system disease**. Brain disease may manifest as altered sense of taste and smell, altered vision, dementia, and psychosis. The psychosis and other central

REVIEW QUESTIONS

1. Which of the following statements about folic acid is **incorrect**?
   A. It is found in fruits and vegetables.
   B. It is absorbed in the jejunum bound to R protein complex.
   C. It is required for conversion of dTMP to dTTP.
   D. Its absorption is blocked by alcohol.

2. Which of the following statements about cobalamin (vitamin B_{12}) is **incorrect**?
   A. Cobalamin is absorbed in the ileum bound to intrinsic factor.
   B. Intrinsic factor deficiency caused by loss of chief cells in atrophic gastritis leads to poor absorption of vitamin B_{12} and development of pernicious anemia.
   C. The neurotoxicity in combined system disease is caused by methionine deficiency and excess methyl malonyl coenzyme A.
   D. In both folate and cobalamin deficiency, incorporation of dUTP into DNA leads to delayed DNA replication.

3. All the following peripheral blood findings are seen in megaloblastic anemia **except**
   A. hypersegmented neutrophils,
   B. thrombocytopenia,
   C. macro-ovalocytes,
   D. schistocytes,

10

Myeloid Cells

KEY POINTS

- Under the influence of specific cytokines, common myeloid progenitors in the marrow undergo differentiation into granulocytes (neutrophils, eosinophils, mast cells, basophils, and monocytes.

- Neutrophils are phagocytic microbicidal cells that contain cytoplasmic granules rich in proteolytic enzymes.

- In response to localized infection, neutrophils collect to form netlike extracellular traps of chromatin and antimicrobial toxins.

- Upon activation, neutrophils produce toxic reactive oxygen species.

- Neutrophils released into the blood from the marrow rapidly migrate to sites of infection or trauma; their accumulation in tissue is indicative of an acute inflammatory reaction.

- Neutropenia and neutrophil defects in adhesion, degranulation, chemotaxis, and microbicidal activity are associated with increased risk of bacterial and fungal infection.

- Eosinophils contain cytoplasmic granules rich in cationic proteins, some of which are highly active against helminthic parasites.

- Eosinophils modulate the allergic response by releasing histaminase, which degrades histamine released by basophils and mast cells.

- Basophils and mast cells are closely related granulocytes that play important roles in the allergic response by releasing histamine in response to allergen–immunoglobulin E immune complexes.

- Mast cells, unlike basophils, do not circulate in blood, contain the anticoagulant heparin, and play a role in maintaining vascular lumen patency.

- Blood monocytes rapidly enter tissues, where they undergo cytokine-mediated differentiation into a variety of cell types, including macrophages, dendritic cells, microglia, and osteoclasts.

Broadly defined, myeloid cells include five cell types—neutrophils, eosinophils, basophils, mast cells, and monocytes—all but one of which (mast cell) is found in normal peripheral blood (Table 10.1 and Fig. 10.1). The term **granulocyte** is commonly used to refer to the nonmonocytic myeloid cells. All myeloid cells derive from undifferentiated bone marrow cells known as common myeloid progenitors (CMPs). Under the influence of specific cytokines, CMPs differentiate into lineage-committed precursors (granulocyte colony-stimulating factor for neutrophils, interleukin [IL]-5 for eosinophils, IL-3 for basophils, **stem cell factor (SCF)** for mast

cells, and **macrophage colony-stimulating factor [M-CSF]** for monocytes). Neutrophils are often the "first responders" to acute inflammation and infection, rapidly migrating from blood into affected tissues. Neutrophils are highly phagocytic cells that kill ingested microorganisms with toxic highly reactive oxygen intermediates. Eosinophils, which home to mucosal sites, play an important role in allergy and parasitic infection by producing histaminase, a modulator of the allergic response, and cationic proteins that are toxic to helminthic parasites. Mast cells, located primarily within highly vascularized connective tissue, produce heparin to

TABLE 10.1 Nucleated Blood Cells

Cell Type	Cell Surface Markers	Granular Constituents	Function
Neutrophil	CD33 (sialic acid lectin)	Myeloperoxidase Lysozyme Defensins	Phagocytic Microbicidal
Eosinophil	CCR3 (eotaxin receptor) FcεR1 (IgE receptor)	MBP Histaminase	Helminth killing Modulation of immediate hypersensitivity
Basophil	CCR3 (eotaxin receptor) FcεR1 (IgE receptor)	Histamine	Immediate hypersensitivity
Monocyte	CD14 (LPS receptor) FcγR1 (IgG receptor)	Lysozyme	Phagocytic (macrophage) Antigen presentation (dendritic cell)
T lymphocyte	CD3 T-cell receptor (αβ, γδ)	Perforin, granzyme, TIA-1 (CD8+ only)	Helper or suppressor (CD4+) Cytotoxic (CD8+)
B lymphocyte	CD20 (B-cell activator) Immunoglobulin	None	Humoral immunity
Natural killer lymphocyte	CD16 (IgG receptor) CD56 (cell adhesion molecule)	Perforin Granzyme	Cytotoxic

Ig, Immunoglobulin; *MBP,* mannose binding protein; *TIA-1,* T-cell-restricted intracellular antigen-1.

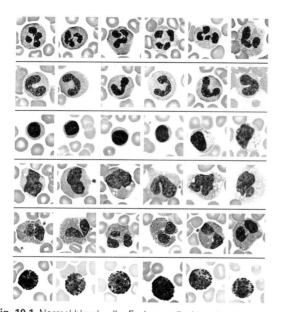

Fig. 10.1 Normal blood cells. Each row displays six examples of each of six cell types (*top to bottom,* segmented neutrophils, band neutrophils, lymphocytes, monocytes, eosinophils, and basophils). Results were obtained on a Micro21 instrument (IMI).

maintain vascular integrity and, along with basophils, release histamine upon allergic challenge. Monocytes enter tissues and rapidly differentiate into macrophages (phagocytic histiocytes), antigen-presenting dendritic cells, osteoclasts, and microglia. As human leucocyte antigen DR–positive antigen-presenting cells (APCs),

monocytes, macrophages, and dendritic cells in particular play a critical role in the immune response by presenting foreign antigen to T cells.

NEUTROPHILS

Neutrophil differentiation in the marrow can be roughly divided into six morphologically distinctive stages: myeloblast, promyelocyte, myelocyte, metamyelocyte, band, and mature neutrophil (Fig. 10.2). Differentiation begins in the marrow with the myeloblast, a relatively large immature cell with oval nucleus, prominent nucleolus, and scanty agranular basophilic cytoplasm. Myeloblasts typically express immature markers CD34 and CD117 and can usually be differentiated from other types of blasts by expression of myeloid cell surface proteins CD13 and CD33 and the granule enzyme **myeloperoxidase (MPO)**. Cytoplasmic differentiation of the myeloblast gives rise to the **promyelocyte**, a large cell with an oval nucleus, small nucleolus, and abundant light blue cytoplasm containing numerous lavender-colored (azurophilic) **primary granules**. Further differentiation yields the **myelocyte**, a medium-sized cell with an oval nucleus, absent nucleolus, and abundant pale cytoplasm with an admixture of azurophilic primary and light pink **secondary granules**. The myelocyte is the last stage in leukocyte differentiation capable of mitotic division. Further differentiation of the myelocyte yields the **metamyelocyte**, a small- to medium-sized cell with

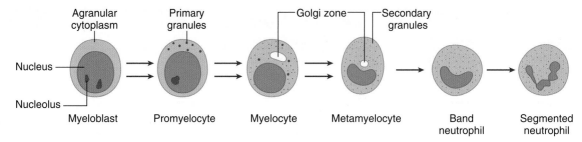

Fig. 10.2 Neutrophil maturation stages.

an oval, indented nucleus and abundant pale-stained cytoplasm with numerous secondary and tertiary granules, followed by the smaller **band neutrophil** with an elongated nonsegmented nucleus and ending with the mature segmented neutrophil (**polymorphonuclear leukocyte**) with a segmented nucleus (typically three or four segments). As myeloid cells mature, secondary and tertiary granules accumulate, and primary granules decline in number.

As mentioned previously, neutrophils contain two major types of granules, primary (azurophilic) and secondary (specific) granules, as well as tertiary granules and secretory vesicles (Fig. 10.3). **Primary granules** are medium-sized, lavender-colored (i.e., azurophilic)

cytoplasmic granules on Wright-stained smears. Primary granules first become apparent at the promyelocyte stage and contain MPO, lysozyme, elastase, and defensins. The enzyme MPO catalyzes the reaction of hydrogen peroxide and chloride ion to form the microbicidal agent hypochlorous acid ("bleach"). **Lysozyme** is an enzyme that hydrolyzes peptidoglycans that make up the cell wall of primarily gram-positive bacteria. **Elastase** is an enzyme that not only cleaves elastic tissue (allowing for movement of neutrophils through connective tissue) but also degrades bacterial membrane proteins. **Defensins** are small, cationic, microbicidal proteins that kill microbes by binding to and forming porelike membrane defects, leading to osmotic lysis.

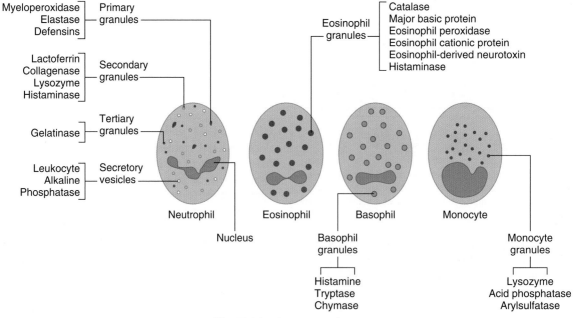

Fig. 10.3 Leukocyte granules.

Secondary granules first become apparent at the myelocyte stage as small, indistinct, light pink cytoplasmic granules on Wright-stained smears. Secondary granules in neutrophils contain lactoferrin, collagenase, histaminase, and lysozyme. The antimicrobial properties of the iron-binding protein **lactoferrin** result from interference with iron bioavailability for bacterial growth, direct damage to microbial cell membranes, and interference with virus binding to cells. Secondary granules in eosinophils also contain **major basic protein (MBP)**, which is toxic to helminthic parasites. Meanwhile, secondary granules in basophils (and mast cells) contain **histamine**, which acts to increase microvascular permeability, allowing for leukocyte migration into inflamed tissues. **Tertiary granules** become most apparent at the metamyelocyte stage and contain **gelatinase** (matrix metalloproteinase), an enzyme that may play a role in neutrophil migration through connective tissue. Neutrophils also contain **secretory vesicles** that contain **leukocyte alkaline phosphatase (LAP)**, an enzyme for which a distinct function has yet to be determined (Box 10.1).

Most neutrophils remain in reserve within the **marrow storage pool**, ready to enter the circulation when triggered by infection or inflammation. Blood neutrophils themselves spend little time in the circulation and instead rapidly enter inflamed tissues. Neutrophils are also found loosely adherent to vascular endothelium, especially in the pulmonary capillary bed and in the **marginal pool**. Neutrophils in the marginal pool rapidly enter the circulation by demarginating in response to physical or emotional stress.

Circulating neutrophils enter inflamed tissues by first rolling along and firmly binding to activated endothelium

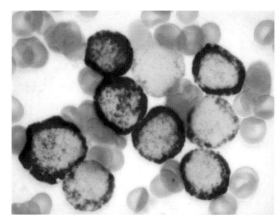

Fig. 10.4 Chloroacetate esterase (red cytoplasmic) staining of granulocyte precursors.

and then passing through postcapillary venules into inflamed tissues (Fig. 10.5). The process begins with inflammatory cytokine-induced expression of **leukocyte adhesion receptors** (E-selectin, P-selectin, intercellular adhesion molecule 1 [ICAM-1]) on endothelial cells. Passing neutrophils first loosely "roll along" the endothelium via **neutrophil L-selectin** interaction with endothelial E- and P-selectins. This is followed by firm binding of neutrophils to endothelium via **neutrophil integrin (leukocyte function-associated antigen 1 [LFA-1])** interaction with endothelial ICAM-1. Firmly bound neutrophils then migrate through **platelet endothelial cell adhesion molecule (PECAM)**–modified endothelium in response to a variety of chemotactic signals (complement C5a and IL-8) arising from inflamed or damaged tissues. Leukocyte response to external signals is mediated by binding of ligands to cell surface receptors for cell adhesion, phagocytosis, chemotaxis, and cell growth (Fig. 10.6). Adhesion to endothelium is mediated by receptors for LFA-1 and ICAM-1. Movement of leukocytes to sites of tissue damage or infection is mediated by binding of **inflammatory chemokines** to leukocyte chemokine receptors. Leukocyte maturation and growth signals are generated by binding of **cytokines** to cytokine receptors. Neutrophils that collect at sites of infection release netlike complexes of chromatin and antimicrobial agents (including myeloperoxidase, elastase, and defensins) that entrap and kill extracellular pathogens. Formation of these **netlike extracellular traps (NET)** is dependent on **peptidyl-arginine deiminase (PAD4)**–mediated nuclear disintegration.

BOX 10.1 Technical Note

Differentiation of granulocytes and precursors from monocytes and precursors on blood and bone marrow smears can be accomplished by staining for either **myeloperoxidase (MPO)** or **chloroacetate esterase (CAE)** activity with a soluble colorless substrate converted to an insoluble colored product that is deposited within the cytoplasm and can easily be seen by light microscopy (Fig. 10.4). Whereas granulocytes are positive for MPO and CAE, monocytes are negative. Monocytes can be positively identified by staining for **alpha naphthyl butyrate esterase (ANBE)**.

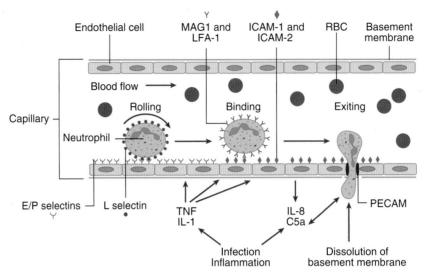

Fig. 10.5 Neutrophil emigration. *ICAM,* Intercellular adhesion molecule 1; *IL,* interleukin; *LFA-1,* leukocyte function-associated antigen 1; PECAM, platelet endothelial cell adhesion molecule; *RBC,* red blood cell; *TNF,* tumor necrosis factor.

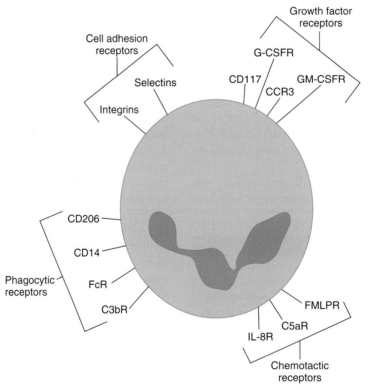

Fig. 10.6 Leukocyte cell surface receptors. *CCR3,* C-C chemokine receptor 3; *FMLPR,* formyl peptide receptor: *G-CSFR,* granulocyte colony-stimulating factor receptor; *GM-CSFR,* granulocyte–macrophage colony-stimulating factor receptor; IL, interleukin.

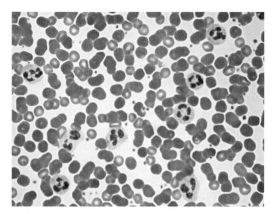

Fig. 10.7 Neutrophilic leukocytosis (no left shift).

Neutrophilia is defined as an increased absolute blood neutrophil count in excess of 11,000 neutrophils per microliter in adults (somewhat higher in children) (Fig. 10.7). Neutrophilia is associated with a range of conditions, including bacterial infections, tissue damage (e.g., myocardial infarction or thermal burns), chronic inflammatory diseases (e.g., rheumatoid arthritis or ulcerative colitis), malignancy, myeloproliferative neoplasms, metabolic disorders (e.g., thyrotoxicosis), drugs (e.g., corticosteroids or lithium), and severe emotional stress (Table 10.2). Although neutrophilia is commonly seen with gram-positive bacterial infection, **neutropenia** sometimes occurs with gram-negative bacteremia or septic shock. Rarely, ingested bacteria may be seen within neutrophils on peripheral smear (Fig. 10.8). Extreme reactive neutrophilia accompanied by increased immature myeloid cells (myeloid left shift) is referred to as a **leukemoid reaction** because these findings may mimic chronic myeloid leukemia. Leukemoid reactions may be seen in acute infections (especially in children), hemolysis, and a variety of solid tumors. Leukemoid reactions can be differentiated from chronic myeloid leukemia by staining for LAP. Whereas leukemoid neutrophils express high LAP, neutrophils in CML are LAP weak to negative (Fig. 10.9). Left-shifted neutrophilia accompanied by numerous nucleated RBCs is termed **leukoerythroblastosis** (Fig. 10.10). This condition usually indicates the presence of an abnormal infiltrative process in the bone marrow, such as metastatic cancer, leukemia, or myelofibrosis.

Several neutrophil function disorders lead to increased susceptibility to infection, most often superficial pyogenic bacterial infections. Neutrophil dysfunction

TABLE 10.2 Common Causes of Leukocytosis	
Neutrophilia	**Basophilia**
Acute infection (bacterial, fungal, tuberculosis)	Myeloproliferative disease
Chronic inflammatory disorders	Hyperthyroidism
Blood loss	
Hypercortisolism	
Stress	
Myeloproliferative disease	
Cancer	
	Monocytosis
	Infection (bacterial, protozoal)
	Inflammatory bowel disease
	Sarcoidosis
	Connective tissue disorders
Eosinophilia	*Lymphocytosis*
Allergic reactions (including drugs)	Infection (bacterial, viral)
Chronic skin diseasesss	Lymphoid leukemia
Parasitic infection	Lymphoma
Hypereosinophilic syndrome	
Cancer	

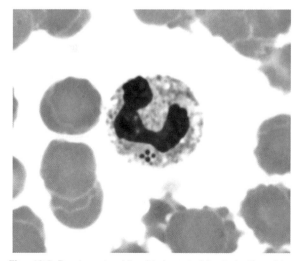

Fig. 10.8 Band neutrophil with ingested bacteria (four blue cytoplasmic inclusions).

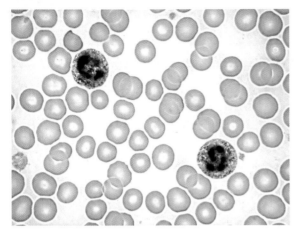

Fig. 10.9 Strong leukocyte alkaline phosphatase staining (red cytoplasmic) of two neutrophils in leukemoid reaction.

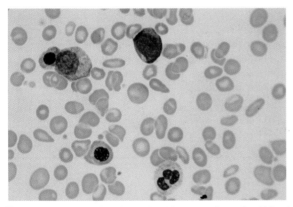

Fig. 10.10 Leukoerythroblastosis with two nucleated red blood cells (RBCs), two immature granulocytes, and a segmented neutrophil. Also note the two teardrop-shaped RBCs (dacrocytes). This additional feature is indicative of chronic idiopathic myelofibrosis.

can arise from defects in adhesion, chemotaxis, degranulation, and bactericidal activity (Fig. 10.11). **Adhesion defects**, such as the autosomal recessive disorder **leukocyte adhesion deficiency** caused by β2-integrin deficiency, prevent the transmigration of circulating neutrophils through vascular endothelium into infected tissues (diapedesis). Patients with leukocyte adhesion deficiency typically present with neutrophilia and recurrent nonsuppurative bacterial infections (without pus formation).

Chemotaxis defects, such as those caused by ethanol intoxication, opsonin (immunoglobulin, complement)

deficiency, and **immune complex disease**, prevent neutrophil migration to areas of infection by interfering with neutrophil response to complement C5a and IL-8 elaborated by inflamed tissue.

Degranulation defects prevent release of bactericidal substances. In the rare autosomal recessive disorder **Chediak-Higashi syndrome**, abnormal lysosomal fusion leads to huge neutrophil granules noted on peripheral smear. Patients with Chediak-Higashi syndrome are usually susceptible to pyogenic infections (especially *Staphylococcus aureus*) because of both neutropenia and various neutrophil defects in chemotaxis, degranulation, and microbicidal activity. The neutropenia appears to result from reduced marrow neutrophil production, that is, ineffective granulopoiesis.

Microbicidal defects lead to recurrent bacterial and fungal infection. Mutations of enzymes nicotinamide adenine dinucleotide phosphate (NADPH) oxidase and myeloperoxidase lead respectively to deficiency of neutrophilic superoxide or hypochlorous acid, tyrosyl radical, and peroxynitrite (Fig. 10.12). **Chronic granulomatous disease (CGD)** is caused by mutations in **NADPH oxidase**, the enzyme responsible for conversion of molecular oxygen (O_2) to microbicidal superoxide (O_2^-). Most cases CGD are X-linked and thus are most common in males. However, up to one-third of cases follow an autosomal pattern of inheritance. Superoxide-deficient neutrophils and monocytes in CGD ingest but do not kill catalase-positive microorganisms, including *S. aureus*, *Aspergillus fumigatus*, and *Candida albicans*. Under normal circumstances, ingested microbes are killed within phagolysosomes by toxic oxidizing agents, including hydrogen peroxide and superoxide. However, by neutralizing hydrogen peroxide, catalase-positive microbes are especially resistant to killing. The diagnosis of CGD can be established by the **nitroblue tetrazolium (NBT) test**. In this test, normal NADPH oxidase–positive neutrophils oxidize the colorless NBT substrate to form an insoluble, dark blue reaction product. In contrast, a negative to weak positive NBT test is seen in CGD.

Acquired neutropenia (absolute neutrophil count <1500/μL) is often seen after viral infections, especially in childhood. Other causes of acquired neutropenia include acquired immunodeficiency syndrome (AIDS), overwhelming sepsis, drugs, autoimmunity, and aplastic anemia (Table 10.3). Patients with an absolute neutrophil count below 500/mL because of marrow failure

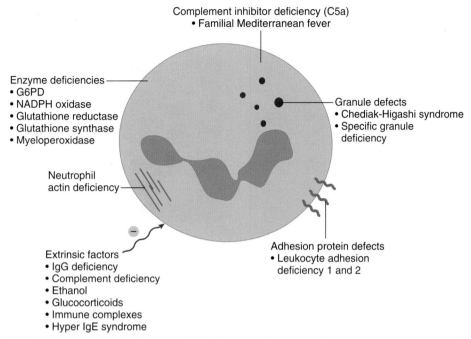

Fig. 10.11 Leukocyte function defects. *G6PD*, Glucose-6-phosphate dehydrogenase; *Ig*, immunoglobulin; *NADPH*, nicotinamide adenine dinucleotide phosphate.

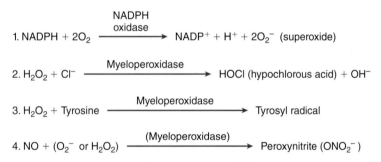

Fig. 10.12 Antimicrobial oxidants produced by leukocytes. *NADPH*, reduced form of nicotinamide adenine dinucleotide phosphate; *NADP*⁺, oxydized form of nicotinamide adenine dinucleotide phosphate.

or chemotherapy have a significantly increased risk of systemic bacterial infection and should be managed as inpatients with intravenous antibiotics. On the other hand, there is poor correlation between neutrophil count and risk of infection in patients with adequate marrow reserve. For example, children with chronic benign neutropenia and many adults with immune neutropenia show no increased risk of serious infection. Chronic neutropenia of any cause may lead to pyoderma caused by *S. aureus*, *Escherichia coli*, or *Pseudomonas aeruginosa* and otitis media caused by *Streptococcus pneumoniae* or *P. aeruginosa*.

EOSINOPHILS

Eosinophils develop in the marrow from the CMP under the influence of IL-3, **granulocyte–macrophage colony-stimulating factor (GM-CSF)**, IL-5, and eotaxin. Eosinophil precursors are distinguished from neutrophil and basophil precursors by the presence of

TABLE 10.3	Causes of Neutropenia
Decreased Production	**Increased Destruction**
Aplastic anemia	Autoimmune (FcγRIIIb
Megaloblastic anemia	autoantigen)
Myelodysplasia	Drug induced (carbimazole,
Acute leukemia	clozapine, dapsone,
Cytotoxic chemotherapy	dipyrone, methimazole,
and radiotherapy	penicillin G, procain-
Neutrophil elastase	amide, propylthiouracil,
defects	rituximab, sulfasalazine,
Congenital neutropenia	ticlopidine)
(Kostmann disease)	Hypersplenism
Cyclic neutropenia	
Chronic infection (HIV,	
EBV, TB)	

EBV, Epstein-Barr virus; *HIV,* human immunodeficiency virus; *TB,* tuberculosis.

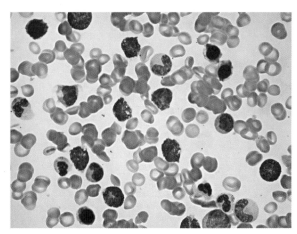

Fig. 10.13 Eosinophilia.

large specific granules that contain catalase and several basic proteins, including MBP, eosinophil peroxidase, eosinophil cationic protein, and eosinophil-derived neurotoxin. Binding of opsonized particles to immunoglobulin (Ig) G, IgA, IgE, and complement receptors can induce eosinophil degranulation and phagocytosis. Eosinophils spend only a brief period in the blood, instead rapidly migrating to the submucosa of the gastrointestinal, respiratory, and urinary tracts, where they serve as a first-line defense against invading parasites by binding IgA immune complexes and releasing toxic granule contents. Primary granules of eosinophils contain the **Charcot-Leyden crystal protein** that is commonly seen as needle-shaped extracellular crystals in eosinophil-rich tissues. The eosinophil granule protein MBP exhibits toxicity against helminthic parasites, particularly schistosomes. MBP toxicity may be mediated by its hydrophobicity, negative charge, and ability to inhibit microbial ATPase. Eosinophils play a role in atopic allergic diseases such as hay fever, atopic dermatitis, and asthma. The severity of asthma is directly related to the number of airway eosinophils. Eosinophils produce **histaminase**, an enzyme that, by inactivating excessive histamine released by basophils and mast cells at the sites of allergic reactions, modulates the allergic response.

Hypereosinophilic syndrome (HES) is a condition marked by chronic sustained blood and tissue eosinophilia that leads to tissue damage (Fig. 10.13). Primary (idiopathic) HES is a rare disorder with no identifiable cause. In idiopathic HES, all known secondary causes of hypereosinophilia (parasitic infection, allergic disease, drug reaction, and underlying neoplasms) must be excluded. Cases of HES marked by a clonal cytogenetic abnormality and peripheral blood cytopenia may best be classified as **chronic eosinophilic leukemia**. Some cases of HES are associated with activating mutations of the tyrosine kinase platelet-derived growth factor receptor alpha *(PDGFRα)* gene and may respond to tyrosine kinase inhibitors such as imatinib. A variety of malignant neoplasms, including carcinoma, acute myeloid leukemia, T-cell lymphoma, and Hodgkin lymphoma, are associated with secondary HES, possibly caused by overproduction of eosinophil growth factors such as IL-5. Whatever the cause of HES, the excessive amount of eosinophil granule proteins (MBP, eosinophil peroxidase, eosinophil cationic protein, and eosinophil-derived neurotoxin) released into tissues such as the heart, lung, and central nervous system leads to end-organ damage. Clinically, HES is marked by congestive heart failure caused by endomyocardial fibrosis, pulmonary disease caused by pulmonary fibrosis, and a variety of neurologic abnormalities (e.g., confusion, coma, blurred vision, and peripheral neuritis). The neurologic damage likely results from the combined toxic effects of eosinophil cationic protein and eosinophil-derived neurotoxin.

BASOPHILS AND MAST CELLS

Despite their many similarities, it is not known whether basophils and mast cells derive from a common marrow allergen with allergen-specific IgE on mast cells and basophils provokes release of histamine (Fig. 10.15). Histamine induces increased capillary permeability and vasodilation, which leads to localized leukocyte recruitment and fluid accumulation (swelling, edema). In some cases, a hyperallergic response to an allergen leads to severe bronchoconstriction and vascular collapse (**anaphylactic shock**).

Basophils promote T-helper 2 (Th2) immune responses and may play an important role in host defense to parasites. Basophilia is a rare condition but can be seen in allergic conditions, autoimmune disease, endocrine disorders, infection, and myeloproliferative disorders. Mast cells, unlike basophils, produce heparin. Endogenous heparin produced by perivascular mast cells likely contributes to the maintenance of vascular patency. **Heparan sulfate**, a ubiquitous heparinlike polysaccharide, plays an important role in transendothelial emigration of leukocytes into tissues. Mast cells do not normally circulate in blood and are seen only in mast cell leukemia, a rare manifestation of systemic mastocytosis.

Urticaria pigmentosa, the most common form of cutaneous mastocytosis, is a benign condition of the skin, usually in young children, caused by accumulations of mast cells within the dermis. Findings include urticaria, pruritus, and raised pigmented skin lesions. **Systemic mastocytosis** is a more serious condition, usually seen in adults who present with urticaria, pruritus, abdominal distress, dyspnea, and hypotension, associated with accumulations of mast cells in multiple organs, including the bone marrow (Fig. 10.16). Systemic

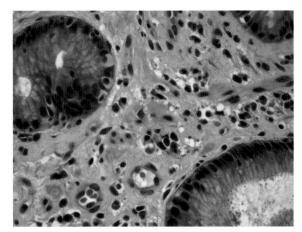

Fig. 10.14 Mast cells (small mononuclear cells with purplish cytoplasm) and eosinophils (nucleated cells with red cytoplasmic granules) in the lamina propria of the gastrointestinal tract.

progenitor. Whereas basophil growth is stimulated by IL-3, mast cell growth is stimulated by SCF (kit ligand). Mast cells, unlike basophils, are not normally seen in the blood and rapidly migrate to connective tissues, where they are relatively long lived and capable of cell division (Fig. 10.14). In contrast, basophils, like eosinophils, briefly circulate in the blood and rapidly enter mucosal tissues during allergic responses. Both basophils and mast cells contain metachromatic granules that contain histamine and the neutral proteases **trypsin** and **chymase**. Both cell types participate in **allergic hypersensitivity reactions** to allergens (exogenous antigens that elicit an IgE antibody response). Cross-linking of

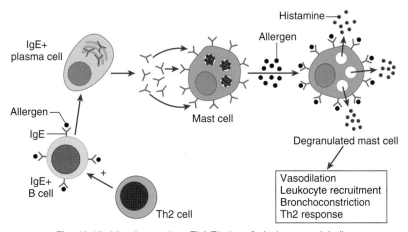

Fig. 10.15 Allergic reaction. *Th2*, T-helper 2; *Ig*, immunoglobulin.

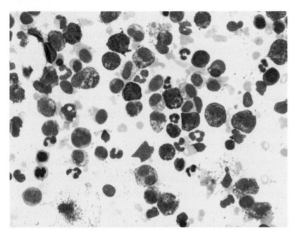

Fig. 10.16 Numerous bone marrow mast cells (cells with prominent purplish granules) in systemic mastocytosis.

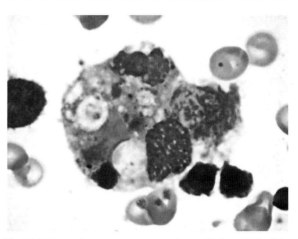

Fig. 10.17 Large bone marrow macrophage with ingested cellular debris.

mastocytosis is associated with activating point mutations of the c-kit gene.

MONOCYTES

Monocytes develop in the bone marrow from myelomonocytic progenitor cells known as colony forming unit–granulocyte monocyte (CFU-GM) under the influence of the cytokines M-CSF and GM-CSF. Mature monocytes are released from the marrow into the circulation, where they circulate with a half-life of 2 to 3 days before entering tissues and body fluids in response to inflammation and infection. Within tissues, monocytes may further differentiate into a wide variety of cell types, including macrophages (histiocytes), dendritic cells, **Langerhans cells** (skin), Kupffer cells (liver), splenic macrophages, alveolar macrophages (lung), serous macrophages (serous spaces), microglia (central nervous system), and osteoclasts. Liver macrophages, also known as **Kupffer cells**, line the hepatic sinusoids, where they clear the blood of opsonized cells and bacteria. **Splenic macrophages** are found within the red pulp sinusoids, where they clear the blood of aged and damaged blood cells, bacteria, and immune complexes. **Bone marrow macrophages** deliver iron to developing erythroid cells and clear the marrow of apoptotic marrow cells and cell debris (Fig. 10.17). In the thymus, macrophages clear the thymic cortex of apoptotic thymocytes. Under the influence of specific cytokines, monocytes within tissues can differentiate into macrophages or dendritic cells (Fig. 10.18). The prime functions of macrophages are phagocytosis and lysosomal degradation of microbes, damaged cells, and immune complexes. In contrast, the prime function of **dendritic cells** is antigen presentation to T cells.

Monocytes are large mononuclear cells with abundant amounts of finely granular cytoplasm and a delicately folded nucleus (Fig. 10.19). Monocytes and macrophages express CD14, the **lipopolysaccharide receptor** that binds to gram-negative bacteria; CD68, a lysosomal sialomucin; CD163, the **hemoglobin–haptoglobin scavenger receptor**; CD206, the **mannose binding protein** that binds to mannose-bearing microbes (bacteria, fungi, parasites); and **immunoglobulin** and complement (C3b) receptors for binding and phagocytosis of antibody- and complement-bound cells. Monocytes express small amounts of MPO and large amounts of alpha naphthyl butyrate esterase and lysozyme. Monocytes are phagocytic cells, and in pathologic body fluids, they may contain a variety of phagocytosed materials, including crystals (urate), hemosiderin, lipid, cells (erythrocytes, neutrophils, and lymphocytes), and infectious agents (bacteria and fungi).

Monocytosis is most commonly seen in clonal hematologic disorders (chronic myelomonocytic leukemia or myelodysplasia), chronic inflammatory conditions, and chronic infections. **Monocytopenia** is often seen in aplastic anemia, hairy cell leukemia, autoimmune disease, and human immunodeficiency virus (HIV) infection. Unlike monocytes, macrophages are seldom found in peripheral blood. Dendritic cells are rarely seen in blood, accounting for less than 1% of circulating leukocytes.

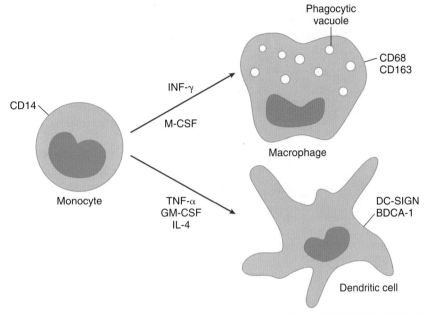

Fig. 10.18 Monocyte differentiation. *BDCA-1,* blastic dendritic cell antigen 1; *DC-SIGN,* dendritic cell-specific ICAM-3-grabbing nonintegrin: *GM-CSF,* granulocyte–macrophage colony-stimulating factor; *IL,* interleukin; *INF-γ,* interferon-γ; *M-CSF,* macrophage colony-stimulating factor; *TNF-α,* tumor necrosis factor-α.

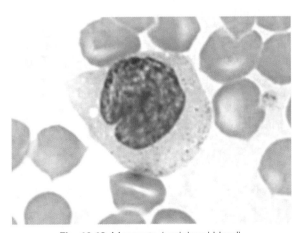

Fig. 10.19 Monocyte (peripheral blood).

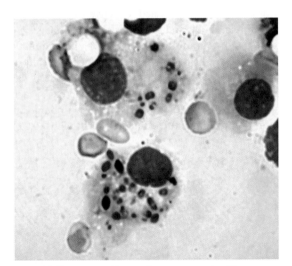

Fig. 10.20 Two macrophages (bone marrow) with numerous ingested yeast forms of *Histoplasma capsulatum* (large blue cytoplasmic inclusions). Note the plasma cell on the *right.*

Macrophages (also known as histiocytes) are produced from monocytes in response to interferon-γ (INF-γ). In contrast, **myeloid dendritic cells**, produced from monocytes in response to tumor necrosis factor-α (TNF-α), are APCs designed for activation of the immune response. Tissue macrophages are large actively phagocytic cells that proteolytically degrade microorganisms and cellular debris within phagolysosomes.

Macrophages are large highly phagocytic cells derived from monocytes, with more abundant, finely granular cytoplasm and often with vacuoles and phagocytic debris (Fig. 10.20). Macrophages can be functionally subclassified as M1 and M2 macrophages. IFN-γ–activated

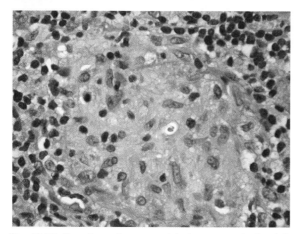

Fig. 10.21 Granuloma (non-necrotizing) composed of a tight nodular collection of histiocytes (macrophages) surrounded by a loose collection of small lymphocytes.

M1 macrophages are bactericidal and produce proinflammatory cytokines (including IL-12 and IL-23), whereas IL-4– or IL-10–activated **M2 macrophages** are scavenger cells that are immunosuppressive and promote tissue repair. Under conditions in which antigen cannot be degraded (digested) effectively (mycobacteria, fungi, foreign body, and sarcoidosis), macrophages congregate to form **granulomas** (Fig. 10.21), in conjunction with CD4+ T-helper cells. Granulomas typically are nodules composed of macrophages, T-helper cells, and fibroblasts, sometimes accompanied by necrosis. Macrophages within granulomas sometimes undergo cell fusion to form **multinucleated giant cells** (Fig. 10.22).

Hemophagocytic syndrome is a life-threatening condition marked by a proliferation of highly activated phagocytic histiocytes (Fig. 10.23). Hemophagocytic syndrome typically presents with fever, hepatosplenomegaly, and peripheral cytopenia. The bone marrow, spleen, and liver contain numerous hemophagocytic histiocytes. The disorder appears to result from an exaggerated proinflammatory response to infection or cancer, marked by high levels of inflammatory cytokines, including IFN-γ and TNF-α. Diagnostic findings may include fever, splenomegaly, bicytopenia, increased ferritin, high triglycerides, low fibrinogen, high IL-2 receptor, low natural killer cell activity, and increased hemophagocytic histiocytes in the marrow. A familial autosomal recessive form of hemophagocytic syndrome termed **hemophagocytic lymphohistiocytosis** is seen in infants. Several disease-associated genetic mutations have been described, including a mutation in the *PRF1* gene that encodes for the cytotoxic protein **perforin**.

Monocytes may enter the skin and mucous membranes and differentiate into immature dendritic cells called **Langerhans cells**. Langerhans cells express markers CD1a and S-100. They contain **Birbeck bodies**, cytoplasmic organelles of obscure function that can be identified by electron microscopy. Upon antigen uptake, Langerhans cells migrate from skin or mucosal sites to regional lymph nodes and differentiate into **interdigitating dendritic cells** that present antigen to T cells within the lymph node paracortex. In chronic dermatitis, the numerous Langerhans cells recruited to regional lymph nodes leads to a form

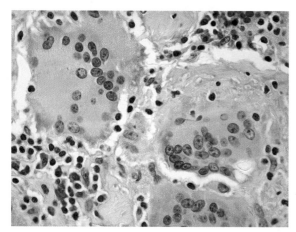

Fig. 10.22 Multinucleated giant cells created by fusion of numerous mononuclear macrophages (>20).

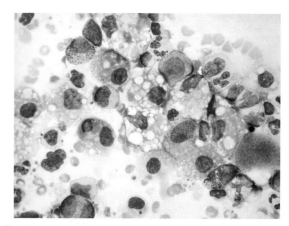

Fig. 10.23 Numerous phagocytic histiocytes (large mononuclear cells with abundant blue vacuolated cytoplasm) in hemophagocytic syndrome.

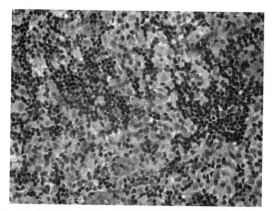

Fig. 10.24 Dermatopathic lymphadenitis. A lymph node with irregular collections of Langerhans cells (cells with abundant pale cytoplasm) and small lymphocytes is shown.

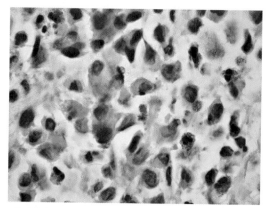

Fig. 10.25 Langerhans cell histiocytosis (bone lesion) with numerous large Langerhans cells (with twisted irregular nuclei) and admixed eosinophils.

of lymph node enlargement termed **dermatopathic lymphadenitis** (Fig. 10.24).

Langerhans cell histiocytosis is a family of neoplastic disorders, seen in children and young adults marked by variable degrees of Langerhans cell proliferation, often involving bone (with lytic lesions), skin, and other sites (Fig. 10.25). In some cases, the disease is localized and indolent; in other cases, the disease is multifocal and malignant.

KEY WORDS AND CONCEPTS

- Acquired neutropenia
- Adhesion defects
- Allergic hypersensitivity reactions
- Anaphylactic shock
- Band neutrophil
- Basophils
- Birbeck bodies
- Charcot-Leyden crystal protein
- Chediak-Higashi syndrome
- Chemotaxis defects
- Chloroacetate esterase (CAE)
- Chronic eosinophilic leukemia
- Chronic granulomatous disease (CGD)
- *C-kit*
- Chymase
- Cytokines
- Defensins
- Degranulation defects
- Dermatopathic lymphadenitis
- Elastase
- Gelatinase
- Granulocyte–macrophage colony-stimulating factor (GM-CSF)
- Granulomas
- Hemoglobin–haptoglobin scavenger receptor
- Hemophagocytic lymphohistiocytosis
- Hemophagocytic syndrome
- Heparan sulfate
- Histaminase
- Histamine
- Hypereosinophilic syndrome (HES)
- Immune complex disease
- Immunoglobulin
- Inflammatory chemokines
- Interdigitating dendritic cells
- Lactoferrin
- Langerhans cell histiocytosis
- Langerhans cells
- Leukemoid reaction
- Leukocyte adhesion deficiency
- Leukocyte adhesion receptors

- Leukocyte alkaline phosphatase (LAP)
- Leukoerythroblastosis
- Lipopolysaccharide
- Lysozyme
- M1 macrophages
- M2 macrophages
- Macrophages
- Macrophage colony-stimulating factor (M-CSF)
- Major basic protein (MBP)
- Mannose binding protein
- Marginal pool
- Marrow storage pool
- Metamyelocyte
- Microbicidal defects
- Monocytopenia
- Monocytosis
- Multinucleated giant cells
- Myelocyte
- Myeloid dendritic cells
- Myeloperoxidase (MPO)

- NADPH oxidase
- Netlike extracellular trap (NET)
- Neutropenia
- Neutrophilia
- Neutrophil integrin (LFA-1)
- Neutrophil L-selectin
- Nitroblue tetrazolium (NBT) test
- Peptidyl-arginine deiminase (PAD4)
- Perforin
- Platelet endothelial cell adhesion molecule (PECAM)
- Polymorphonuclear leukocyte
- Primary granules
- Promyelocyte
- Secondary granules
- Secretory vesicles
- Stem cell factor (SCF)
- Systemic mastocytosis
- Tertiary granules
- Trypsin
- Urticaria pigmentosa

REVIEW QUESTIONS

1. All of the following are enzymes in neutrophil granules **except**
   A. myeloperoxidase.
   B. catalase.
   C. elastase.
   D. lysozyme.

2. All of the following are antimicrobial oxidants in neutrophils **except for**
   A. superoxide.
   B. hydrochloric acid.
   C. tyrosyl radical.
   D. peroxynitrite.

3. Chronic granulomatous disease is caused by
   A. superoxide deficiency.
   B. abnormal lysosomal fusion.

   C. integrin defects.
   D. MPO deficiency.

4. Which of the following mast cell molecules is not present in basophils?
   A. Histamine
   B. IgE receptor
   C. Heparin
   D. Chymase

5. Which of the following is **not** a consequence of eosinophil toxins in hypereosinophilic syndrome?
   A. Congestive heart failure
   B. Peripheral neuritis
   C. Pulmonary fibrosis
   D. Pancreatic insufficiency

11

Immune System and Related Disorders

KEY POINTS

- Immune system organs include the bone marrow, thymus, lymph nodes, spleen, tonsils, as well as gut-, skin-, and bronchial-associated lymphoid tissues.

- The major types of immune system cells are lymphocytes, plasma cells, and antigen-presenting cells (APCs).

- The four major lymphocyte types are T cells, B cells, natural killer (NK), and natural killer T cells (NKT cells).

- APCs include dendritic cells and macrophages.

- Lymphocytes and dendritic cells (excluding follicular dendritic cells) derive from bone marrow progenitors.

- Immature T cells migrate from the marrow to the thymus and with the help of thymic epithelial cells and dendritic cells undergo maturation into antigen-specific CD4+ and CD8+ T cells and dual CD4/CD8− T cells.

- CD4+ and CD8+ T cells recognize antigens in association with human leukocyte antigen (HLA) molecules (class II and class I, respectively) via cell surface heterodimeric alpha-beta T-cell receptors ($\alpha\beta$TCRs).

- Dual CD4/CD8 negative T cells recognize conserved bacterial antigens via $\gamma\delta$TCRs independent of HLA molecules.

- A variety of CD4+ T-cell subsets have been described; some are helper cells (e.g., Th1, Th2, and Th17), and others are suppressor cells (e.g., regulatory T cells and Th3).

- NK cells exit the marrow fully mature and recognize abnormal or foreign cells by their decreased expression of HLA class I molecules.

- CD8+ T cells and NK cells kill target cells by forming membrane pores (perforin) and injecting toxic proteins (granzyme B or TIA1) that induce apoptosis-like DNA fragmentation.

- B cells recognize antigens directly (without prior lysosomal digestion) via cell surface immunoglobulin receptors.

- Immature B cells are released form the bone marrow, migrate to lymphoid organs, react with antigen-bearing dendritic cells and T-helper cells, undergo proliferation, and mature into either antigen-specific memory B cells or antibody-secreting plasma cells.

- Immune complexes, composed of antigen, antibody, and complement, are cleared from the circulation by phagocytic cells bearing receptors for immunoglobulin (Fc fragment) and complement C3b.

- Antibody and complement binding to bacteria leads to neutralization of infectivity and phagocytosis by neutrophils and macrophages.

- Complement activation by microbes and senescent or apoptotic cells leads to opsonization and membrane attack complex–mediated osmotic lysis.

- Lymph nodes consist of a cortical region with B cell–rich lymphoid follicles, a T cell–rich paracortical zone, a central medullary region rich in plasma cells, and macrophage-rich lymphatic sinusoids.

- Primary (unstimulated) lymphoid follicles consist of small resting B cells, follicular dendritic cells, and T follicular helper (Tfh) cells.

- Secondary (stimulated) lymphoid follicles consist of a central germinal center—with proliferating

Continued

antigen-specific B cells, antigen-bearing follicular dendritic cells, and Tfh cells—and a circumferential mantle zone of small resting B cells.

- The spleen is a large abdominal lymphoid organ that serves two overlapping functions: that of blood filter (in the vascular red pulp) and that of immune responder to bloodborne antigens (in the lymphoid white pulp).

- The tonsils and adenoids are submucosal lymphoid organs in the oral and nasopharyngeal cavity (Waldeyer's ring) that respond to ingested or inhaled antigens.

- Peyer's patches are lymphoid aggregates in the submucosa of the terminal ileum that respond to ingested intestinal antigens.

All lymphocytes derive from bone marrow progenitors. T-cell progenitors complete their maturation in the **thymus** before entering lymphoid tissues, and B-cell and natural killer (NK) cell progenitors complete their maturation in the bone marrow. Early B-cell precursors can be identified by cell surface expression of the **CD19** antigen, and T and NK cell precursors can be identified by cell surface expression of the **CD7** antigen.

Expression of the recombination-activating genes *(RAG1, RAG2)* and terminal deoxynucleotidyl transferase (TdT) herald the initiation of immunoglobulin heavy chain gene rearrangement on chromosome 14 in B cell precursors and T-cell receptor (TCR) gene rearrangement on chromosomes 7 and 14 in T cell precursors. During this process, a variable (V) gene segment, a diversity (D) gene segment, and a joining (J) gene segment, which in the germline are widely separated by intronic DNA, are cut by RAG-1 and RAG-2, altered by DNA polymerase and TdT, and spliced together by DNA repair enzymes to form a VDJ segment. TdT specifically catalyzes the addition of random nucleotides to the ends of V, D, and J gene segments before ligation. RAG components of the V(D)J recombinase complex catalyze the formation of double-strand breaks at the ends of the V, D, and J gene segments of immunoglobulin and TCR loci. NK cells do not express polymorphic antigen receptors; thus, TdT and RAG are not expressed.

The complex process of **immunoglobulin gene rearrangement** yields tremendous variability in antigen binding. There are about 45 V region segments, 23 D segments, and 6 J segments from which to choose, yielding a **combinatorial diversity** of approximately 6210 antigen-binding domains (Fig. 11.1). Additional diversity known as **junctional diversity** is derived from random

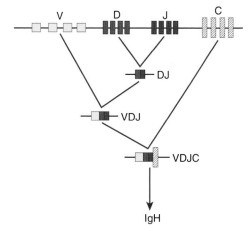

Fig. 11.1 VDJH recombination. *Ig,* Immunoglobulin.

additions of nucleotides at the regions between segments by the enzymes DNA polymerase and TdT. The total potential antigen-binding diversity generated by the immunoglobulin heavy and light chain loci is estimated to be 10^{11}. A similar process takes place in precursor T cell (thymocyte) VDJ (or VJ) gene loci on chromosome 7 (beta and gamma chains) and chromosome 14 (alpha and delta chains) to generate even greater antigen-binding diversity (10^{16}–10^{18} potential antigenic specificities) in heterodimeric αβTCRs (and γδTCRs).

T CELLS

T cells begin life in the bone marrow and complete their maturation in the **thymus**, a lymphoid organ located in the anterior mediastinum (Fig. 11.2). Immature CD7/TdT+ CD3− **precursor T cells** migrate from the bone

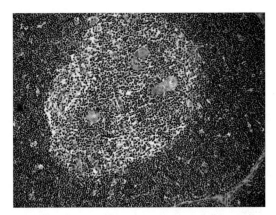

Fig. 11.2 The thymus. Note the central medullary region and the peripheral cortical zone. Immature naïve T cells from the marrow enter the cortex and pass into the medulla only after successful acquisition of non–self-antigen specificity. The medullary thymic epithelial cells (MTECs) form whorls known as Hassall corpuscles. Recent evidence suggests that these structures play a role in the maturation of regulatory (suppressor) T cells.

marrow to the outer **thymic cortex** (Fig. 11.3). At this stage, the precursor T cells (**cortical thymocytes**) undergo rearrangement of the βTCR, γTCR, and δTCR genes. In most cases (95%), beta-chain rearrangement occurs first and leads to expression of a heterodimeric **pre-TCR** composed of beta chain complexed with an invariant pre-alpha chain. This is followed by alpha chain rearrangement and suppression of gamma and delta chain rearrangement. Expression of the mature heterodimeric alpha/beta TCR (**TCRαβ**), along with accessory molecules CD3, CD4, and CD8, allows interaction of cortical thymocytes with common self-antigens expressed by endoderm-derived **cortical thymic epithelial cells** and marrow-derived thymic **dendritic cells**. Both thymic cell types present self-antigens in association with self-**MHC** (**major histocompatibility complex**) protein. The terms *MHC* and *HLA* are often used interchangeably. However, strictly speaking, MHC (major histocompatibility complex) refers to the gene complex, and **HLA** (**human leukocyte antigen**) refers to the proteins encoded by MHC genes. Whereas **cortical T cells** that bind to these specialized antigen-presenting cells (APCs) via their TCR complexes are positively selected for further development in the **thymic medulla**, T cells that fail to bind to self-antigen undergo **apoptosis** (cell death). T cells with no interaction with self-antigen are deleted because they are unlikely to recognize foreign antigen bound to self-MHC ("altered self").

Positively selected cortical T cells that bind to self-antigen in association with HLA class I lose expression of CD4 to become mature CD8+ T cells, and positively selected T cells that bind to self-antigen in association with HLA class II lose expression of CD8 to become mature CD4+ T cells. Whereas CD4 stabilizes the TCR complex by binding to the invariant backbone of the HLA class II molecule, CD8 stabilizes the invariant backbone of the HLA class I molecule. Both subsets (CD4+ and CD8+) of positively selected cortical T cells migrate into the thymic medulla.

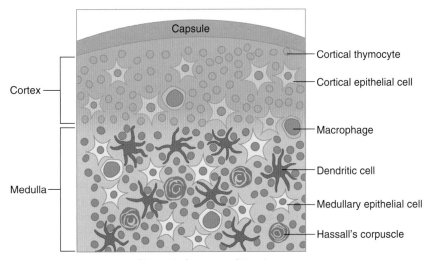

Fig. 11.3 Structure of the thymus.

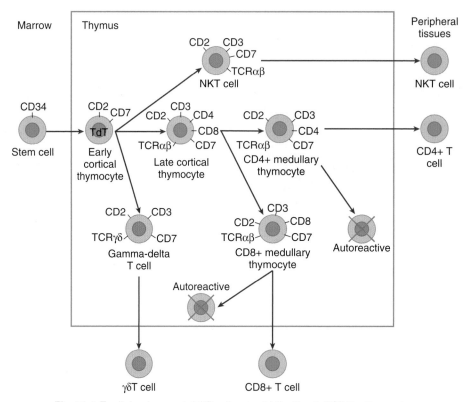

Fig. 11.4 T-cell development. *NKT cell*, natural killer T cell; *TCR*, T-cell receptor.

Within the medulla, the developing T cells encounter a greatly expanded universe of more restricted, often organ-specific self-antigens expressed by **medullary thymic epithelial cells (MTEC)** and **medullary thymic dendritic cells** (Fig. 11.4). Expression of organ-specific antigens by MTEC is mediated by the transcription factor **autoimmune regulator**. Thymic T cells with receptors that bind weakly to self-antigen proliferate through the process of **positive selection**, and thymic T cells that express receptors with no affinity for self-antigen die of neglect. In a process termed **negative selection**, thymic T cells that bind avidly to self-antigens undergo apoptosis, are rendered anergic (unresponsive) or are converted to **FoxP3+ regulatory T (Treg) cells**. Treg cells suppress immune responses in an antigen-specific fashion and provide a second line of defense against self-reactive T cells that escape thymic deletion.

The relatively few cortical thymocytes that undergo productive gamma-delta rearrangement (5%) express CD3 but unlike the more common alpha-beta T cells do not express CD4 or CD8. These double-negative **gamma-delta T cells** respond directly to antigen in an HLA-unrestricted fashion. Gamma-delta T cells express cell surface antigens CD16 (a low-affinity immunoglobulin Fc [fragment crystallizable] receptor) and CD56 (a homophilic adhesion receptor), proteins that are also expressed by NK cells. Many antigens recognized by gamma-delta T cells are unconventional phosphoantigens, endogenous metabolites of cholesterol biosynthesis produced by bacteria. Gamma-delta T cells home primarily to mucocutaneous sites (the skin, genital tract, and gastrointestinal tract), where they serve as first responders to commonly encountered bacteria.

From the thymic medulla, most mature T cells are released into the peripheral circulation and migrate to secondary lymphoid tissues: the lymph nodes, spleen, **mucosa-associated lymphoid tissue (MALT)**, **bronchial-associated lymphoid tissue (BALT)**, and so on. After antigen encounter, naïve CD4+ T cells differentiate into Th1, Th2, Th3, Th17, Treg, or Tfh cells. Antigen-activated **Th1 cells** drive proinflammatory T cell–mediated immune responses by secreting proinflammatory cytokines (**interferon-γ [IFN-γ]** and transforming growth factor β [TGF-β]) that induce activation of CD8+ **cytotoxic T cells (CTLs)**. Antigen-activated **Th2 cells**, on the other hand, drive antiinflammatory T cell–mediated immune responses by secreting interleukin (IL)-10 and humoral-mediated immune responses by secreting cytokines IL-4, IL-6, and IL-21 that induce B-cell activation and **plasma cell** maturation. **Th3 cells** present in **gut-associated lymphoid tissues (GALT)** contribute to oral tolerance to food antigens by producing antiinflammatory cytokines IL-10 and TGF-β. IL-10 inhibits proinflammatory Th1 responses, and TGF-β favors production of noninflammatory immunoglobulin (Ig) A. By secreting IL-17, proinflammatory **Th17 cells** recruit neutrophils to sites of infection. Similar to Th3 cells, FoxP3+ Treg cells inhibit T-cell immune responses by inhibiting IL-2–mediated T cell growth factor IL-2 and producing antiinflammatory IL-10 and TGFβ. **Follicular T-helper (Tfh) cells** are specialized memory T cells that provide growth signals to germinal center B cells. Tfh home to CXCL13+ lymphoid follicles via receptor–ligand interaction between the chemokine receptor CXCR5, expressed by Tfh, and the chemokine CXCL13, expressed by **follicular dendritic cells (FDCs)**.

B CELLS

The earliest identifiable B-cell precursor, the **progenitor B cell**, is characterized by expression of B cell–specific cell surface proteins CD19 and CD10 and immunoglobulin genes in germline configuration (Fig. 11.5). Expression of the enzymes RAG1, RAG2, and TdT heralds initiation of immunoglobulin heavy chain gene rearrangement. Synthesis of mu heavy chain and marked reduction in RAG and TdT activity define the **precursor B-cell** stage. At this stage, most mu heavy chain is found in the cytoplasm, with only a small amount expressed on the cell surface in association with an invariant surrogate light chain to form the **pre-B cell receptor (pre-BCR)**. Signaling through the pre-BCR triggers light chain rearrangement, leading to the next stage of B cell maturation, the **immature B cell** stage. Immature B cells express cell surface IgM, which associates with the **invariant Igαβ heterodimer** (**CD79**a/CD79b). B-cell activation induced by antigen cross-linking of IgM is mediated by intracellular signaling through the invariant Igαβ heterodimer. Immature B cells that bind avidly to self-antigen in the bone marrow undergo receptor editing, deletion by apoptosis, or functional inactivation, also known as **anergy**. If successful, **receptor editing**, triggered

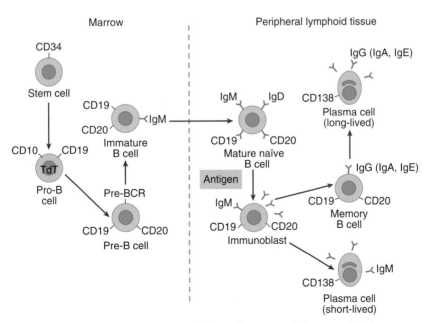

Fig. 11.5 B-cell development. *BCR*, B-cell receptor; *Ig*, immunoglobulin.

by reactivation of light chain gene rearrangement, leads to the expression of non–self-reactive immunoglobulin. The phenomenon of negative selection of immature B cells in the marrow, somewhat analogous to negative selection of immature T cells in the thymus, is important in deletion of potentially pathogenic self-reactive (autoimmune) B cells from the immature B-cell pool.

Surviving marrow B cells exit the marrow as **mature naïve B cells** that, through a process of differential mRNA splicing of the primary mu-delta transcript, co-express both surface IgM and IgD. At this stage, RAG expression is terminated. The function of membrane IgD, although not entirely understood, may be to prevent antigen-induced apoptosis or anergy of naïve B cells by providing T cell co-stimulation by IgD receptor-bearing T-helper cells. Naïve B cells are drawn to lymphoid follicles via interaction between **CXCR5** expressed by B cells and **CXCL13** released by follicular dendritic cells. Soluble antigen that binds to surface IgM or IgD of naïve antigen-specific B cells is internalized, proteolytically degraded to small peptides, and presented on the B cell surface by HLA class II.

Meanwhile, naïve CD4+ T cells released from the thymus migrate from the blood, through high endothelial venules and into lymph node paracortical T zones, where they encounter soluble antigen presented by **interdigitating dendritic cells (IDCs)** in association with HLA class II. IL-12 released by activated IDCs also provides an additional T-cell proliferative stimulus.

Antigen-primed B cells migrate from the lymphoid follicle into the paracortical T zone, where they cross-present HLA class II-bound molecules to activated T-helper cells, which then signal the B cells to proliferate and differentiate into **extrafollicular B cell blasts** in a small region called the primary focus (Fig. 11.6). Although some antigen-activated B cells develop into **short-lived IgM-secreting plasma cells** (the primary humoral immune response), most B blasts in the primary focus return to the lymphoid follicle to form a prominent secondary focus called the **germinal center**. With help from Tfh cells and antigen-bearing FDCs, germinal center B cells undergo multiple rounds of proliferation and somatic (Ig variable region) hypermutation. Somatic hypermutation of the immunoglobulin variable region genes is dependent on activity of **activation-induced cytidine deaminase**, an enzyme that converts deoxycytidine (in DNA) to uracil, which triggers processing by uracil DNA glycosylase (UNG) and endonucleases, leading to error-prone DNA repair and hypermutation. Germinal center B cells that produce antibody of high affinity are positively selected—a process known as **affinity maturation**—and B cells that fail to develop high-affinity antibody undergo apoptosis. Under the influence of T-helper cells, positively selected

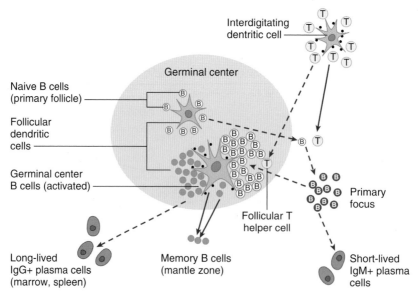

Fig. 11.6 Germinal center reaction. *Ig,* Immunoglobulin.

IgM- and IgD-positive germinal center B cells undergo heavy chain class switching or **isotype switching** from IgM/IgD to IgG, IgA, or IgE. Whereas B cells in lymph nodes most often switch to IgG expression, B cells in MALT often switch to IgA production for transport into body secretions. Whereas IgG binding to microbes leads to complement activation and phagocytosis, IgA binding to microbes leads to neutralization. IgE+ B cells are most often found in mast cell- and basophil-rich sites such as the dermis. In these sites, allergens that bind to IgE-bearing mast cells and basophils induce degranulation, with release of histamine. Thus, IgE imbues allergic (hypersensitivity) reactions with antigen specificity.

Some germinal center B cells differentiate into long-lived plasma cells, and others differentiate into memory B cells. **Long-lived plasma cells** migrate to the marrow and spleen, where they secrete low-level antibody for months to years. **Memory B cells** are quiescent long-lived IgG+ B cells that recirculate in lymph node mantle zones, splenic marginal zones, and MALT located in the skin (skin-associated lymphoid tissue [SALT]), lung (BALT), conjunctiva, and gastrointestinal tract (GALT). Memory B cells activated by antigen within germinal centers provide a rapid secondary IgG-predominant immune response to previously encountered antigen.

Control of the secondary humoral immune response is mediated by an **antibody feedback mechanism**. Antigen–antibody immune complexes that simultaneously bind IgG Fc receptors (e.g., CD32) and surface immunoglobulin block B-cell activation, thus preventing further development of memory and plasma cells.

IMMUNOGLOBULIN STRUCTURE AND FUNCTION

The genes that encode for the immunoglobulin polypeptides are located on chromosomes 14 (heavy chain), 2 (kappa light chain), and 22 (lambda light chain). Under normal circumstances, Ig protein expression is restricted to B cells and plasma cells. In each Ig-producing cell, pairs of identical **Ig heavy chains (Igμ, Igδ, Igγ, Igα, and Igε)** are linked to each other by a pair of disulfide bonds. Identical **Ig light chains (Igκ or Igλ)** then bind to each heavy chain pair by a single disulfide bond to form the complete immunoglobulin molecule. Every Ig molecule produced by a single cell expresses identical variable regions, one contributed by the heavy chain and

one by the light chain. Membrane Ig alone is incapable of delivering an activating signal to the B cell. B-cell signaling by antigen requires interaction with the **BCR complex** expressed on the B-cell surface. The BCR complex is composed of membrane Ig and the signaling invariant Igαβ heterodimer (CD79a/CD79b) as well as the co-receptor complex composed of CD19, CD21 (C3d receptor), and CD81 (Fig. 11.7). Binding of antigen to the BCR leads to tyrosine phosphorylation of Igαβ and CD19. The BCR signaling threshold is significantly reduced when antigen is bound to both immunoglobulin and complement.

Five major classes, or **isotypes**, of Ig are defined by the invariant heavy chain polypeptide:

- **IgM** cell surface expression is limited to immature B cells and mature naïve B cells, and IgM production by plasma cells is characteristic of a primary immune response.
- **IgD** cell surface expression is limited to mature naïve B cells, and IgD is rarely produced by plasma cells.
- **IgG** is expressed on the cell surface of most mature B cells and plasma cells and is the major antibody isotype in plasma.
- **IgA** is expressed by a small fraction of memory B cells and plasma cells, many of which are located in the lamina propria of mucosal tissues. Secretory IgA is the major Ig type in body fluids.
- **IgE** is expressed by a very small fraction of memory B cells and plasma cells, often in mucosal sites rich in mast cells and basophils. Allergen-specific IgE produced by plasma cells in allergic reactions triggers release of histamine by mast cells and basophils.

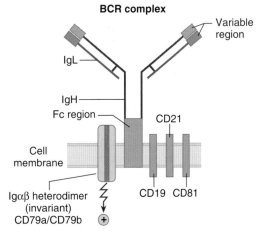

Fig. 11.7 B-cell receptor (BCR) complex. *Ig,* Immunoglobulin.

All membrane-bound Ig molecules are expressed as monomers composed of four disulfide-linked polypeptide chains (two heavy chains and two light chains). Although the secreted forms of IgD, IgG, and IgE are monomers, the secreted forms of IgM and IgA are polymers formed in association with a small invariant polypeptide known as the **J chain**. Polymeric IgM is a pentamer composed of five IgM monomers linked together by disulfide bonds with one molecule of J chain. Polymeric IgA is a dimer composed of two IgA monomers linked with one molecule of J chain. For polymeric IgA to be secreted into the lumen of the gut, bronchi, mammary gland, or salivary gland, it must first pass through the mucosa. After binding to the **polymeric Ig receptor** expressed on the basolateral aspect of mucosal epithelial cells, dimeric IgA is released from transport vesicles into the lumen bound to a fragment of the polymeric Ig receptor referred to as **secretory component**. After secretion into the lumen, the secretory component serves no further purpose and is released from IgA.

The Ig isotypes vary in function. IgM and IgG (excluding the IgG4 subclass) are effective in **complement fixation**. Complement fixation leads to recruitment and activation of inflammatory cells and target cell cytolysis. IgG1, IgG3, and IgA antibodies are effective in virus and toxin neutralization. IgG1, IgG3, and IgM are effective in opsonization for phagocytosis and NK cell–mediated killing. IgA and IgE are effective in binding to **crystallizable fragment (Fc)** receptor–bearing phagocytic cells. Proteolytic cleavage of monomeric Ig yields two fragments, an **antigen-binding fragment (Fab or F(ab)′2)** and an **Fc fragment**. The antigen-binding fragment includes the variable (antigen-binding) regions of the heavy and light chains, and Fc consists of the transmembrane and cytoplasmic tail of the molecule. The Fc portion of the Ig molecule binds to cell membrane Fc receptors expressed by phagocytes including neutrophils, eosinophils, basophils, mast cells, NK cells, and macrophages. Fc receptors vary in affinity for Ig isotypes. For example, the high-affinity **IgE receptor** is expressed only by mast cells, basophils, and eosinophils, and the **IgA receptor** is expressed only by macrophages, neutrophils, and eosinophils. A key factor in phagocyte activation is binding and cross-linking of multiple Fc receptors by opsonized pathogens (Ig, complement-bound, or both types of pathogens). In contrast, binding of free Ig to Fc receptors does not trigger phagocyte activation. The effectiveness of Ig-mediated phagocytosis is further enhanced by binding of complement-bound pathogens to **C3b receptors** expressed by phagocytes.

COMPLEMENT

The complement system (Fig. 11.8) includes nine circulating proteins (C1–C9) and three alternative pathway co-factors (B, D, and **properdin**). The complement proteins are zymogens, circulating in an inactive form, and requiring sequential activation by proteolysis, similar to the coagulation cascade. Complement activation is triggered by microbes (virus, bacteria, fungi, parasites) and senescent or apoptotic cells that are recognized by antigen–antibody complexes, abnormal membrane carbohydrates (mannose, N-acetyl glucosamine), or spontaneous hydrolysis of membrane-bound C3 [C3(H$_2$O)]. The three pathways of complement activation are the classical pathway, the lectin pathway, and the alternative pathway.

The **classical pathway** is initiated by antigen–antibody complexes. Complement protein C1 binds to the antibody molecule. The **C1q** fragment converts C4 to fragments C4a and C4b and C2 to C2a and C2b. C4b binds to C2a to form the C4b2a (**C3 convertase**) complex that converts C3 to C3a and C3b. C3b binds to the C4b2a complex to form the **C5 convertase** C4b2a3b that converts C5 to C5a and C5b. The **anaphylatoxins** C3a and C5a induce vasoconstriction, increased vascular permeability, and recruitment of neutrophils and monocytes. Membrane-bound C5b forms a molecular complex with C6-C8 followed by assembly of several C9 molecules to form a pore-shaped poly-C9 channel through the cell wall or membrane called the **membrane attack complex (MAC)**. The poly-C9 pore allows free flow between cell contents and extracellular fluid that induces cell death by osmotic cytolysis.

The **lectin pathway** is initiated by binding of lectins to membrane carbohydrate expressed by microbes and senescent or apoptotic cells. **Mannose-binding lectin (MBL)** and **ficolin** are lectins that bind to carbohydrates expressed by microbes and senescent or apoptotic cells. MBL binds to terminal mannose residues and ficolin binds to bacterial N-acetyl glucosamine (GlcNAc). Binding of MBL or ficolin induces C4 and C2 activation by **MASP** (MBL-associated serine protease), with formation of C3 convertase C4b2a, and ultimately to MAC-mediated cytolysis.

The **alternative pathway** requires no antibody or lectin to trigger complement activation. Instead, activation begins with spontaneous hydrolysis of membrane-bound

Complement pathways

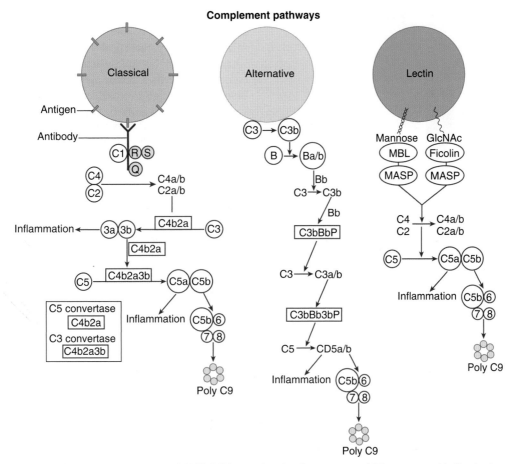

Fig. 11.8 Complement pathways. *MASP*, MBL-associated serine protease; *MBL*, mannose-binding lectin.

C3—termed C3(H₂O)—activation of factor B to Ba and Bb, and formation of an unstable **alternative C3 convertase** (C3(H₂O)Bb). The alternative C3 convertase generates a limited but sufficient amount of C3b for formation of a C3 convertase C3bBbP stabilized by properdin (P). Alternative pathway C5 convertase is formed by addition of a terminal C3b to C3 convertase (C3bBb3bP), leading to formation of the MAC.

Complement also serves to enhance phagocytosis of antibody-bound (opsonized) antigens. C3b binding to complement receptor 1 (CR1, **CD35**) expressed by leukocytes (neutrophils, monocytes) enhances antibody-mediated phagocytosis. Also, CR1 expressed by dendritic cells plays a critical role in antigen presentation to germinal center B cells.

C3b (CD35) C3b bound to antigen–antibody complexes binds to complement receptor CR1 (CD35) that is expressed by phagocytes. In conjunction with Ig binding to the phagocyte Fc receptor, phagocytosis is initiated. Complement receptor CR2 (CD21) binds to C3d.

T-CELL RECEPTOR SIGNALING

The clustering of receptors by polyvalent antigen-antibody complexes on the surface of phagocytes or lymphocytes leads to tyrosine kinase-mediated activation of secondary messengers; phosphorylation and activation of nuclear transcription factors **nuclear factor (NF) κB, AP-1**, and **nuclear factor of activated T cells (NFAT)**; and ultimately cell activation. T-cell signaling through the TCR is enhanced approximately 100-fold by simultaneous binding of MHC I or MHC II by **CD4** or **CD8** co-receptors, respectively. B-cell signaling through Ig is enhanced about thousandfold

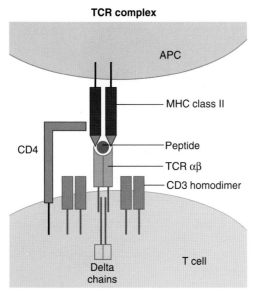

Fig. 11.9 T-cell receptor (TCR) complex. *APC,* Antigen-presenting cell; *MHC,* major histocompatibility complex.

by simultaneous binding of C3d to BCR-associated C3d receptor **CD21.**

The **TCR complex** (Fig. 11.9) in alpha-beta T cells is composed of alpha-beta heterodimer associated with CD3, CD4 or CD8, and **zeta chain.** Binding of antigen-MHC complex to alpha-beta and CD4 (or CD8) induces phosphorylation of tyrosine residues in the cytoplasmic tails of CD3 and zeta chain; activation of the **zeta-associated protein (ZAP-70)** tyrosine kinase; and downstream activation of transcription factors such as NFAT, AP-1, and NFκB that ultimately lead to T-cell activation.

Most antigens are proteins that after proteolytic digestion are presented to immune cells by APCs as small peptides complexed to either MHC I or MHC II. These antigens, collectively referred to as **T cell–dependent antigens**, require T-cell help to elicit an effective immune response. In contrast, **T cell-independent antigens** are large multivalent molecules (mostly bacterial polysaccharides) that can bind and activate B cells by cross-linking multiple antigen receptors without the need for antigen presentation or T-cell help. Specialized B cells with specificity for T cell–independent antigens, including **splenic marginal zone B cells** and **peritoneal CD5+ B cells**, continually produce low levels of low-affinity IgM antibody termed *natural* antibodies to common bacterial antigens (e.g., anti-ABO blood group).

Memory T cells are composed of central memory and effector memory subsets. **Central memory T cells** migrate to the paracortical T zones of lymph nodes, where they may be rapidly activated by antigen to become effector cells. **Effector memory T cells** circulate in blood and through mucosal sites and are rapidly activated to eliminate antigen. Long-lived memory T cells are maintained by IL-7. Memory T cells can be distinguished from naïve T cells by high expression of the RO isoform of CD45 (CD45RO), a tyrosine phosphatase that enhances TCR-mediated signaling.

T-CELL SUBSETS

Four separate lineages of T-helper cells are currently described: Th1, Th2, Th17, and Tfh cells (Table 11.1). All four types of T-helper cells express CD3 and the TCR-associated membrane protein CD4. Activation of naïve T-helper cells is induced by simultaneous binding of HLA class II–complexed molecules by the TCR and binding of specific cytokines to cytokine receptors. Th1 cells are coactivated by antigen and IFN-γ, Th2 cells by antigen and IL-4, and Th17 cells by antigen and TGFβ. Th1 cells are stimulated by IL-12 to produce and secrete

TABLE 11.1	T-Cell Subsets	
Cell Subset	**Phenotype**	**Function**
Th1 cell	CD4 IFN-γ TNF-α	Proinflammatory
Th2 cell	CD4 IL-4 IL-10	Anti-inflammatory
Th3 cell	CD4 IL-4 IL-10 TGF-β	Suppression (gut)
Th17 cell	CD4 IL-17	Proinflammatory
Tfh cell	CD4 CD10 CD57	Germinal center B-cell help
Tr1 cell	CD4 TGF-β	Suppression (gut)
Cytotoxic T cell	CD8 perforin granzyme	Cell-mediated cytotoxicity
Treg cell	CD4 CD25 FoxP3 IL-10 TGF-β	Suppression
NKT cell	CD8 CD16 CD56 perforin granzyme	Antigut bacteria (liver)
Gamma-delta T cell	CD4−/CD8− γδTCR perforin granzyme	Intraepithelial surveillance

IFN-γ, Interferon-γ; *IL,* interleukin; *TGF-β,* transforming growth factor β; *TNF-α,* tumor necrosis factor α; *TCR,* T-cell receptor.

IFN-γ and tumor necrosis factor α (TNF-α). The major role of **Th1 cells** appears to be control of intracellular pathogen infections via direct antiviral effects, NK cell activation by IFN-γ, and macrophage activation by TNF-α. Th2 cells are stimulated by IL-4 to produce and secrete IL-4, IL-5, IL-10, and IL-13. The major role of **Th2 cells** appears to be control of parasitic infections. The eosinophilia and elevated IgE seen in allergic conditions and asthma result from excessive Th2 cell activity. Th17 cells are stimulated by IL-23 to produce and secrete IL-17. The major role of **Th17 cells** seems to be control of the acute inflammatory response to extracellular bacterial infections via the proinflammatory actions of IL-17, including recruitment of neutrophils. The immunosuppressive cytokine TGFβ activates Th17 cells while suppressing production of IFN-γ and IL-4 by Th1 and Th2 cells and inhibiting B-cell growth and macrophage activation. **Tfh cells**, located within germinal centers, act to promote proliferation and differentiation of antigen-specific germinal center B cells. Native unprocessed antigen bound to B-cell surface Ig (BCR) is degraded into peptides and presented on the B-cell surface with MHC class II to antigen-specific T helper cells. This B cell–T helper cell interaction leads to T-cell release of B cell growth factors IL-4 and IL-21, proliferation of antigen-specific T and B cells, and plasma cell production of antibody (Fig. 11.10).

Another category of CD3+/CD4+ T cells is the **regulatory (suppressor) T-cell group**. This group includes classic CD25+/FoxP3+ Treg cells, Th3 cells, and Tr1 cells. CD25+/FoxP3+ **Treg cells** suppress T-cell immune responses by secreting the immunosuppressive cytokines IL-10 and TGF-β. Th3 and Tr1 are CD4+ CD25− suppressor cells found primarily in the gut. **Th3 cells** suppress by production of IL-4, IL-10, and TGF-β, and **Tr1 cells** suppress by production of TGF-β alone. These cells may normally function to suppress immune reactions in the gut to foodborne antigens.

Cytotoxic T cells (CTL) are CD3+/CD8+ T cells that respond to peptide antigens expressed on the surface of abnormal cells (of all types) in association with self-MHC I molecules (Fig. 11.11). CTLs kill target cells by binding, formation of an immunologic synapse (TCR antigen–MHC complex with B7/CD28 co-stimulation), releasing perforin with formation of target cell membrane pores, and injecting of granzymes and the intracellular antigen that induce target cell apoptosis. **Perforin**, structurally similar to the complement protein C9, forms plasma membrane pores in target cells that are remarkably similar

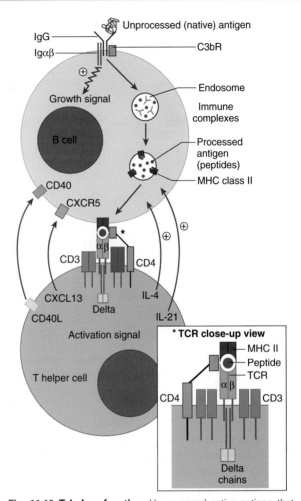

Fig. 11.10 T helper function. Unprocessed native antigen that binds and cross-links surface immunoglobulin (sIg) expressed by antigen-specific B cells can generate a humoral response without need for T cell help (T cell independent). Antigens may also be absorbed and transported to acidic endosomes for proteolysis into small peptide fragments and binding to class II major histocompatibility (MHC) protein. Peptide–MHC class II complexes displayed by B cells bind to the T-cell receptor (TCR) of peptide-specific T helper cells (T cell dependent). Accessory signaling is achieved by binding of B cell CD40 with T-cell CD40L and B-cell CD80 with T-cell CD28. Also, release of the cytokine CXCL13 by activated T cells attracts CXCR5 receptor-bearing B cells. Positive signals provided to B cells by activated T helper cells include interleukin (IL)-4 (B-cell growth), and IL-21 (plasma cell differentiation).

to those produced by the membrane attack complex complement (C5-C9). **Granzymes** are serine proteases that trigger caspase-induced DNA fragmentation, leading to apoptosis. Granzyme-mediated apoptosis is inhibited by **Bcl-2** (B-cell lymphoma 2) protein. Granzyme

Cytotoxic T-cell killing

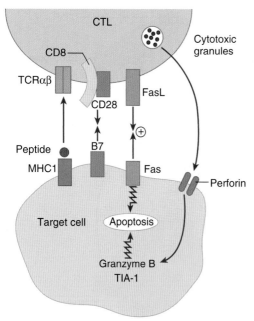

Fig. 11.11 Cytotoxic T-cell function. *CTL,* Cytotoxic T cell; *FasL,* Fas ligand; *MHC,* major histocompatibility complex; *TCR,* T-cell receptor; *TIA-1,* T-cell intracellular antigen 1.

expression by CD8+ T cells is induced upon activation, whereas in gamma-delta T cells and NK cells, it is constitutively expressed. **T-cell intracellular antigen 1 (TIA-1)** is an RNA-binding translational repressor that suppresses cell proliferation.

Gamma-delta T cells are CD3+ dual CD4/CD8− intraepithelial T cells that home to the gut, skin, and genital tract, where they rapidly respond to MHC I–like molecules (**MIC-A and MIC-B**) expressed by damaged epithelial cells, heat shock proteins, and glycolipid bacterial antigens.

NKT cells are cytotoxic CD3+ CD8+ T cells that express NK markers (CD16 and CD56), as well as TCRαβ heterodimers that recognize highly conserved glycolipid bacterial antigens in association with CD1, an invariant MHC I–like protein. After leaving the thymus, most of these cells home to the liver, where they likely are an important first-line response to gut bacteria that enter the portal circulation.

Natural killer (NK) cells are CD3− CD8+ CD16/CD56+ bone marrow–derived lymphoid cells that express both activating and **inhibitory receptors**. Engagement of activating receptors **NKG2D** (which recognizes stress-related MHC I-like proteins expressed by abnormal virus-infected or malignant cells) and **CD16** (a low-affinity IgG receptor) induces tyrosine phosphorylation of secondary intracellular messengers, leading to cell activation and proliferation. In contrast, engagement of inhibitory receptors such as **killer Ig-like receptor (KIR)**, an HLA class I receptor, induces tyrosine phosphatase activity that blocks cell activation and proliferation. Virus-infected cells and tumor cells that do not express HLA class I are susceptible to NK cell–mediated killing (Fig. 11.12). Activated NK cells release cytotoxic granule proteins **perforin** and **granzyme B** that form membrane channels and induce apoptosis, respectively, in target cells. NK cells also activate macrophages by producing IFN-γ. NK cells provide a first-line antigen-nonspecific mechanism for cell-mediated killing of abnormal (virus-infected or tumor) cells.

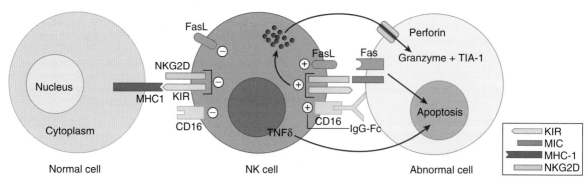

Fig. 11.12 Natural killer (NK) cell function. *KIR,* Killer immunoglobulin-like receptor; *MHC,* major histocompatibility complex *TIA-1,* T-cell intracellular antigen 1.

IMMUNODEFICIENCY

Immune deficiency disorders can be caused by either inherited genetic defects (primary forms) or acquired defects (secondary forms). Primary and secondary immune deficiency disorders can be roughly divided into those caused by defects in B cells and those caused by defects in T cells. T-cell defects can be further subdivided into Th1 and Th2 defects. **B-cell defects** are marked by increased susceptibility to extracellular bacterial and fungal infections. **Th1 defects** are marked by increased susceptibility to infection with intracellular microorganisms, including *Mycobacteria* and *Babesia* spp. and viruses. **Th2 defects** are marked by increased susceptibility to extracellular bacterial and fungal infections. The difference in types of infection seen in Th1 and Th2 defects results from differences in Th1 and Th2 function.

Secondary **(acquired) immunodeficiency** may be caused by a variety of primary conditions. Some of the more common causes of secondary immunodeficiency include diabetes, uremia, aplastic anemia, chronic viral infection (herpesviruses and human immunodeficiency virus), malnutrition, autoimmune disease, and drugs (anticonvulsants, corticosteroids, immunosuppressants, and cytotoxic drugs).

Primary (inherited) immunodeficiency disorders are classified into disorders of B cells, T cells, NK cells, complement proteins, phagocytic function, and both B and T cells.

Primary **B-cell disorders**, which comprise the largest group of primary immune deficiency diseases (50%–60%), are often marked by recurrent gram-positive bacterial infections, allergies, and diarrhea. Examples of these disorders include X-linked agammaglobulinemia, hyper-IgM syndrome, and common variable immunodeficiency disease. Patients with **common variable immunodeficiency disease** are at increased risk for development of lymphoma. The most common inherited B-cell defect is **selective IgA deficiency**. Patients with selective IgA deficiency are at risk of serious anaphylactic transfusion reactions caused by reaction between recipient anti-IgA antibody and donor blood IgA. Known patients are provided with washed donor red blood cells to reduce the amount of IgA transfused.

Primary T-cell disorders, comprising only 5% to 10% of primary immunodeficiency diseases, predispose to infection with viruses, *Pneumocystis jirovecii,* and fungi. The most common primary T cell disorders are

DiGeorge syndrome (thymic hypoplasia), **ZAP-70 deficiency**, and **X-linked lymphoproliferative disorder (XLD)**. Patients with XLD often develop fatal Epstein-Barr virus (EBV)–associated infectious mononucleosis.

Primary combined B- and T-cell disorders account for about 20% of immunodeficiency disorders. These conditions include **severe combined immunodeficiency disease (SCID)**, Wiskott-Aldrich syndrome, and ataxia telangiectasia. SCID results from a variety of mutations, including those involving the common cytokine receptor gamma chain, adenosine deaminase, and IL-7Ra. Mutations of **TCR gamma chain** or **IL-7 receptor (IL-7Ra)** lead to defective lymphocyte signaling. **Adenosine deaminase deficiency** causes a buildup of adenosine in T lymphocytes, leading to apoptosis. **Wiskott-Aldrich syndrome (WAS)** is an X-linked disorder characterized by eczema, thrombocytopenia, and recurrent gram-positive bacterial infection caused by an impaired immune response to polysaccharide antigens. Patient with WAS often succumb to EBV-associated lymphoproliferative disease.

Primary NK cell deficiency is a rare disorder that is associated with increased susceptibility to viral infections and tumors.

Primary **complement deficiency** accounts for fewer than 2% of primary immunodeficiency disorders. These disorders, characterized by deficient opsonization and clearance of infectious agents and immune complexes, are marked by recurrent infection and autoimmune disease.

Phagocytic defects are characteristic of patients with **chronic granulomatous disease (CGD)**, Chediak-Higashi syndrome, and leukocyte adhesion deficiency. These conditions are marked by recurrent bacterial and fungal infections. CGD results from a variety of defects leading to an inability of phagocytic cells (neutrophils, monocytes, and macrophages) to produce reactive oxygen intermediates that are toxic to ingested bacteria and fungi. **Nicotinamide adenine dinucleotide phosphate (NADPH) oxidase** deficiency prevents the formation of **reactive oxygen species**, including superoxide (O_2^-), hydrogen peroxide (H_2O_2), hydroxide radical (OH^-), and hypochlorite (OCl^-), leading to the inability to kill intracellular microbes within macrophage phagolysosomes and to the formation of nodular aggregates of macrophages (**granulomas**) in affected tissues.

Given the defective ability to produce **peroxide**, it is perhaps not surprising that the most common bacteria encountered in CGD are those that are catalase positive.

Catalase is a bacterial enzyme that converts peroxide to water and oxygen. In CGD, catalase-positive bacteria (e.g., *Staphylococcus aureus*) are able to neutralize the small amounts of peroxide produced by the defective phagocytes of CGD and survive within the intracellular compartment. **Chediak-Higashi syndrome**, which is caused by defective phagolysosome formation, is characterized by large abnormal primary granules in neutrophils. The inability to fuse phagosomes with lysosomes (packed with bactericidal compounds) prevents bacteriolysis. **Leukocyte adhesion deficiencies** prevent the transmigration of blood leukocytes through the vascular wall into foci of infection.

WHIM syndrome is an immune deficiency disorder caused by mutations of the CXCR4 homing receptor that impacts myeloid and lymphoid function. The syndrome consists of warts, hypogammaglobulinemia, infections, and **myelokathexis** (with abnormal chromatin) of myeloid and lymphoid cells.

LYMPHOID TUMORS

There is a remarkable correspondence between normal lymphocyte subsets and malignant lymphoid tumors (Tables 11.2 and 11.3). In most cases, these tumors appear to have retained the phenotype of their lymphocyte subset origin. This remarkable correspondence has not only informed our understanding of pathogenesis but also has allowed the development of precise diagnostic criteria that have proved of value in predicting clinical behavior, response to therapy, and prognosis (see the section on lymphoma).

TABLE 11.2   B Lymphocyte Subsets and Related Tumors

Cell Subset	Phenotype	Related Tumors
Precursor B lymphoblast	TdT CD19	Precursor B lymphoblastic leukemia or lymphoma
Naïve B cell	IgM/IgD CD5 CD19 CD23	Chronic lymphocytic leukemia or small lymphocytic lymphoma
Plasmacytoid B cell	cIgM CD20	Lymphoplasmacytic lymphoma
Centroblast	IgM/IgG CD10 CD20 Bcl-6	Follicular lymphoma, Burkitt lymphoma, diffuse large B-cell lymphoma
Centrocyte	IgM/IgG CD10 CD20 Bcl-6	Follicular lymphoma
Mantle zone B cell	IgM/IgD CD5 CD20 (CD23−)	Mantle cell lymphoma
Marginal zone B cell	IgM/IgD CD20 CD21 CD35	Marginal cell (MALT) lymphoma
Plasma cell	cIgG (CD20−) CD138	Myeloma or plasmacytoma

Ig, Immunoglobulin; *MALT,* mucosa-associated lymphoid tissue.

TABLE 11.3   T-Cell or Natural Killer Cell Subsets and Related Tumors

Cell Subset	Phenotype Markers	Related Tumors
Precursor T lymphoblast	TdT cCD3 CD7	Precursor T lymphoblastic leukemia or lymphoma
Helper T cell	CD3 CD4 (CD10− CD57−)	Peripheral T-cell lymphoma, mycosis fungoides, adult T-cell leukemia or lymphoma
Tfh cell	CD3 CD4 CD10 CD57	Angioimmunoblastic T-cell lymphoma
Cytotoxic T cell	CD3 CD8 (CD16−)	Subcutaneous panniculitis-like T-cell lymphoma, T-cell large granular lymphocytic leukemia
Gamma-delta T cell	CD3 (CD4− CD8−)	Hepatosplenic T-cell lymphoma
NKT cell	CD3 CD8 CD16	Not well described
NK cell	(CD3−) CD8 CD16/CD56	Extranodal NK or T-cell lymphoma, NK cell leukemia, chronic NK cell lymphocytosis
Treg cell	CD3 CD4 CD25 FoxP3	Adult T-cell leukemia or lymphoma

NK, Natural killer; *NKT cell,* natural killer T cell; *Tfh,* T follicular helper; *Treg,* T regulatory.

Lymphoid Organs

The lymphoid system is composed of a branching system of lymphatic channels lined by specialized lymphatic endothelial cells and interconnected lymph nodes. **Lymph** is a lymphocyte-rich interstitial fluid that collects into thin-walled lymphatic vessels from all parts of body except the central nervous system, globe of the eye, and spleen. After passing through regional lymph nodes, efferent lymph passes into progressively larger lymphatic channels, ultimately emptying into the superior vena cava via the thoracic duct. About 1.5 L of lymph enters the bloodstream every 24 hours.

Lymph nodes are composed of distinct microanatomic compartments (Fig. 11.13). The outer cortex contains small aggregates of B cells termed **lymphoid follicles** that are separated by a T cell–rich zone termed the **interfollicular (or paracortical) zone**. The inner **medullary region** contains a branching collection of lymphatic channels (sinuses) and blood vessels with numerous associated histiocytes and plasma cells. Lymphatic fluid enters the lymph node through afferent lymphatics that pierce the lymph node capsule. The lymph passes into the subcapsular sinus, moves down through the paracortical and medullary sinuses, and exits through the efferent lymphatic in the hilum. In contrast, blood enters the lymph node through the hilar artery, branches into arterioles and capillaries in the cortex, and returns in the hilar vein after passing through highly specialized **postcapillary venules** that allow for lymphocyte transmigration. The prominent postcapillary venules noted during immune responses caused by endothelial cell hypertrophy are sometimes referred to as **high endothelial venules**. Up to 50% of the blood lymphocytes that enter the node via the hilar artery pass into the nodal parenchyma through the high endothelial venules.

Immature dendritic cells that reside in peripheral tissues (e.g., **Langerhans cells** in skin) carry antigen to lymph nodes via afferent lymphatics. Within the lymph node, the immature dendritic cells enter the T cell–rich paracortical zone and differentiate into IDCs. Antigen-specific B cells and T cells that encounter antigen expressed by IDC form a **primary focus** within the lymph node paracortical zone. Naïve B cells that undergo activation-induced proliferation in the primary focus either differentiate into IgM+ plasma cells or migrate to the germinal center, where interactions with antigen-positive follicular dendritic cells and antigen-specific

Tfh cells induce proliferation, somatic hypermutation, and isotype switching. This intrafollicular focus of B cell proliferation leads to the formation of an ovoid microanatomic structure known as the germinal center (Figs. 11.14 to 11.16). Follicular B cells that do not participate in the germinal center immune reaction form an outer mantle of small B cells called the mantle zone. Most mantle zone B cells, such as circulating B cells, are mature naïve IgM+ or IgD+ B cells, with an admixture of mature IgG+ memory B cells.

The **spleen** is an abdominal organ in the left upper quadrant that serves as a blood filter and immune organ (Fig. 11.17). As a blood filter, the spleen removes microparticulates, bacteria, immune complexes, and damaged blood cells. This filtration take place in the **red pulp** of the spleen, a complex network of low-pressure venous cords and sinusoids through which arteriolar blood enters and slowly percolates before returning the venous system (Figs. 11.18 and 11.19). During this transit, the blood encounters a loose array of intrasinusoidal **splenic macrophages** armed with an array of receptors for Ig, complement, and desialylated carbohydrates. Immune complexes and damaged or aged cells are ingested and degraded by the splenic macrophages. The **splenic white pulp**, located along splenic arterioles, is composed of lymphoid tissue. Surrounding the arterioles is a T cell–rich **periarteriolar lymphoid sheath (PALS)**. Adjacent to the PALS are B cell follicles. Splenic B-cell follicles are composed of three compartments—the germinal center, mantle zone, and marginal zone (Fig. 11.20). (In contrast to splenic follicles, lymph node follicles consist only of a germinal center and a mantle zone.) The **splenic marginal zone** is composed of mature B cells and macrophages. Marginal zone B cells express a unique phenotype (with expression of **complement receptors** CD21 and CD35) and appear to be restricted in antigen specificity. Although their exact function is not clear, some investigators have suggested that marginal zone B cells provide a rapid innate response to highly conserved common bloodborne antigens.

A ring of lymphoid tissue known as **Waldeyer's ring** surrounds the back of the oral cavity. Waldeyer's ring is composed of the tonsils and adenoids, lymph node–like structures in the oropharynx that provide immune responses to microbes and other antigens that enter the oral cavity. The **adenoids** are covered by respiratory epithelium, and the **tonsils** are covered by oral squamous epithelium. The tonsil epithelium contains scattered

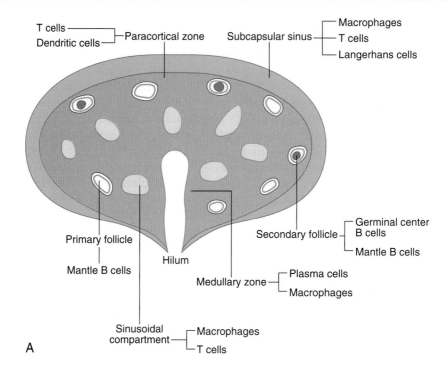

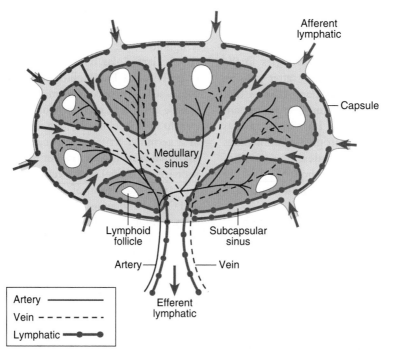

Fig. 11.13 A, Lymph node cellular compartments. **B,** Lymph node vascular compartments.

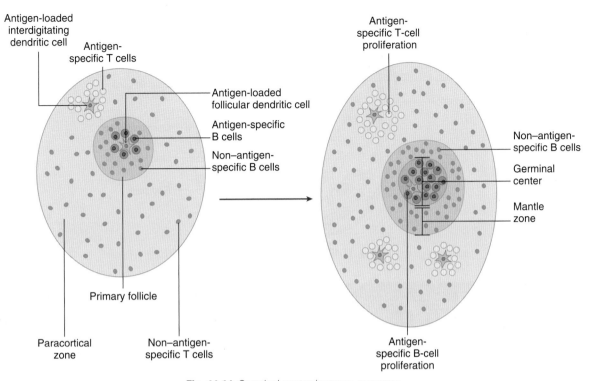

Antigen-loaded interdigitating dendritic cell
Antigen-specific T cells
Antigen-loaded follicular dendritic cell
Antigen-specific B cells
Non–antigen-specific B cells
Primary follicle
Paracortical zone
Non–antigen-specific T cells

Antigen-specific T-cell proliferation
Non–antigen-specific B cells
Germinal center
Mantle zone
Antigen-specific B-cell proliferation

Fig. 11.14 Germinal center immune response.

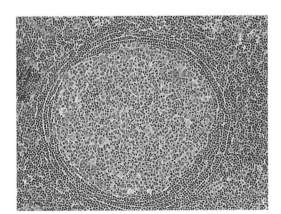

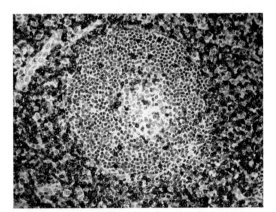

Fig. 11.15 Lymph node secondary follicle. The central region, the germinal center, contains mostly large B cells, with a few small follicular T helper cells, follicular dendritic cells, and macrophages. The large cells are antigen-specific B cells proliferating in response to antigen displayed by follicular dendritic cells. Immediately surrounding the germinal center is a narrow band of small B lymphocytes that seem to form a few concentric rings of cells. This is the mantle zone. Just outside the mantle zone is the T cell–rich paracortical (interfollicular) zone.

Fig. 11.16 CD3 immunostain of a secondary lymphoid follicle. Numerous CD3+ T cells (*brown* stain) of the paracortical T zone surround the follicle. A few CD3+ follicular T helper cells are present within the germinal center. Few T cells are seen within the follicle mantle zone.

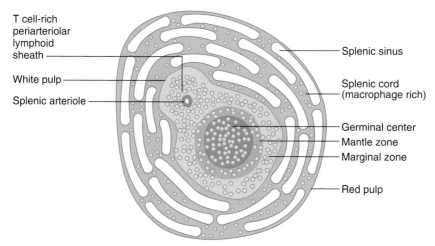

T cell-rich periarteriolar lymphoid sheath

White pulp

Splenic arteriole

Splenic sinus

Splenic cord (macrophage rich)

Germinal center

Mantle zone

Marginal zone

Red pulp

Fig. 11.17 Structure of the spleen.

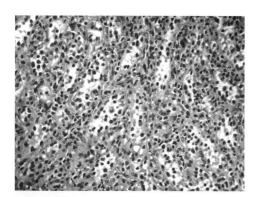

Fig. 11.18 Splenic red pulp. Shown are numerous venous sinusoids with patent lumens lined by splenic macrophages and marginating lymphoid cells. In the process of passing through the cords and venous sinusoids, damaged cells and debris are removed from the blood.

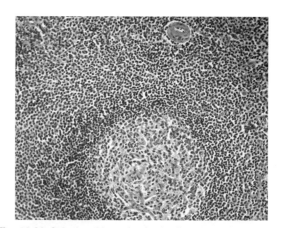

Fig. 11.20 Splenic white pulp. At the *lower center* is an oval-shaped germinal center surrounded by a thin band of small lymphocytes—the mantle zone. The mantle zone is surrounded by a wider margin of slightly larger paler-staining lymphocytes—the marginal zone, which imperceptibly merges into the periarteriolar lymphoid sheath that surrounds the arteriole *(upper center).* Memory B cells in the marginal zone are primed to quickly respond to bloodborne antigens.

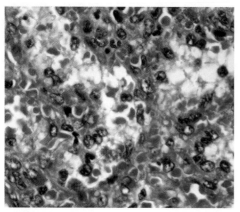

Fig. 11.19 Splenic sinusoid (high-magnification image) lined by numerous splenic macrophages.

specialized epithelial cells known as **microfold cells** capable of rapid uptake and transport of oral cavity antigens to the underlying lymphoid tissue. Secretory IgA, produced by plasma cells in these sites, neutralizes many microbes in the oral cavity.

Peyer's patches are small nodular aggregates of lymphoid tissue in the submucosa of the terminal ileum. These structures are covered by specialized follicle-associated epithelium that contains scattered microfold cells similar to those found in the tonsil. These cells, via transcytosis, take up and deliver gut antigens to the underlying lymphoid tissue. Peyer's patch lymphoid tissue resembles that of lymph nodes, with nodular B cell follicles, T cells, and antigen-presenting dendritic cells. Antigen-activated lymphocytes in Peyer's patches can migrate to mesenteric lymph nodes via efferent lymphatic channels.

KEY WORDS AND CONCEPTS

- Activation-induced cytidine deaminase
- Adenoids
- Adenosine deaminase deficiency
- Affinity maturation
- Alternative C3 convertase
- Alternative pathway
- Anergy
- Anaphylatoxins
- Antibody feedback mechanism
- Antigen-binding fragment (Fab or F(ab)$'_2$)
- AP-1
- Apoptosis
- Autoimmune regulator
- B-cell defects
- B cell disorders
- BCR complex
- Bronchial-associated lymphoid tissue (BALT)
- Catalase
- C1q
- C3 convertase
- C3 convertase
- C3b receptors
- CD4
- C5 convertase CD8
- CD7
- CD16
- CD19
- CD21 (C3d receptor)
- CD35
- CD79
- Central memory T cell
- Chediak-Higashi syndrome
- Chronic granulomatous disease (CGD)
- Classical pathway
- Combinatorial diversity
- Common variable immunodeficiency disease
- Complement deficiency
- Complement fixation
- Complement receptors
- Cortical T cell
- Cortical thymic epithelial cell
- Crystallizable fragment (Fc)
- CXCL13
- CXCR5
- Cytotoxic T cell (CTL)
- Dendritic cell
- DiGeorge syndrome
- Effector memory T cell
- Extrafollicular B cell blast
- Fc fragment
- Ficolin
- Follicular dendritic cell (FDC)
- Follicular T-helper cell (Tfh)
- FoxP3+ regulatory T cell (Treg)
- Gamma-delta T cell
- Germinal center
- Granulomas
- Granzymes
- Gut-associated lymphoid tissues (GALT)
- High endothelial venule
- HLA (human leukocyte antigen)
- Ig heavy chains (Igμ, Igδ, Igγ, Igα, and Igε)
- Ig light chains (Igκ or Igλ)
- IgA
- IgA receptor
- IgD
- IgE
- IgE receptor
- IgG
- IgM
- Immature B cell
- Immature dendritic cells

- Immunoglobulin gene rearrangement
- Immunoglobulin heavy chains
- Inhibitory receptors
- Interdigitating dendritic cell (IDC)
- Interferon-γ (IFN-γ)
- Interfollicular (paracortical) zone
- Invariant Igαβ heterodimer
- Isotype switching
- Isotypes
- J chain
- Junctional diversity
- Killer Ig-like receptor (KIR)
- Langerhans cell
- Lectin pathway
- Leukocyte adhesion deficiencies
- Long-lived plasma cell
- Lymph
- Lymph nodes
- Lymphoid follicles
- Mannose-binding lectin (MBL)
- MASP
- Mature naïve B cell
- Medullary region
- Medullary thymic dendritic cell
- Medullary thymic epithelial cell (MTEC)
- Membrane attack complex (MAC)
- Memory B cell
- MHC (major histocompatibility complex)
- MIC-A and MIC-B
- Microfold cell
- Mucosa associated lymphoid tissue (MALT)
- Natural killer (NK) cell
- Negative selection
- Nicotinamide adenine dinucleotide phosphate (NADPH) oxidase
- NKG2D
- NKT cell
- Nuclear factor (NF) κB
- Nuclear factor of activated T cells (NFAT)
- Perforin
- Periarteriolar lymphoid sheath (PALS)
- Peritoneal CD5+ B cell
- Peroxide
- Peyer's patches
- Phagocytic defects
- Plasma cell
- Polymeric Ig receptor
- Positive selection
- Postcapillary venule
- Pre-B cell receptor (pre-BCR)
- Precursor B cell
- Precursor T cell
- Pre-TCR
- Primary combined B- and T-cell disorders
- Primary complement deficiency
- Primary focus
- Primary NK cell deficiency
- Primary T-cell disorders
- Progenitor B cell
- Properdin
- Reactive oxygen species
- Receptor editing
- Recombination-activating gene (RAG1, RAG2)
- Red pulp
- Regulatory (suppressor) T-cell group
- Secondary (acquired) immunodeficiency
- Secretory component
- Severe combined immunodeficiency disease
- Selective IgA deficiency
- Short-lived IgM-secreting plasma cell
- Spleen
- Splenic macrophage
- Splenic marginal zone
- Splenic marginal zone B cell
- Splenic white pulp
- T cell–dependent antigens

- T cell–independent antigens
- T-cell intracellular antigen 1 (TIA-1)
- T-cell receptor (TCR) complex
- TCR complex
- TCR gamma chain IL-7 receptor (IL-7Ra)
- TCRαβ
- Terminal deoxynucleotidyl transferase (TdT)
- Th1 cell
- Th1 defects
- Th17 cell
- Th2 cell
- Th2 defects
- Th3 cell
- Thymic cortex
- Thymic epithelial cells
- Thymic medulla
- Thymus
- Tonsils
- Tr1 cell
- Treg cells
- Waldeyer's ring
- WHIM syndrome
- Wiskott-Aldrich syndrome (WAS)
- X-linked lymphoproliferative disorder (XLD)
- Zeta chain
- ZAP-70 deficiency
- Zeta-associated protein (ZAP-70)

REVIEW QUESTIONS

1. Which Ig isotype is specifically modified for secretion into body fluids?
   A. IgE
   B. IgA
   C. IgD
   D. IgM

2. Which of the following chemicals is **not used** by T cells or NK cells to kill target cells?
   A. Perforin
   B. Granzyme B
   C. Tryptase
   D. TIA-1

3. Germinal centers contain which one of the following B-cell types?
   A. Centrocytes

   B. Naïve B cells
   C. Memory B cells
   D. Plasma cells

4. Which statement regarding complement is **false**?
   A. The classical pathway of activation begins with binding of C3b to antibody-bound antigen.
   B. C3a and C5a fragments are chemotactic and anaphylatoxic.
   C. The MAC induces osmotic lysis.
   D. Bacterial lipopolysaccharide and mannose can directly activate complement without antibody.

12

Genetic Basis of Hematologic Neoplasia

KEY POINTS

- The cell cycle is controlled at two steps, the G1 and G2 restriction points, by cyclin-dependent protein kinases (CDKs).

- CDKs are subject to control by cyclin proteins, cyclin-CDK inhibitors such as cell damage-sensing protein (p53) and retinoblastoma (RB) protein, and cyclin-CDK activators such as c-Myc protein.

- Growth factors stimulate hematopoietic cell growth and differentiation by binding to growth factor receptors, which activate the JAK-STAT pathway, leading to cell growth- or differentiation-related gene expression.

- Apoptosis is a form of programmed cell death triggered by extracellular tumor necrosis factor (TNF)–like signals through TNF receptors and by intracellular

- signals (reactive oxygen intermediates, gamma radiation, or DNA damage) through mitochondria.

- Apoptosis can also be triggered by c-Myc and p53, presumably (in the case of c-Myc) to balance c-Myc proliferative effects and (in the case of p53) in response to DNA damage.

- Apoptosis is induced by activation of intracellular caspases, enzymes that lead to cell death by cleaving proteins and DNA.

- Malignant transformation can follow acquisition of growth factor independence, inactivation of suppressor oncogenes such as *TP53* and *RB*, activation of activator oncogenes such as *c-Myc*, or resistance to apoptosis (as with Bcl-2 overexpression).

Two common features of hematologic malignancy are **uncontrolled cell proliferation** and **resistance to apoptosis** caused by defects (mutations, deletions, or translocations) of genes involved in cell growth and death.

CELL PROLIFERATION

Cell division requires that cells first replicate their DNA and then divide into two daughter cells. These two phases of the **cell cycle**, termed the synthesis phase (**S phase**) and the mitosis phase (**M phase**), are separated by two preparatory **gap phases** (G1 and G2) (Fig. 12.1). Cells that are not actively dividing are in a resting state termed G0. Nonproliferating cells activated to proliferate first transit from the quiescent G0 phase to the G1 phase, during which time synthesis of enzymes required for DNA replication takes place. DNA replication that is

completed during the S phase is followed by synthesis of enzymes required for mitotic cell division during the G2 phase. During the M phase, the tetraploid DNA is partitioned into two diploid daughter cells. The daughter cells may either continue to proliferate by directly passing into the G1 phase or cease cell division by passing into the G0 phase.

Regulation of the cell cycle is governed by the concerted actions of two families of proteins, the cyclins and the cyclin-dependent protein kinases (CDKs). **Cyclins**, each specific for the G1 or the G2 checkpoint, accumulate during either G1 or G2 and trigger activation of CDKs. Activated **CDKs** phosphorylate specific substrates that regulate transcription of genes involved in DNA synthesis or mitosis. One of the substrates phosphorylated by the G1-specific cyclin D–CDK4/6 complex is the **retinoblastoma (RB) protein**. RB is normally bound to the E2F

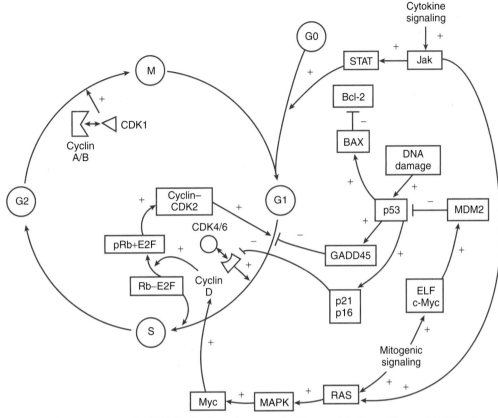

Fig. 12.1 Cell cycle control. *CDK*, Cyclin-dependent protein kinase; *Jak*, Janus kinase; *MAPK*, mitogen-activated protein kinase; *STAT*, signal transducer and activator of transcription; *MDM2*, mouse double minute 2 homolog; *GADD45*, Growth Arrest and DNA Damage Inducible Alpha.

transcription factor in a complex that represses transcription of E2F target genes. After phosphorylation, RB dissociates from E2F, allowing E2F to enter the nucleus and activate transcription of target genes involved in DNA synthesis, including DNA polymerase and thymidine kinase.

Important checkpoints in the cell cycle are strictly governed by the CDKs, in particular the **restriction point** in late G1. Before this point is reached, normal cells respond to extracellular proliferative and antiproliferative cytokines. After this point is passed, the cells no longer respond to extracellular signals, instead proceeding inexorably through cell division. Cancer cells often carry mutations in cell cycle regulatory genes that make them refractory to restriction point control, leading to unregulated cell proliferation. **RB mutations** that interfere with binding to E2F allow unregulated E2F transcriptional activity. Mutations in several other regulatory proteins that inhibit the cyclin

D–CDK4/6 complex have been discovered in cancer cells. The most common mutations of this sort are those involving the *TP53* gene that encodes the **p53 protein**. p53 regulates transcription of several genes involved in G1 or G2 cell cycle control, including the proapoptotic **BAX** gene and the **WAF1/CIP1** complex that inhibits the cyclin D–CDK4/6 complex. Mutations in p53 lead to both unregulated cell proliferation and resistance to apoptosis.

Entry of hematopoietic cells into the cell cycle (G0 and G1) is stimulated by diffusible extracellular growth factors (**cytokines**) that bind to growth factor receptors. Most of these hematopoietic growth factor receptors are expressed on the cell surface and are composed of a ligand (cytokine)-binding extracellular domain, a transmembrane domain, and an intracellular signaling domain. Binding of ligand to the extracellular domain leads to activation of CDKs that are loosely bound to the intracellular domain of the receptor. The activated kinases detach from the receptor and activate specific transcription factors by phosphorylation of either their tyrosine residues or their serine and threonine residues. The activated transcription factors then migrate to the nucleus and activate transcription by binding to regulatory regions of specific genes. The **JAK-STAT pathway** is particularly important in hematopoietic cells. Cytokine receptor-mediated activation of **Janus (JAK) kinase** leads to phosphorylation of the transcription factor **signal transducer and activator of transcription (STAT)**, which induces cellular growth and differentiation through its effect on gene expression.

Neoplastic cells are characterized by gene mutations that lead to uncontrolled proliferation—often caused by dysregulation of cell cycle checkpoints in G1 and G2, growth factor independence, and resistance to apoptosis. Dysregulation of cell cycle checkpoints may be caused by inactivating mutations in **cyclin-CDK inhibitors** (including RB, p53, INK4, and CIP/KIP proteins) or, in the case of mantle cell lymphoma, activating translocation of the **cyclin D1 gene**. Growth factor dependence may be caused by a variety of mechanisms, including the following:

1. Autocrine production of growth factors by tumor cells

2. Increased sensitivity to growth factors caused by the increased number of receptors on tumor cells
3. Constitutive ligand-dependent activation by mutant growth factor receptors
4. Functional inactivation of tumor suppressor proteins, leading to cell activation by minute quantities of growth factors not normally sufficient to drive cell proliferation

APOPTOSIS

Apoptosis, or programmed cell death, is a normal physiologic mechanism used for control of cell numbers and prevention of abnormal cell growth. For example, most developing lymphocytes, both T and B cells, undergo apoptosis within the thymus and bone marrow, respectively, because of expression of dysfunctional antigen receptors. Apoptosis is triggered by a variety of extracellular and intracellular signals, including Fas ligand, tumor necrosis factor α (TNF-α), p53, and c-Myc, and inhibited by *Bcl-2*.

Two distinct pathways of apoptosis have been described, the death-receptor pathway and the mitochondrial pathway (Fig. 12.2). The **death-receptor pathway** is triggered by members of the TNF superfamily—Fas, TNF,

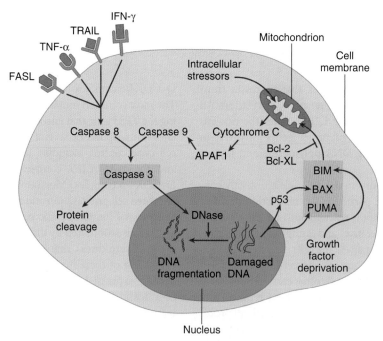

Fig. 12.2 Apoptosis pathways. *APAF1*, apoptotic peptidase activating factor 1; *FASL*, Fas ligand; *IFN-γ*, interferon-γ; *TNF-α*, tumor necrosis factor α; *TRAIL*, tumor necrosis factor–related apoptosis inducing ligand.

and TNF-related apoptosis inducing ligand (TRAIL)—that bind to cell surface receptors and trigger activation of **caspase 8**. **Fas ligand** is a membrane protein expressed by activated T cells that induces caspase-mediated apoptosis of Fas-expressing target cells upon binding to and trimerization of the receptor Fas. Genetic defects of Fas and Fas ligand are characteristic of the hereditary condition known as **autoimmune lymphoproliferative syndrome**, a childhood condition characterized by massive lymphadenopathy, splenomegaly, and autoimmune cytopenia caused by autoreactive lymphoid cells. ALPS T cells express neither CD4 nor CD8, an unusual double-negative phenotype. **TNF-α** is a protein with pleotropic effects that is produced by activated macrophages. In some situations, TNF-α induces apoptosis upon binding to TNF-α receptor–bearing target cells, including hematopoietic progenitors. In addition to apoptosis, TNF-α can induce a variety of proinflammatory effects, including neutrophil activation, cytokine production by endothelial cells, and **interferon-γ (IFN-γ)** production by lymphocytes. The proapoptotic effects of **Fas** and TNF-α signaling are mediated by activation of the caspase cascade. TNF-α signaling is complex and may lead to nuclear factor (NF) κB transcription factor activation with pleiotropic (including antiapoptotic) effects.

Mitochondrial-mediated apoptosis can be initiated by a variety of intracellular stressors, including toxic reactive oxygen intermediates, DNA damage, the unfolded protein response, and growth factor deprivation. These stressors all induce increased mitochondrial permeability, with release of **cytochrome c** into the cytoplasm. Cytochrome c binds to the cytoplasmic protein **Apaf-1**, which activates **caspase 9**, culminating in protein cleavage and **deoxyribonuclease (DNase)** activation. DNase cleaves target cell DNA into 200 base-pair fragments. Members of the Bcl-2 protein family control mitochondrial-mediated apoptosis. The Bcl-2 protein family includes proapoptotic (BAX, BAK, BIM, and PUMA) and antiapoptotic (Bcl-2 and Bcl-XL) members. The proapoptotic members directly increase mitochondrial permeability, and the antiapoptotic members block the actions of the proapoptotic members. **BIM** is specifically involved in triggering apoptosis caused by growth factor deprivation, and **PUMA** is specifically involved in apoptosis triggered by DNA damage. During lymphocyte development, BIM plays a critical role in the deletion of autoreactive T and B cells in the thymus and bone marrow, respectively.

The oncoproteins p53 and c-Myc can also trigger apoptosis. **p53,** activated in response to DNA damage, forms DNA-binding tetramers that regulate transcription of genes that promote cell cycle arrest (CDK4 inhibitor *WAF1/Cip1*) and apoptosis *(BAX)*. Thus, in some circumstances, p53 induces cell cycle arrest to allow for DNA repair; in other circumstances, p53 induces apoptosis. In this manner, p53 prevents the growth of abnormal, potentially oncogenic, cells. **Myc** protein, the production of which is triggered by cell growth factors, forms heterodimers with **Max** protein that activate gene transcription and promote both cell proliferation (by enhancing the G1-to-S transition) and apoptosis. This dual proliferative–apoptotic effect of c-Myc is particularly well illustrated in **Burkitt lymphoma**, a B-cell lymphoma characterized by chromosome translocations between the *Myc* gene and the immunoglobulin (Ig0 genes. The high level of Myc protein in Burkitt tumor cells leads to both rapid proliferation and apoptosis (Fig. 12.3).

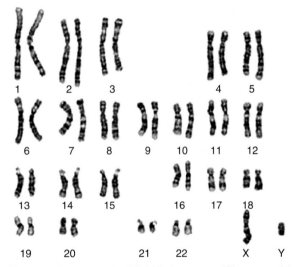

Fig. 12.3 Normal male (diploid) karyotype (Giemsa stain). These are metaphase chromosomes (46 total) from a single cell arranged according to chromosome number. There are 22 pairs of autosomes, 1 X chromosome, and 1 Y chromosome. Giemsa staining of trypsin-digested (protein-depleted) metaphase chromosomes yields characteristic alternating light and dark regions representing adenine/thymine (AT)-rich euchromatin and guanine/cytosine (GC)-rich heterochromatin, respectively. Chromosomes are typically arranged with the short arms up and long arms down, separated by a prominent dark centromeric band. Numeric and structural abnormalities can be readily identified with this approach.

SPECIFIC GENETIC DEFECTS IN HEMATOLOGIC CANCER

Hematologic cancers can roughly be divided into five categories: myelodysplastic syndromes (MDSs), myeloproliferative diseases, leukemias, lymphomas, and histiocytic and dendritic cell tumors. Hematologic cancer types are often characterized by highly specific genetic defects, including translocations, inversions, deletions, and point mutations (Table 12.1).

Common genetic defects in MDS include deletions of specific regions of chromosomes 5, 7, and 20. These deletions presumably lead to loss of so-far-unidentified tumor suppressor genes. The MDS subtype known as

TABLE 12.1 Major Cytogenetic Defects in Leukemia and Lymphoma

PRECURSOR B-ALL			
Marker	**Genes**	**Frequency (Pediatric) (%)**	**Prognosis**
Hyperdiploidy >50	Unknown	25–30	Favorable
t(12;21)(p13;q22)	TEL/RUNX1	20	Favorable
t(1;19)(q23;p13)	E2A/PBX1	5	Favorable
t(9;22)(q34;q11)	BCR-ABL	4	Unfavorable
t(4;11)(q21;q23)	AF4/MLL	2	Unfavorable
AML			
Marker	**Genes**	**Subtype**	**Prognosis**
t(15;17)(q22;q21)	PML-RARα	AML-M3	Favorable
t(8;21)(q22;q22)	ETO/RUNX1	AML-M2	Favorable
inv16(p13;q22)	CBFβ/MYH11	AML-M4Eo	Favorable
t(9;11)(p21;q23)	MLL	AML-M4 or AML-M5	Unfavorable
−5/del(5q), −7/del(7q)	Unknown	AML with myelodysplasia	Unfavorable
NON-HODGKIN LYMPHOMA			
Marker	**Genes**	**Lymphoma Subtype**	
t(8;14)(q24;q32)	Myc/IGH	Burkitt	
t(2;8)(q12;q24)	IGκ/Myc	Burkitt	
t(8;22)(q24;q11)	IGλ/Myc	Burkitt	
t(14;18)(q32;q31)	IGH/Bcl-2	Follicular	
t(11;14)(q13;q32)	CCND1/IGH	Mantle cell	
t(11;18)(q21;q21)	API2/MALT1	Extranodal marginal cell (MALT)	
t(14;18)(q32;q21)	IGH/MALT1	Extranodal marginal cell (MALT)	
t(1;14)(p22;q32)	Bcl-10	Extranodal marginal cell (MALT)	
t(9;14)(p13;q32)	PAX5/IGH	Lymphoplasmacytic	
t(2;5)(q23;q35)	ALK-1/NPM	Anaplastic large T cell	
t(1;2)(q25;p23)	TPM3/ALK-1	Anaplastic large T cell	
3q27 mutations	Bcl-6	Diffuse large B cell	
13q14 deletions	Unknown	Chronic lymphocytic leukemia	
BRAF V600E mutation	BRAF kinase	Hairy cell leukemia	
iso7q	Unknown	Hepatosplenic T cell	
inv14	TCL1	T-cell prolymphocytic	

AML, Acute myeloid leukemia; API2, apoptosis inhibitor; CCND1, cyclin D1 (induces transition from G1 to S phase of cell cycle); del-, chromosome deletion; IGH, immunoglobulin heavy chain; IGκ, immunoglobulin kappa light chain; IGλ, immunoglobulin lambda light chain; inv-, chromosome inversion; iso-, duplication of one chromosome arm with loss of the other; MALT1, paracaspase (binds to Bcl-10, leading to nuclear factor κB activation); PML-RARα, promyelocytic leukemia-retinoic acid receptor alpha; TPM3, nonmuscular tropomyosin.

refractory anemia with excess blasts is frequently associated with point mutations of the gene for *RUNX1*, a transcription factor important in stem cell development.

Chronic myelogenous leukemia (CML) is marked in nearly all cases by a translocation between chromosome 9 and chromosome 22 that yields a hybrid **BCR-ABL fusion gene.** The *BCR-ABL* fusion gene encodes for a hybrid BCR-ABL protein with constitutive tyrosine kinase activity that leads to unrestrained myeloid cell growth and resistance to apoptosis. The myeloproliferative neoplasms polycythemia vera, essential thrombocythemia, and primary myelofibrosis are often marked by a specific point mutation of the *JAK2* gene (V617F) that leads to a valine to phenylalanine switch at position 617. This change renders affected marrow cells hypersensitive to the proliferative effects of hematopoietic growth factors.

Acute myeloid leukemia (AML) is marked by a variety of genetic defects, including t(8;21) involving the *RUNX1* gene (encodes the alpha subunit of core binding factor), inv(16) and t(16;16) involving the **CBFβ** gene (encodes the beta subunit of core binding factor), t(15;17) involving the **RARα** gene (encodes the alpha subunit of the retinoic acid receptor), 11q23 defects involving the **MLL** gene (encodes a DNA-binding histone methylator), mutations of the nucleophosmin (**NPM**) gene that encodes for a multifunctional nucleolar protein, and mutations of the **FLT3** tyrosine kinase gene.

Acute lymphoblastic leukemia is also marked by a variety of genetic defects, including t(12;21) involving the *RUNX1* gene, t(9;22) with production of a hybrid BCR-ABL tyrosine kinase (similar to CML), 9p13 defects involving the **PAX5** gene (involved in B cell differentiation), and mutations of the **NOTCH1** gene (involved in T-cell differentiation).

B-cell lymphomas are marked by many specific gene defects, including 13q deletions in chronic lymphocytic leukemia/small lymphocytic lymphoma, t(14;18) translocation (involving the gene for apoptosis inhibitor Bcl-2) in follicular lymphoma, activating **Bcl-6** mutations (with inhibition of p53 expression) in diffuse large B-cell lymphoma, translocations between *c-Myc* and *Ig* genes [t(8;14), t(2;8), t(8;22)] that lead to c-Myc overexpression in Burkitt lymphoma, t(11;14) involving the **cyclinD1** and *Ig* heavy chain genes (leading to unrestricted cyclin D1-mediated cell cycle progression) in mantle cell lymphoma, and activating translocations involving the **MALT1** gene [t(11;18), t(14;18)] or the *Bcl-10* gene [t(1;14)] in extranodal marginal zone B-cell (MALT) lymphoma. MALT1 and Bcl-10 apparently cooperate in activating the NFκB pathway.

T-cell lymphomas are also marked by several specific genetic defects, including activating translocations of the **ALK-1** tyrosine kinase gene [t(2;5), t(1;2)] in anaplastic large cell lymphoma, and activation of the **TCL-1** gene (encodes an AKT kinase coactivator) via inv(14) in T cell prolymphocytic leukemia. In some cases, such as peripheral T-cell lymphoma and Hodgkin lymphoma, the bewildering variety of genetic defects has so far frustrated attempts to understand their molecular pathogenesis.

MOLECULAR AND CYTOGENETIC TECHNIQUES

Acquired neoplastic and inherited hematologic disorders are characterized by a variety of genetic lesions, ranging from single point mutations to chromosome deletions and duplications. Detection of submicroscopic point mutations and deletions require molecular genetic techniques such as **polymerase chain reaction (PCR)** and **restriction fragment length polymorphism (RFLP).** Larger genetic defects, including chromosome translocation, duplication, deletion, inversion, and gene amplification, can be detected by karyotype analysis or fluorescence in situ hybridization (FISH). These latter techniques are the domain of cytogenetics.

Karyotype analysis requires fresh viable cells that, in the presence of the mitotic spindle inhibitor colchicine, arrest in metaphase. Metaphase chromosomes are highly condensed bodies that can easily be identified by light microscopy after staining with the basophilic dye Giemsa. Giemsa staining of chromosomes yields an alternating banded pattern of dark and light stained regions called **G-banding** that allows for identification of the 22 pairs of autosomes and the 2 sex chromosomes (see Fig. 12.3). About 550 G-bands can be identified in the normal diploid genome. The darkly stained regions are composed of tightly coiled inactive **heterochromatin,** and the lightly stained regions are composed of loosely coiled transcriptionally active **euchromatin.** With this technique, changes in chromosome number (duplication or deletion) are easily identified after pairing the autosomes and sex chromosomes. Translocations are identified as differences in length or banding pattern of autosome pairs. Inversions are identified as inverted banding patterns. Gene amplifications are

identified as enlarged **homogenous staining regions**
(**HSR**), enlarged regions of light or dark G-banding. A
limitation of karyotype analysis is the requirement for
fresh viable cells of interest that can be induced to proliferate. Nonviable tumor cells with outgrowth of proliferating normal cells yield a false-negative karyotype.

Fluorescence in situ hybridization (FISH) is a useful
technique when a specific genetic defect is sought. FISH
is performed by hybridizing fluorochrome-labeled oligonucleotide probes to metaphase chromosomes, cells,
or tissue sections in which the DNA has been denatured
(Fig. 12.4). The advantage of FISH over karyotyping is
that there is no need for fresh viable cells. Although
FISH can be used to specifically identify single genes or
entire chromosomes on traditional metaphase prepara-
tions, it can also be used on cell smears or tissue sections
to identify specific genes or chromosomes in cells in all
stages of the cell cycle, including interphase. Also, in
contrast to karyotype analysis, multicolor FISH with
gene-specific probes can identify specific genes involved
in translocations (e.g., *BCR* and *ABL* genes in CML).

Dual-labeled FISH probes allow for detection of
chromosome translocations. For example, cells of interest
can be simultaneously hybridized with both an orange
FISH probe to one gene target and a green FISH probe to
another gene target. Whereas a normal diploid cell displays four separate signals (two orange and two green), a
cell with a translocation involving the target genes displays three signals (one orange, one green, and one hybrid yellow [orange-green]) (Fig. 12.5). Dual FISH with
break-apart probes allows for detection of translocations
involving gene segments. In this technique, dual-colored
probes are designed to hybridize to two separate regions
of the target gene of interest (Fig. 12.6). A normal diploid

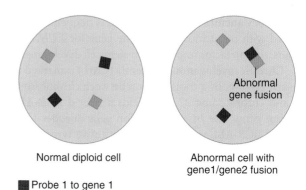

Fig. 12.5 Dual fluorescence in situ hybridization gene.

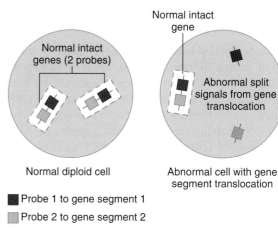

Fig. 12.6 Break-apart fluorescence in situ hybridization.

cell displays two hybrid yellow (orange-green) signals,
and a cell with a translocation that takes place within the
gene and between the two probe targets displays three
signals—one normal hybrid yellow signal, one abnormal
orange signal, and one abnormal green signal. The advantage of break-apart FISH over dual gene FISH is that
the translocation partner need not be specified (as with
Bcl-2); the advantage of dual gene FISH over break-apart
FISH is that the specific partner gene can be identified, as
with *BCR* and *ABL* in t(9;22).

Polymerase chain reaction (PCR) is a technique for
the rapid amplification of targeted nucleic acid sequences.
In DNA PCR, a small amount of purified sample DNA
is added to a reaction tube with the following:
1. Two short, single-stranded oligonucleotide primers
   designed to hybridize to the 5′ and 3′ ends of a particular DNA sequence of interest

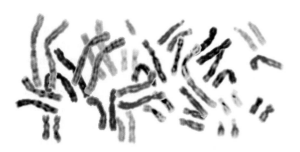

Fig. 12.4 Spectral karyotyping. In this technique, a set of
chromosome-specific fluorescent probes are used to uniquely
label each set of chromosomes.

2. Taq DNA polymerase enzyme
3. Four deoxynucleotides (deoxyadenosine triphosphate, dTTP, deoxyguanosine triphosphate, and deoxycytidine triphosphate)

The contents of the tube are subjected to a series of carefully timed heating and cooling cycles in a thermal cycler. Theoretically, a typical series of 40 cycles yields an enormous amplification (2^{40}) of the PCR product. After completion of the cycling, the PCR product is subjected to horizontal gel electrophoresis for separation of DNA fragments by molecular size, stained with a DNA-binding fluorescent dye, and visualized with ultraviolet light.

DNA PCR has been widely used to detect clonal **antigen receptor gene rearrangements** in lymphoma. In this case, two primers, one to the V region and one to the J region, are designed to yield a PCR product by spanning across rearranged DNA of either the **Ig heavy chain locus** on chromosome 14 in B cells or the **T-cell receptor-γ locus** on chromosome 7 in T cells. In nonlymphoid cells, the DNA at these loci is unrearranged; that is, they are in a so-called **germline configuration**. If the DNA in these loci is in the germline configuration, then the molecular distance between the primer binding sites is too great for a PCR product to be formed. In the case of polyclonal lymphocytosis, the DNA from multiple cell clones contains many different PCR-amplifiable gene rearrangements of various molecular size. In this case, gel electrophoresis or column chromatography of the PCR product demonstrates a smear of multiple DNA bands, each of which represents the amplified product of a single clone. In the case of a B- or T-cell lymphoma, the DNA from a single clone of tumor cells contains one or two clonal gene rearrangements. Electrophoresis or chromatography of this PCR product demonstrates one or two prominent (monoclonal) DNA bands (Fig. 12.7). As the process of antigen receptor gene rearrangement begins, only one of the two diploid loci undergoes rearrangement (**allelic exclusion**). If this rearrangement is productive, that is, if it leads to synthesis of functional antigen receptor protein, then the other locus will remain in the germline configuration. If this clone becomes malignant, then all the tumor cells will contain one single clonal rearrangement (one band). If, on the other hand, the first rearrangement is nonproductive, rearrangement of the second locus will be activated. Lymphoid tumors that arise from cells that have undergone two antigen receptor

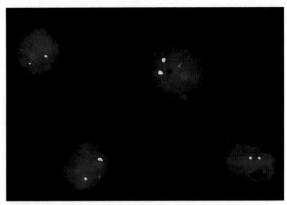

Fig. 12.7 Fluorescence in situ hybridization. In this image, three cells are hybridized with two nonoverlapping gene probes to the *Bcl-2* gene on chromosome 18. All three cells display three signals—one normal polychromatic signal (orange-green, or yellow), representing an intact *Bcl-2* gene, and two monochromatic split signals (one orange and one green) caused by translocation and fusion of a portion of the *Bcl-2* gene to the immunoglobulin heavy chain locus on chromosome 14, or t(14;18). This translocation is characteristic of follicular lymphoma.

gene rearrangements will yield two clonal rearrangements (two bands).

For **reverse transcription PCR (RT-PCR)**, highly labile sample RNA is first converted to stable complementary DNA by the enzyme reverse transcriptase and then subjected to PCR amplification with primers designed to hybridize to complementary DNA sequences of interest. An RT-PCR assay for detection of the BCR-ABL fusion transcripts has proved useful in diagnosis and monitoring of patients with CML.

More recently, **real-time detection** of PCR products as they are produced in the tube (without the need for gel electrophoresis) has been made possible with the use of special dual-labeled (Taqman) probes that fluoresce only after binding to target DNA. These probes are labeled with a fluorochrome at the 5′ end and a fluorescence quencher at the 3′ end. The quencher blocks fluorochrome-mediate fluorescence in the intact probe. During the process of amplification, DNA polymerase cleaves probe that has bound (hybridized) to the target sequence, releasing the bound fluorochrome from the quencher. The accumulation of free fluorochrome during thermal cycling leads to an exponential increase in fluorescence. The rate of increase in fluorescence intensity is directly proportional to the amount of initial

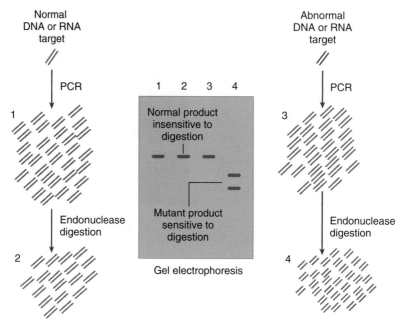

Fig. 12.8 Polymerase chain reaction (PCR) restriction fragment length polymorphism analysis.

target sequence in the sample. This method has been adapted to allow for real-time quantification of target sequences, or **real-time quantitative PCR**. This method of quantification has been particularly useful in monitoring viral load in patients with chronic viral infection and tumor burden in patients with leukemia.

PCR techniques can also be used to detect mutant genes with single nucleotide substitutions. **PCR-RFLP (PCR restriction fragment length polymorphism)**, is performed by amplification of the target sequence of interest by conventional PCR followed by digestion of the amplified product with a DNA restriction enzyme. After digestion, the resulting DNA fragments are separated based on molecular size by gel electrophoresis or column chromatography. By using a restriction enzyme that cleaves DNA at only a specific site marked by the sought-after nucleotide substitution, mutant product can be detected as two short fragments of specific length and unmutated product is detected as a single, larger, uncut fragment (Fig. 12.8). A confirmatory test for the presence of the **factor V Leiden mutation** that is associated with thrombophilia is a PCR-RFLP test.

Automated DNA and RNA sequencing is carried out by sequential cleavage and nucleotide identification of a specific sequence that has been amplified by PCR.

KEY WORDS AND CONCEPTS

- Acute lymphoblastic leukemia (ALL)
- Acute myeloid leukemia (AML)
- ALK-1
- Allelic exclusion
- Antigen receptor gene rearrangements
- Apaf-1
- Apoptosis
- Autoimmune lymphoproliferative syndrome (ALPS)
- BAX
- B-cell lymphomas
- Bcl-10
- Bcl-2
- Bcl-6
- *BCR-ABL* fusion gene
- BIM
- Break-apart probes
- Burkitt lymphoma
- Caspase 8
- Caspase 9

- CBFβ
- Chronic myelogenous leukemia (CML)
- c-Myc
- Cyclin-CDK inhibitors
- Cyclin D1
- *Cyclin D1 gene*
- Cyclin-dependent protein kinases (CDKs)
- Cyclins
- Cytochrome c
- Cytokines
- Death-receptor pathway
- Deoxyribonuclease (DNase)
- Dual-labeled FISH
- E2F transcription factor
- Euchromatin
- Factor V Leiden mutation
- Fas
- Fas ligand (FasL)
- Fluorescence in-situ hybridization (FISH)
- G-banding
- Germline configuration
- Heterochromatin
- Homogenous staining regions (HSR)
- Ig heavy chain locus
- Janus (JAK) kinase
- *JAK2*
- JAK-STAT pathway
- Karyotype analysis
- M phase

- MALT1
- Max
- *MLL*
- Myc
- *NOTCH1*
- *NPM*
- p53
- p53 protein
- *PAX5*
- PCR-RFLP
- Polymerase chain reaction (PCR)
- PUMA
- *RARα*
- *RB mutations*
- Real-time detection
- Real-time quantitative PCR
- Refractory anemia with excess blasts
- Resistance to apoptosis
- Restriction point
- Retinoblastoma (RB) protein
- Reverse transcription PCR (RT-PCR)
- *RUNX1*
- S phase
- Signal transducer and activator of transcription (STAT)
- T-cell lymphoma
- *TCL-1*
- T-cell receptor-γ locus
- *WAF1/CIP1*

REVIEW QUESTIONS

1. Which of the following statements regarding p53 is **false**?
   A. Activated by DNA damage
   B. Competes with Rb for binding to E2F
   C. Inhibits cyclin-dependent kinase 4/6
   D. Activates the proapoptotic *BAX* gene

2. Which of the following statements regarding apoptosis is **false**?
   A. *FASL*-positive T cells bind to *Fas*-positive target cells and induce caspase 8 activation.
   B. *Fas/Fas ligand* mutations lead to autoimmune lymphoproliferative disorder.
   C. Mitochondrial damage induces increased permeability, leakage of cytochrome c and activation of caspase 9.

   D. Growth factor deprivation induces apoptosis mediated by PUMA.

3. Which one of the following statements regarding gene defects is **false**?
   - **A.** A tyrosine kinase fusion gene leads to unrestrained growth in CML.
   - **B.** *JAK2* mutations render myeloproliferative neoplasms hyperresponsive to growth factors.
   - **C.** *BCL-2* gene translocation blocks apoptosis in AML.
   - **D.** *c-myc* translocation leads to unrestrained cell proliferation in Burkitt lymphoma.

4. All of the following are required for PCR **except**
   - **A.** DNA or RNA substrate.
   - **B.** restriction endonuclease.
   - **C.** Taq DNA polymerase or reverse transcriptase.
   - **D.** primers.

13

Leukemia and Related Disorders

INTRODUCTION

The term **leukemia** refers to a family of malignant neoplasms of the bone marrow characterized by clonal proliferation of hematopoietic cells and often accompanied by circulating immature cells in the peripheral blood. Leukemia is often accompanied by suppression of normal hematopoiesis, leading to pancytopenia. Neutropenia (<500 neutrophils per microliter of blood) and thrombocytopenia (<20,000 platelets per microliter of blood) increase the risk of life-threatening sepsis and bleeding in patients with leukemia. Leukemic infiltration of vital organs can lead to life-threatening organ failure.

Leukemia may be subclassified as acute or chronic, and myeloid or lymphoid (Table 13.1). Myeloblasts and lymphoblasts can be recognized by their expression of specific markers (Fig. 13.1). Whereas in acute leukemia, there is a predominance of immature cells (lymphoblasts, myeloblasts, promyelocytes, or promonocytes), in chronic leukemia, there is a predominance of more mature cells (lymphocytes, myelocytes, metamyelocytes, bands, or neutrophils). In acute myelogenous leukemia (AML), the proliferating tumor cells may be myeloblasts, promyelocytes (in acute promyelocytic leukemia), promonocytes (in acute monocytic leukemia), erythroblasts (in acute erythroid leukemia), or megakaryoblasts (in acute megakaryoblastic leukemia). In acute lymphoblastic leukemia (ALL), the proliferating cells may be B lymphoblasts or T lymphoblasts. In **chronic myeloid leukemia (CML)**, the proliferating cells range from myeloblasts (<20%) to myelocytes. In **chronic myelomonocytic leukemia (CMML),** the proliferating cells include a preponderance of promonocytes and monocytes. In B-cell **chronic lymphocytic leukemia (CLL)**, the proliferating cells are CD5+ B lymphocytes.

The **myelodysplastic syndromes (MDSs)** and myeloproliferative neoplasms (MPNs) are myeloid neoplasms with leukemia-like features (Table 13.2). MDSs are characterized by peripheral blood cytopenia (anemia, neutropenia, and/or thrombocytopenia), a variable number of myeloblasts (<20%), and dysplastic maturation. MPNs are characterized by peripheral blood cytosis (erythrocytosis, leukocytosis, and/or thrombocytosis) and a variable number of myeloblasts (<20%). Transformation to AML is seen in both MDS and MPN.

Leukemia is a genetic disease associated with mutations of cellular **oncogenes** (Table 13.3). Cellular oncogenes are genes that, when expressed under normal

TABLE 13.1	General Features of Common Leukemia Types			
	Acute Myeloid Leukemia	**Acute Lymphoblastic Leukemia**	**Chronic Myelogenous Leukemia**	**Chronic Lymphocytic Leukemia**
Pathology	>20% myeloblasts in blood or marrow	>20% TdT+ lymphoblasts in blood or marrow	Increased myeloid cells with left shift but <20% myeloblasts	Lymphocytosis with >5000 CD5+ B cells per μL of blood
Clinical course	Rapid progression with pancytopenia, bleeding, infection, and organ failure		Indolent chronic phase followed by progression to acute leukemia (CML) or aggressive lymphoid leukemia/lymphoma (CLL)	

CML, Chronic myeloid leukemia; *CLL,* chronic lymphocytic leukemia; *TdT,* terminal deoxynucleotidyl transferase.

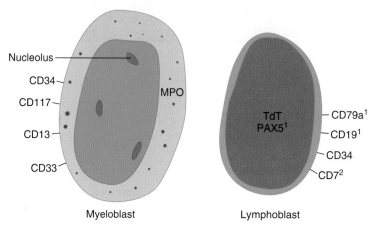

Fig. 13.1 Basic leukemia blast types. *MPO,* Myeloperoxidase; *PAX5,* paired box 5; *TdT,* terminal deoxynucle-otidyl transferase.

TABLE 13.2 General Features of Myeloid Neoplasms

	Acute Myeloid Leukemia	Myelodysplastic Neoplasm	Myeloproliferative Neoplasm	Myelodysplastic/ Myeloproliferative Neoplasm
Blood counts	Low-high	Low	High	High
Blast count (%)	20–100	0–19	0–19	0–19
Dysplasia	Sometimes	Always	Never	Always
Marrow cellularity	Usually increased	Usually increased	Increased	Increased
Common genetic defects	inv(16)/t(16;16), t(15;17), +8, t(8;21); *NPM1, RUNX1, FLT3, CEBPA, KIT* mutations	-7/del(7q), -5/del(5q), +8, del(20q)	t(9;22)[BCR-ABL1], JAK2 mutation, +8, del(20q)	+8, -7/del(7q), del(20q)

TABLE 13.3 Functional Groups of Gene Mutations in Acute Myelogenous Leukemia

Group	Function	Gene Example
I	Cell signaling	*FLT3*
II	Differentiation	*RARA*
III	Epigenetic modifiers	*DNMT3A*
IV	Cell adhesion	*RAD21*
V	DNA repair	*TP53*
VI	Spliceosome	*SRSF2*
VII	Transcription	*CEBPA*

circumstances, support essential cellular functions such as mitosis and cell death inhibition. However, when expressed inappropriately, these same oncogene products drive mitosis or block apoptosis in an unregulated fashion. Leukemia develops as a result of uncontrolled cellular proliferation induced by inappropriate expression of growth-promoting or apoptosis-inhibiting (suppressor) oncoproteins. In some cases, oncogenes are created by translocation of cell cycle– or apoptosis-related genes into transcriptionally active regions, for example, *c-Myc* gene translocation into immunoglobulin gene loci in some cases of B cell (Burkitt type) ALL. In other cases, oncogenes are created by fusion of two genes that yield hybrid fusion proteins with unusual oncogenic activities, such as BCR-ABL protein in CML and promyelocytic leukemia-RARα (PML-RARα) protein in acute promyelocytic leukemia.

Leukemic infiltration of the bone marrow leads to reduction in normal hematopoiesis, leading in turn to reduction in normal blood cell counts (cytopenia). The combination of decreased erythrocyte, neutrophil, and platelet count in peripheral blood is referred to as **pancytopenia**. Symptoms commonly associated with pancytopenia include pallor, fatigue, and weakness caused by anemia; bacterial or fungal infection caused by neutropenia; and mucocutaneous bleeding caused by thrombocytopenia. Acute promyelocytic leukemia is often accompanied by the bleeding disorder known as **disseminated intravascular coagulation** (**DIC**). Acute monocytic and myelomonocytic leukemias are sometimes associated with leukemic infiltrates of extramedullary sites, including the gums. ALL may involve the central nervous system (CNS) and often involves lymph nodes and anterior mediastinum. CML, actually classified as an MPN, characteristically involves the spleen, leading to massive splenomegaly.

Patients with leukemia are treated most often with **cytotoxic chemotherapeutic drugs** followed in many cases by **bone marrow stem cell transplantation**. The rationale for chemotherapy is that chemotherapeutic suppression of the neoplastic clone allows for repopulation of the marrow by normal residual stem cells. The rationale for stem cell transplantation is that, for some chemoresistant tumors, the high dose of chemotherapy required for tumor eradication leads to loss of normal marrow stem cells

(**myeloablative therapy**). Bone marrow stem cell transplantation provides a sufficient number of normal residual stem cells to repopulate the marrow.

Pharmacologic classes of drugs used in leukemia include alkylating agents (cyclophosphamide and busulfan), cell cycle inhibitors (anthracyclines and cytosine arabinoside), cell maturation agents (retinoids), interferons, lymphocytotoxic agents (corticosteroids), and small molecule inhibitors (imatinib). Treatment usually consists of a short course of high-dose **induction** chemotherapy designed to induce **remission** (absence of detectable residual disease) followed by a longer course of low-dose maintenance (or **consolidation**) therapy to ensure complete tumor cell eradication and long-term remission. Because chemotherapeutic agents administered intravenously do not effectively cross the blood–brain barrier, patients with ALL are often treated with intrathecal chemotherapy to prevent CNS relapse. Some leukemias are treated with drugs that specifically target genetic lesions. Examples include the BCR-ABL inhibitor **imatinib** for chronic myelogenous leukemia and the vitamin A derivative **all-*trans* retinoic acid** (**ATRA**) for acute promyelocytic leukemia.

Allogeneic (or autologous) stem cell transplantation after induction of remission and high-dose, marrow-toxic intensification designed to eradicate all tumor cells may lead to cure. Typically, relapsed leukemia is highly resistant to chemotherapy. Patients who develop pancytopenia caused by leukemic replacement of the bone marrow may require supportive transfusions of red blood cells (RBCs) and platelets to reduce the associated symptoms. Neutropenia is not usually treated as such by leukocyte transfusions or cytokines, but infection risk may be reduced with prophylactic antibiotics.

ACUTE MYELOID LEUKEMIA

KEY POINTS

- Acute myelogenous leukemia (AML) is the most common acute leukemia in adults (80%) and neonates.
- Known causative factors include ionizing radiation, benzene exposure, and cytotoxic chemotherapy.
- The incidence is increased in young children with some inherited diseases, including Down syndrome (acute megakaryoblastic leukemia) and Fanconi anemia.

- Most cases of AML are associated with acquired chromosomal abnormalities involving translocations, inversions, and deletions leading to oncogene activation.
- Gene mutations in AML have been classified into five functional groups, with defects in proliferation, differentiation, epigenetics, cell adhesion, and DNA repair.

- Common presenting symptoms include those caused by anemia (pallor, weakness, fatigue, or exertional dyspnea), neutropenia (minor pyogenic skin infections), thrombocytopenia (petechiae, ecchymoses, or epistaxis), systemic effects (fever, anorexia, or weight loss), disseminated intravascular coagulation in acute promyelocytic leukemia, and gum infiltration in acute monocytic leukemia.
- Diagnostic subtypes are based on the morphology, phenotype, and cytogenetics of tumor cells.
- AML can nearly always be differentiated from acute lymphoblastic leukemia by expression of the granulocyte enzyme myeloperoxidase, the monocyte enzyme nonspecific esterase, the granulocyte cell surface antigens CD13 and CD33, the monocyte cell surface antigen CD14, the proerythroblast cell surface antigen glycophorin A, the megakaryocytic antigens CD41 and CD61, or a combination of these.
- The goal of initial treatment with a combination of cytotoxic chemotherapeutic agents is eradication of tumor cells and restoration of normal hematopoiesis—a state referred to as complete remission.
- After induction of remission, long-term, disease-free survival may be achieved by consolidation chemotherapy or stem cell transplantation.

Several AML subtypes are defined by an association with a specific chromosomal defect. AML with **t(8;21)** translocation is morphologically distinctive, is marked by hypergranular myeloblasts and dysplastic myeloid cells and carries a favorable prognosis. Structural abnormalities of chromosome 16 [**inv(16), t(16;16)**] are seen in a type of AML composed of myeloid and monocytic blasts (myelomonocytic) with numerous abnormal eosinophils. This type of AML also carries a favorable prognosis. **AML with 11q23 abnormalities** involving the *MLL* gene (histone methyltransferase) most often resembles acute myelomonocytic or acute monocytic leukemia. **Acute promyelocytic leukemia (AML-M3)**, with numerous abnormal promyelocytes in marrow (and often blood) (Fig. 13.2), is defined by the presence of the t(15;17) translocation that gives rise to the PML-RARα fusion protein (Fig. 13.3). The fusion protein acts by preventing RAR-mediated induction of promyelocyte differentiation. This defect can be overcome by administration of the compound ATRA, which bypasses the defective RAR and induces downstream signaling that leads to cell differentiation beyond the promyelocyte stage. However, because ATRA does not induce leukemia cell death, it must be used with other cytotoxic chemotherapeutic agents.

Nearly half of all AML cases have a normal karyotype, with no chromosome defects detected by classical cytogenetic analysis. In these cases, several recurrent gene mutations have been described, including those of *nucleophosmin (NPM1)*, *CEBPA*, *KIT*, and *Fms-like tyrosine kinase (FLT3)*. Nucleophosmin is a multifunctional protein that serves as a molecular chaperone, shuttling molecules from nucleus to cytoplasm. *CEBPA*

Fig. 13.2 Promyeloblasts with prominent cytoplasmic granularity (acute promyelocytic leukemia [AML-M3]).

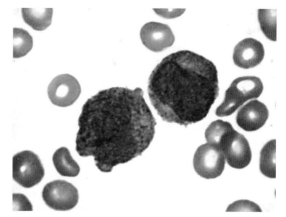

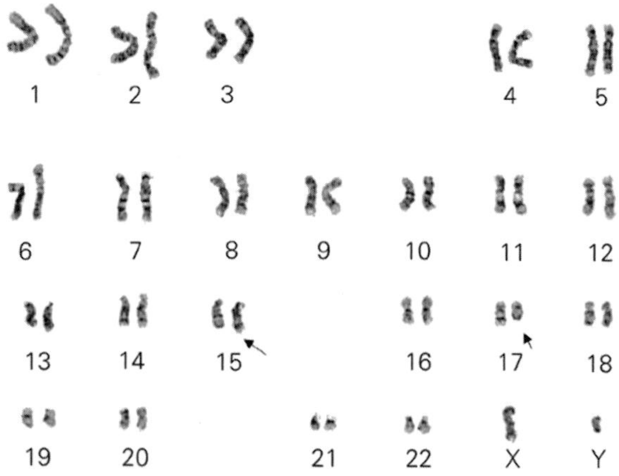

Fig. 13.3 Translocation between chromosomes 15 and 17, i.e., t(15;17) *(arrows)* in acute promyelocytic leukemia (AML-M3) (Giemsa banded karyotype).

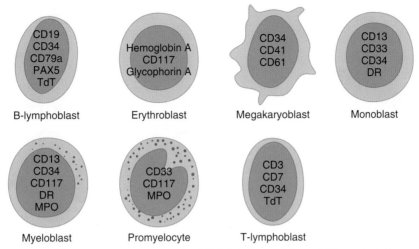

Fig. 13.4 Acute leukemia blast cell phenotype. *MPO,* Myeloperoxidase; *TdT,* terminal deoxynucleotidyl transferase.

encodes for a myeloid transcription factor involved in myeloid differentiation. *KIT* and *FLT3* encode for receptor tyrosine kinases that induce cellular proliferation.

The mutations in AML can be broadly classified into 5 functional groups. Class I mutations enhance proliferation and survival, class II mutations inhibit cell differentiation, class III (epigenetic) mutations modify gene expression, class IV mutations interfere with cell adhesion and cell-cell interaction, and class V mutations inhibit DNA repair and RNA splicing (Fig. 13.4).

One form of AML is defined by its occurrence following treatment with **alkylating agents** or **topoisomerase type II inhibitors**. This type of AML is marked by numerous cytogenetic defects and a poor prognosis. Another AML subtype that is characterized by a poor prognosis is **AML with multilineage dysplasia**. Presumably, many of these tumors arise by progression from preexisting but clinically unrecognized myelodysplasia.

Remaining AML subtypes are defined by the morphology and immunophenotype of the blasts. The marrow in **AML with minimal differentiation (AML-M0)** contains more than 19% CD13/CD33+, myeloperoxidase (MPO)-negative agranular myeloblasts (Fig. 13.5). Given the lack of cellular differentiation, this tumor is morphologically difficult to differentiate from ALL. In contrast to ALL, this form of AML expresses the myeloid cell surface antigen CD13, CD33, or both (see Fig. 13.4).

The marrow in **AML without maturation (AML-M1)** contains more than 19% faintly granular blasts that

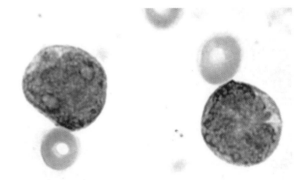

Fig. 13.5 Minimally differentiated (agranular) myeloblasts in acute myelogenous leukemia.

express small amounts of the primary granule enzyme MPO, as well as the myeloid antigen CD13, CD33, or both. In some cases of AML-M1, aggregated primary granules can be seen as Auer rods (Fig. 13.6).

The marrow in **AML with maturation (AML-M2)** contains more than 19% granular blasts that are strongly positive for MPO (Fig. 13.7) and myeloid antigen CD13, CD33, or both. The presence of a t(8;21) translocation is associated with a favorable prognosis.

The marrow in AML-M3 contains more than 19% abnormal promyelocytes that are strongly positive for MPO, positive for CD13 and/or CD33, and human leukocyte antigen (HLA)-DR negative. A translocation between the *PML* and *RARα* genes [t(15;17)] is highly characteristic. Patients with AML-M3 often present

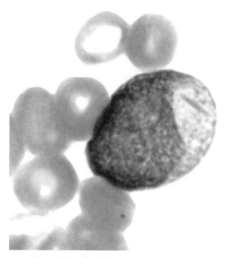

Fig. 13.6 Myeloblasts with a cytoplasmic Auer rod.

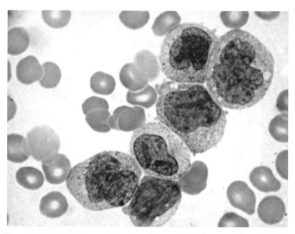

Fig. 13.8 Admixture of blasts with myeloid (two cells with light pink cytoplasm) and monocytic (four cells with more basophilic cytoplasm) features in acute myelomonocytic leukemia (AML-M4).

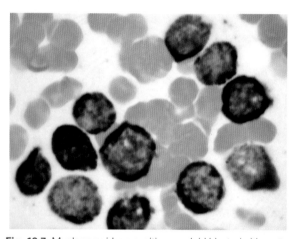

Fig. 13.7 Myeloperoxidase-positive myeloid blasts (with maturation) in acute myelogenous leukemia.

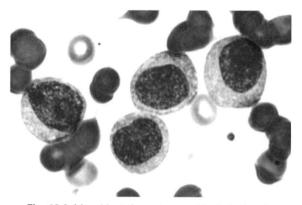

Fig. 13.9 Monoblasts in acute monoblastic leukemia.

with DIC caused by release of thrombogenic substances by the tumor cells. Initial cytotoxic chemotherapy is supplemented with ATRA, a vitamin A derivative that, by bypassing the defective retinoic acid receptor, induces maturation of the abnormal promyelocytes to more mature, less proliferative myeloid cells.

The marrow in **acute myelomonocytic leukemia (AML-M4)** contains an admixture of MPO-positive myeloblasts and nonspecific esterase-positive monoblasts (Fig. 13.8). AML-M4 with marrow eosinophilia (AML-M4Eo) is associated with chromosome 16 defects—inv(16), t(16;16)—and has a more favorable prognosis.

Acute monoblastic/monocytic leukemia (AML-M5) is composed of monoblasts with or without promonocytes. Monoblasts and promonocytes are nonspecific, esterase positive, and MPO negative and have weak CD4+. The mature monocyte antigen CD14 is expressed by promonocytes but only weakly and variably by monoblasts. Whereas the AML-M5a variant is composed of monoblasts only (Fig. 13.9), the AML-M5b variant is composed of both monoblasts and promonocytes (Fig. 13.10). Extramedullary disease is common, with infiltration of the gums, skin, and lymph nodes.

Acute erythroid leukemia (AML-M6) encompasses two distinct entities. The marrow in the more common erythroid/myeloid variant (AML-M6a) contains increased myeloblasts (>19%) in an otherwise markedly

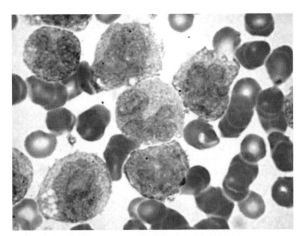

Fig. 13.10 Promonocytes and monocytes in acute monocytic leukemia.

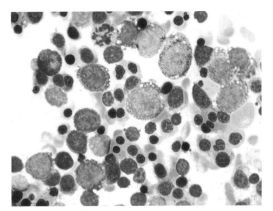

Fig. 13.12 Numerous erythroblasts with vacuolated basophilic cytoplasm in acute erythroid leukemia (AML-M6).

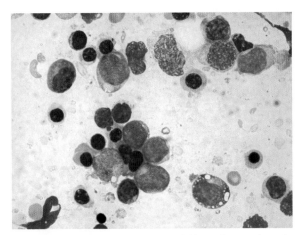

Fig. 13.11 Numerous agranular myeloblasts in an otherwise erythroid-predominant marrow (acute erythroid leukemia erythroid/myeloid variant [AML-M6a]).

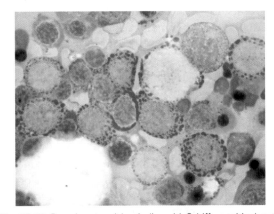

Fig. 13.13 Prominent red (periodic acid–Schiff –positive) cytoplasmic vacuoles in acute erythroid leukemia (AML-M6).

erythroid-predominant marrow (Fig. 13.11). The marrow in the rare variant known as pure erythroid leukemia (AML-M6b) contains abnormal proerythroblasts (>19%) in a markedly erythroid-predominant marrow (Fig. 13.12). Myeloblasts are not increased in the AML-M6b variant. The abnormal proerythroblasts in AML-M6b often contain large periodic acid–Schiff–positive vacuoles in the cytoplasm (Fig. 13.13).

The marrow in **acute megakaryoblastic leukemia (AML-M7)** contains numerous abnormal megakaryoblasts, often with extensive myelofibrosis (Fig. 13.14). Megakaryoblasts express platelet glycoprotein antigens CD41 and CD61 yet are negative for MPO by immunohistochemistry.

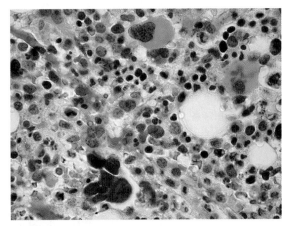

Fig. 13.14 Acute megakaryoblastic leukemia (AML-M7) (marrow biopsy) with numerous undifferentiated blasts and large abnormal megakaryocytes.

AML-M7 is the most common AML subtype in Down syndrome.

Acute eosinophilic and basophilic leukemias are very rare and are not discussed here.

The CMLs (chronic myelogenous leukemia, chronic neutrophilic leukemia, and chronic eosinophilic leukemia) are discussed in the section on myeloproliferative neoplasms.

ACUTE LYMPHOBLASTIC LEUKEMIA (PRECURSOR LYMPHOBLASTIC LEUKEMIA)

KEY POINTS

- Defined as a clonal proliferation of neoplastic lymphoblasts (precursor B or precursor T) in bone marrow (and anterior mediastinum in the T cell type).
- Cases that present with a mass lesion and less than 20% blasts in blood and marrow are classified as lymphoblastic lymphoma.
- Precursor B-cell acute lymphoblastic leukemia (ALL) is more common in children than adults (75% younger than 6 years of age).
- Precursor T-cell ALL (T-ALL) is more common in adolescents than children or adults.
- The clinical presentation of ALL may include fatigue, fever, petechiae, bone pain, hepatosplenomegaly,
lymphadenopathy, central nervous system involvement, and mediastinal mass (in precursor T-ALL).
- Both precursor B and T lymphoblasts express terminal deoxynucleotidyl transferase (intranuclear).
- Whereas precursor B lymphoblasts express CD19 (cell membrane) and CD22 (cytoplasmic), precursor T lymphoblasts express CD7 (cell membrane) and CD3 (cytoplasmic).
- Cytogenetic abnormalities in precursor B-ALL include those associated with a favorable prognosis, such as hyperdiploidy, or t(12;21), and those associated with an unfavorable prognosis, such as hypodiploidy or t(9;22), t(4;11), or t(1;19).

Precursor B-cell ALL (B-ALL) is more common in children than in adults. Patients may present with pallor and fatigue (caused by anemia), fever, petechiae and ecchymosis (caused by thrombocytopenia), bone pain (caused by marrow involvement), hepatosplenomegaly, and lymphadenopathy. The complete blood count often reveals pancytopenia, with lymphoblasts often noted on blood smears (Fig. 13.15). Lymphoblasts account for at least 20% of nucleated cells in blood or marrow. Precursor B-ALL can be subclassified based on cellular differentiation into three subtypes: early precursor B-ALL, common B-ALL, and pre-B-ALL. The prognosis in children ages 2 to 10 years with progenitor B type is excellent. **Early precursor B-ALL** is composed of CD10− CD19+ terminal deoxynucleotidyl transferase (TdT)+ immunoglobulin-negative lymphoblasts. **Common B-ALL** is composed of CD10+ CD19+ TdT+ immunoglobulin-negative lymphoblasts that express cytoplasmic mu heavy chain. **Pre-B-ALL** is composed of CD10+/− CD19+ TdT+/− cytoplasmic mu heavy chain-positive lymphoblasts.

Whereas the cell of origin of **B-cell lymphoblastic lymphoma (B-LBL)** is identical to that of B-ALL, B-LBL presents as a mass lesion rather than as leukemia.

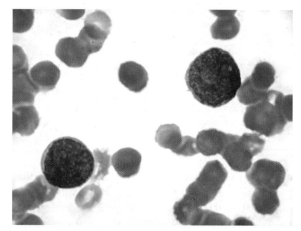

Fig. 13.15 Lymphoblasts in acute lymphoblastic leukemia with finely granular chromatin and nucleoli (peripheral smear).

Patients with B-LBL often present with lymphadenopathy of the head and neck region, as well as anterior mediastinum. In contrast to B-ALL, B-LBL is seen most commonly in older children and adolescents. Nevertheless, B-ALL and B-LBL are now classified together as **B-cell lymphoblastic leukemia/lymphoma.**

In rare cases, Burkitt lymphoma may present as an acute leukemia (Burkitt leukemia or lymphoma) with B lymphoblastic features. In contrast to precursor B-ALL, the Burkitt tumor cells are TdT negative, express membrane immunoglobulin (Ig) M, and display deeply basophilic cytoplasm with numerous small lipid vacuoles. Like Burkitt lymphoma (and unlike precursor B-ALL), Burkitt leukemia is associated with c-Myc translocations: t(8;14), t(2;8), t(8;22) (Figs. 13.16 and 13.17).

T-cell ALL (T-ALL) occurs more commonly in older children and adolescents than B-ALL and more commonly in males. Patients with T-ALL often present with an anterior mediastinal mass that, if bulky, can lead to superior vena cava or mediastinal syndrome, with cough, dyspnea, dysphagia, stridor, cyanosis, and facial edema. In contrast to B-ALL, marrow involvement by T-ALL is less likely to be associated with pancytopenia. T-ALL is composed of CD7, cytoplasmic CD3(cCD3), TdT-positive lymphoblasts.

The cell of origin of **T-cell LBL (T-LBL)** is identical to that of T-ALL, the major difference being the mode of presentation. T-LBL is more common than B-LBL, is often seen in male adolescents, and commonly presents as a mediastinal mass. Genetic defects in T-LBL often involve translocations between TCR genes and homeobox (**HOX**) genes.

Treatment of patients with ALL consists of combination chemotherapy with transfusion for management of life-threatening cytopenia, aggressive antibiotic treatment of infections, and vigorous hydration and allopurinol (xanthine oxidase inhibitor) or rasburicase (recombinant urate oxidase) for control of tumor lysis syndrome. **Tumor lysis syndrome** is an adverse condition that may occur after initial cytotoxic chemotherapy of highly proliferative lymphoid tumors (ALL or Burkitt lymphoma). Massive death of tumor cells leads to release of intracellular contents with increased potassium (hyperkalemia), phosphate (hyperphosphatemia), and **uric acid** (hyperuricemia) and decreased calcium (hypocalcemia). Precipitation of uric acid and calcium phosphate in the kidneys leads to acute renal injury. This complication can be avoided by treatment with allopurinol and rasburicase. **Allopurinol**

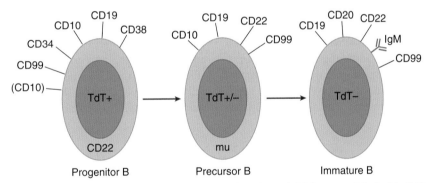

Fig. 13.16 B-cell acute lymphoblastic leukemia phenotypic subset. *IgM*, Immunoglobulin M; *TdT*, terminal deoxynucleotidyl transferase.

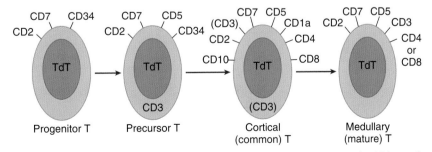

Fig. 13.17 T lymphoblastic leukemia phenotypic subset. *TdT*, Terminal deoxynucleotidyl transferase.

(xanthine oxidase inhibitor) blocks uric acid production, and **rasburicase** converts uric acid to **allantoin**, which is more soluble than uric acid and excreted in urine without precipitation. To prevent relapse of disease in the CNS, patients with ALL also receive **intrathecal chemotherapy**. Given the overall success rate with chemotherapy, especially in children, allogeneic bone marrow transplantation is often limited to patients with ALL in relapse (recurrent disease after chemotherapeutic remission).

Several genetic defects in B-ALL affect the overall prognosis. Genetic defects associated with favorable prognosis include **hyperdiploidy** (>50 chromosomes), *TEL-AML1* fusion t(12;21), and *HOX11* overexpression. Genetic defects associated with poor prognosis include hypodiploidy (<45 chromosomes), *BCR-ABL* fusion t(9;22), *ETA-PBX1* fusion t(1;19), and *MLL-AF4* fusion t(4;11).

CHRONIC LYMPHOCYTIC LEUKEMIA

Chronic lymphocytic leukemia, the most common leukemia in adults, is a low-grade malignancy that usually occurs after the age of 50 years, with an incidence that increases with age. Patients are often asymptomatic at presentation, with the diagnosis based on peripheral blood lymphocytosis (Fig. 13.18) with marrow involvement. Patients may present with fatigue caused by anemia, lymphadenopathy, splenomegaly, hypogammaglobulinemia, autoimmune hemolytic anemia, and autoimmune thrombocytopenia. The abnormal B cells in CLL exhibit a highly characteristic CD5+ CD23+ immunophenotype. Although overall the long-term prognosis is excellent (>6–12 years), a variety of factors negatively influence overall prognosis. These negative prognostic factors include extensive lymphadenopathy; anemia; thrombocytopenia; tumor cell expression of CD38, ZAP-70, or both; and presence of an abnormal karyotype. CD38 and **zeta-associated protein (ZAP-70)** expression marks CLL cells with nonmutated (germline) variable region immunoglobulin (IgV_H) genes. Cells with nonmutated IgV_H genes are immature in comparison to cells with mutated IgV_H genes and are associated with more aggressive disease.

Given the relatively good prognosis and incurability of CLL, asymptomatic disease is often untreated. Symptomatic disease is treated with specific cytotoxic agents, including deoxyadenosine analogs, alkylating agents, and glucocorticoids. Other agents include monoclonal antibodies directed against CD52 (alemtuzumab) and CD20 (rituximab), both of which are usually expressed on the surface of CLL tumor cells. With time, CLL may acquire additional mutations and transform to more aggressive disease. **Prolymphocytic transformation** of CLL is marked by increased prolymphocytes in blood and marrow with progressive splenomegaly. Prolymphocytes are large lymphoid cells with moderate amounts of cytoplasm and prominent central nucleoli (Fig. 13.19). Transformation of CLL to diffuse large B cell lymphoma (termed **Richter transformation**) is marked by rapidly enlarging lymph nodes and spleen.

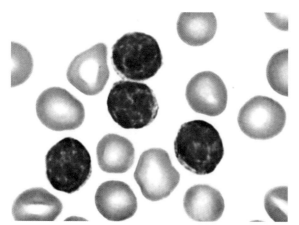

Fig. 13.18 Small lymphocytes in chronic lymphocytic leukemia with coarse irregular chromatin and absence of nucleoli staining (peripheral smear).

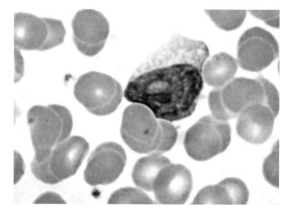

Fig. 13.19 A large immunoblast with a prominent nucleolus in large cell transformation of chronic lymphocytic leukemia.

In either case, transformation of CLL is associated with a poor outcome.

Hairy cell leukemia is a rare low-grade B-cell malignancy of the bone marrow and spleen. The tumor cells carry a point mutation in the ***BRAF* kinase gene (*BRAF-V600E*)**. This disease is seen in older men (median age, 52 years) who present with pancytopenia, abnormal *circulating* lymphocytes, and massive splenomegaly. The abnormal lymphocytes seen on peripheral smear are small, mature B cells with highly characteristic "hairy"

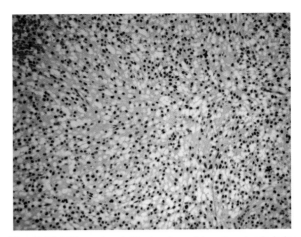

Fig. 13.22 Diffuse, lacy infiltrate of small lymphocytes in hairy cell leukemia (bone marrow biopsy).

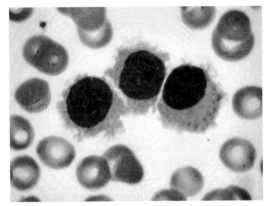

Fig. 13.20 Small mature lymphoid cells with hairy cytoplasmic projections in hairy cell leukemia.

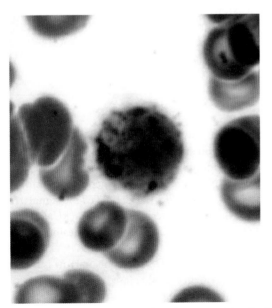

Fig. 13.21 Tartrate-resistant acid phosphatase staining *(red)* in hairy cell leukemia.

cytoplasmic projections (Fig. 13.20). Hairy cells express high levels of **tartrate-resistant acid phosphatase (TRAP)** (Fig. 13.21) as well as CD11c, CD25, CD103, and annexin A1. Although lymphocytes normally express acid phosphatase, acid phosphatase isoenzyme 5 is expressed only by hairy cells. Acid phosphatase isoenzyme 5 is the only acid phosphatase isoenzyme that is resistant to inhibition by tartrate. Hairy cells produce large amounts of tumor necrosis factor α, a cytokine that stimulates growth of hairy cells and inhibits normal hematopoiesis. The marrow space is extensively, if not completely, replaced by a diffuse, lacy infiltrate of small lymphoid cells (Fig. 13.22). The splenomegaly results from diffuse red pulp infiltration by hairy cells. The leading cause of death in hairy cell leukemia is infection. The high risk of infection likely results from a combination of neutropenia, monocytopenia, and decreased natural killer (NK) cell function. Treatment consists of purine analogs that interfere with DNA synthesis.

Large granular lymphocytic (LGL) leukemia consists of two distinct diseases that share one morphologic feature: the presence in blood of numerous large lymphocytes with abundant granular cytoplasm (Fig. 13.23). **T-cell LGL leukemia** is composed of clonal CD3+ CD8+ cytotoxic T cells that coexpress the NK cell marker CD16. T-cell LGL leukemia is a generally indolent condition most often seen in older adults and marked by chronic neutropenia, recurrent infections, and splenomegaly, as well as a variety of autoimmune

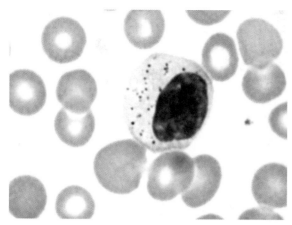

Fig. 13.23 Large granular lymphocyte (LGL) in large granular lymphocytic leukemia (peripheral smear).

conditions, including rheumatoid arthritis, pure red cell aplasia, and autoimmune hemolytic anemia. **NK cell LGL leukemia** is composed of clonal CD3− CD8+ NK cells that are infected by Epstein-Barr virus. NK cell LGL leukemia is a rare, highly aggressive condition most often seen in adolescents and young adults and marked by fever, anemia, thrombocytopenia, hepatosplenomegaly, coagulopathy, and hemophagocytic syndrome. **Indolent NK cell lymphocytosis** is a condition most often seen in adults and marked by chronic non-progressive NK cell lymphocytosis (CD3− CD8+ CD16+) without fever, lymphadenopathy, or hepatosplenomegaly.

MYELODYSPLASTIC SYNDROMES

KEY POINTS

- Myelodysplastic syndrome (MDS) is a family of primary neoplastic conditions of the bone marrow characterized by ineffective dysplastic hematopoiesis, leading to peripheral blood cytopenia.
- Cytogenetic defects include chromosome loss and gene promoter hypermethylation with loss of function of suppressor oncogenes.
- Mutations involve genes for RNA splicing and epigenetic modification.
- Secondary myelodysplasia is a reactive, reversible condition associated with human immunodeficiency syndrome infection, autoimmune conditions, toxins, and drugs.
- MDS is largely subclassified based on the degree of dysplasia (unilineage or multilineage) and the blast count in the blood and marrow.
- High-grade MDS (refractory cytopenia with excess blasts), with marrow blast counts ranging from 5% to 19% in marrow (2%–19% in blood), is associated with a high risk of transformation to AML.

Myelodysplastic syndrome is a neoplastic leukemia-like condition of the bone marrow characterized by peripheral cytopenia (anemia, neutropenia, thrombocytopenia, or a combination of these) and disordered (dysplastic) hematopoiesis (Figs. 13.24 and 13.25). A common finding on peripheral smear is the presence of abnormal neutrophils with dumbbell-shaped bilobed nuclei, a finding referred to as **acquired Pelger-Huët anomaly** (Fig. 13.26). The primary Pelger-Huët anomaly is a benign autosomal dominant condition of terminal neutrophil differentiation caused by defects in the *lamin B receptor* gene.

Common chromosome defects in MDS include del(5q), monosomy 5, trisomy 8, monosomy 7, and loss of the Y chromosome. Chromosome deletion likely leads to haploinsufficiency or loss of tumor suppressor genes. Common mutations in MDS occur in genes involved in **RNA splicing** (*SF3B1*), **epigenetic modification** (*ASXL1, DNMT3A, EZH2, TET2*), **signal transduction** (*JAK2*), **transcription factors** (*RUNX1*), **DNA damage response** (*TP53*), and **cohesion complex** (*STAG2*).

In most cases of MDS, the bone marrow is hypercellular with evidence of increased apoptosis. The paradoxical phenomenon of marrow hyperplasia and blood cytopenia results from high rates of both cell proliferation and cell death within the marrow, a process termed

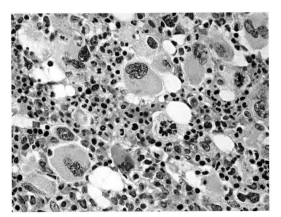

Fig. 13.24 Hypercellular marrow with numerous dysplastic megakaryocytes in an erythroid-predominant background (myelodysplastic syndrome).

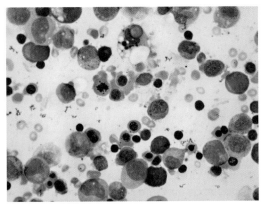

Fig. 13.25 Marrow smear with dysmyelopoiesis and dyserythropoiesis (myelodysplastic syndrome).

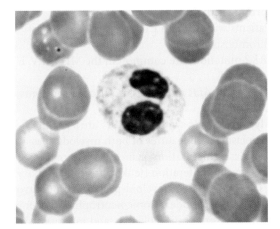

Fig. 13.26 Abnormal neutrophil with hypogranular cytoplasm and bilobed nucleus (pseudo-Pelger-Huët anomaly in myelodysplastic syndrome).

ineffective hematopoiesis. Blasts (nonlymphoid) in MDSs may range from normal (<5% in marrow and 0% in blood) to increased (5%–19% in blood, marrow, or both). In contrast, blast counts of more than 19% in blood or marrow trigger a diagnosis of AML.

In contrast to primary MDS, **secondary myelodysplasia** is a nonclonal disease, lacks any cytogenetic abnormality, and is associated with a primary condition, such as human immunodeficiency syndrome infection, autoimmune disease, toxin exposure, or certain drugs. Unlike primary MDS, secondary myelodysplasia is a potentially reversible condition if the primary condition is controlled. Other conditions to be excluded include **congenital dyserythropoietic anemia** (in infants and young children) and megaloblastic anemia caused by folate or vitamin B_{12} deficiency. These two conditions, like primary MDS, are marked by dyserythropoiesis.

Primary MDS is primarily subclassified based on the degree of dysplasia, the blast count, and the presence of specific gene mutations or chromosome deletions. MDS with no increase in blasts (<1% in blood and <5% in marrow) is termed **MDS with unilineage or multilineage dysplasia.** Some cases are marked by increased ringed sideroblasts (Fig. 13.27), nucleated RBCs in marrow that contain numerous ferritin-laden mitochondria that form rings around the nuclei. **MDS with increased ring sideroblasts** is associated with mutations of the **SF3B1** gene, which encodes for an RNA splicing factor.

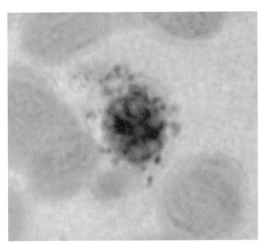

Fig. 13.27 Nucleated RBC with multiple perinuclear iron-positive *(blue)* granules (ringed sideroblast) in myelodysplastic syndrome (bone marrow aspirate).

Ringed sideroblasts are seen in a variety of conditions known collectively as the sideroblastic anemias. **Sideroblastic anemia** is marked by anemia, increased ringed sideroblasts, and decreased heme biosynthesis. Sideroblastic anemia is seen not only in MDS but also secondary to drugs (e.g., ethanol, isoniazid, chloramphenicol), toxins (lead, zinc), and nutritional deficiency (pyridoxine, copper). Some rare hereditary forms of sideroblastic anemia are also described. The most common of these is the X-linked form caused by defects in ALA synthase, the enzyme that catalyzes the rate-limiting step in heme biosynthesis.

Myelodysplastic syndrome with increased blasts (2%–19% in blood and 5%–19% in marrow) is termed **MDS with excess blasts**. The prognosis of primary MDS largely rests on the severity of the cytopenia (and risk of bleeding and sepsis) and the probability of progression to AML. The risk of progression to AML varies from less than 10% for refractory cytopenia to 30% to 40% for refractory cytopenia with excess blasts. The term **clonal hematopoiesis of undetermined significance (CHUS)** is applied to cases with a clonal genetic abnormality but with no evidence of a hematologic neoplasm (including dysplasia and cytopenia). Cases of chronic sustained cytopenia (>6 months) without dysplasia and MDS-related cytogenetic defects are termed **idiopathic cytopenia of undetermined significance (ICUS)**. Some clonal neoplastic myeloid disorders express both myelodysplastic and myeloproliferative features. These disorders, termed **MDS/MPN neoplasms**, are characterized by myeloid-predominant hypercellularity of the marrow with less than 20% blasts in blood and bone marrow, dysplastic maturation, high leukocyte count (often monocytosis), and thrombocytosis. These diseases are covered under the discussion of MPN.

MYELOPROLIFERATIVE NEOPLASMS

KEY POINTS

- Myeloproliferative neoplasms (MPNs) are a family of clonal neoplastic bone marrow stem cell disorders associated with hyperproliferation of marrow cells and increased blood cell counts.
- They are most commonly seen in older adults.
- Four major subtypes are defined by the predominant peripheral blood findings of polycythemia (polycythemia vera [PV]), left-shifted leukocytosis (chronic myelogenous leukemia), thrombocytosis (essential thrombocythemia [ET]), or leukoerythroblastosis and marrow fibrosis (chronic idiopathic myelofibrosis [CIMF]).
- The clinical presentation is often vague and nonspecific but may include plethora, headaches, and pruritus in PV; fatigue and fever in chronic myelogenous leukemia and CIMF; and bleeding in ET.
- Massive splenomegaly is common in chronic myelogenous leukemia and CIMF.
- The risk of progression to acute leukemia ranges from very low in ET to very high in chronic myelogenous leukemia; acute leukemia after chronic myelogenous leukemia may be myeloid or lymphoid.
- Chronic myelogenous leukemia is associated with the specific chromosomal translocation t(9;22) involving the PML gene on chromosome 9 and the *ABL* gene on chromosome 22 with production of a hybrid BCR-ABL tyrosine kinase protein with transforming activity.
- Patients with PV and ET have increased risk of thrombosis.
- *JAK2* mutations are common in the MPNs PV, ET, and CIMF.
- *MPL* and *CALR* mutations are also seen in some cases of MPN.
- Myelodysplastic syndrome/MPN are a group of neoplasms with features of both myelodysplasia (dysplastic maturation or ineffective hematopoiesis) and myeloproliferation (leukocytosis, thrombocytosis, or hypercellular myeloid-predominant marrow).
- Rare MPNs include chronic neutrophilic leukemia, chronic eosinophilic leukemia, and mastocytosis.

The MPNs are a family of clonal neoplastic diseases of the bone marrow most often encountered in middle-aged to older adults who present with symptoms related to marked increase in RBC, leukocyte, or platelet count. Patients with **polycythemia vera (PV)** often present with plethora, headaches, and pruritus that are related to increased blood viscosity caused by increased RBC mass. Patients with chronic myelogenous leukemia and **primary myelofibrosis (PMF)** often present with fatigue, fever, and abdominal discomfort caused by splenomegaly. Patients with **essential thrombocythemia (ET)** may present with platelet-type bleeding (mucosal bleeding or petechiae) or thrombosis caused by abnormal platelet function.

In contrast to MDS, the clonal stem cell defects in the MPNs lead to nondysplastic cell maturation with production of increased numbers of blood cells, that is, polycythemia, leukocytosis, or thrombocythemia. The increased apoptosis of marrow precursors leading to ineffective hematopoiesis characteristic of myelodysplasia is not seen in the MPNs. However, like MDS, MPN may progress to acute leukemia.

The most common MPN is **chronic myelogenous leukemia**. This neoplasm nearly always presents with marked neutrophilic leukocytosis with left shift (increased numbers of immature neutrophil precursors), basophilia, and absence of monocytosis (Fig. 13.28). The bone marrow is markedly hypercellular and myeloid predominant with increased numbers of small (dwarf) megakaryocytes (Fig. 13.29). The diagnosis is established by cytogenetic detection of the **Philadelphia**

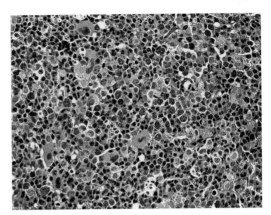

Fig. 13.29 Markedly hypercellular marrow with striking myeloid predominance in chronic myelogenous leukemia.

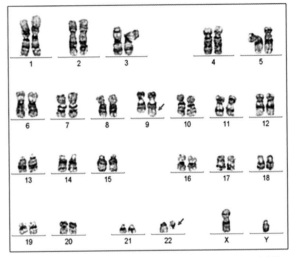

46,XY,t(9;22)(q34.12;q11.23)

Fig. 13.30 Karyotype with a t(9;22) translocation characteristic of chronic myelogenous leukemia. (Provided by Dr. Peining Li of the Yale University Department of Genetics.)

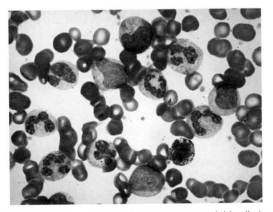

Fig. 13.28 Peripheral smear with numerous myeloid cells (neutrophils, metamyelocytes, and myelocytes) and rare blasts *(lower middle of field)* in chronic myelogenous leukemia.

chromosome, an abnormally shortened chromosome 22 caused by translocation of a portion of chromosome 22 to chromosome 9, in pluripotential stem cells (Fig. 13.30). The t(9;22) translocation creates a ***BCR-ABL*** fusion gene whose 210-kDa protein product is a potent tyrosine phosphokinase with transforming activity. Inhibition of the BCR-ABL protein by the drug imatinib mesylate often contributes to early remission of the disease when administered with standard cytotoxic agents.

It is important to distinguish a **leukemoid reaction**—marked reactive leukocytosis associated with infection, inflammation, or nonhematologic malignancy—from chronic myelogenous leukemia. Unlike chronic myelogenous leukemia, leukemoid reactions are not associated with significant peripheral blood myeloid immaturity (myelocytes or promyelocytes), basophilia, or splenomegaly. Whereas the neutrophils in leukemoid reaction express high levels of **leukocyte alkaline phosphatase (LAP)** (Fig. 13.31), the neutrophils in chronic myelogenous leukemia are LAP negative. Although the clinical setting usually distinguishes these two disorders, absence of the Philadelphia chromosome excludes chronic myelogenous leukemia.

After several years, nearly all cases of chronic myelogenous leukemia undergo transformation to acute leukemia (with >20% blasts) caused by acquisition of additional somatic mutations by the chronic myelogenous leukemia clone. This event, termed **blast crisis**, is often accompanied by new onset of fever, weight loss, and lymphadenopathy. In many cases, the progression to blast crisis is gradual and preceded by a period when the blast count varies between 5% and 19%, a stage of chronic myelogenous leukemia termed the **accelerated phase**. Chronic myelogenous leukemia blast crisis yields AML in 80% of cases and acute lymphoid leukemia in 20% of cases. A mainstay of initial treatment for chronic myelogenous leukemia is the synthetic BCR-ABL inhibitor **imatinib mesylate**. Inhibition of the BCR-ABL tyrosine kinase oncoprotein by imatinib markedly inhibits growth of the neoplastic myeloid clone, leading to a complete hematologic response in nearly all (96%) newly diagnosed cases of chronic myelogenous leukemia. However, imatinib is not a curative agent because fewer than 10% of treated patients sustain a complete molecular response, defined as undetectable levels of *BCR-ABL* mRNA (by nested reverse transcription polymerase chain reaction). Other chemotherapy agents useful in chronic myelogenous leukemia include interferon-α, hydroxyurea, and cytarabine.

Chronic neutrophilic leukemia is a rare neoplasm characterized by sustained peripheral blood and marrow neutrophilia without significant left shift; hepatosplenomegaly; absence of Philadelphia chromosome or *BCR-ABL* fusion gene; absence of *PDGFR* or fibroblast growth factor receptor (*FGFR*) rearrangements; and no evidence of a chronic infectious or inflammatory disorder, myelodysplasia, or other MPN.

Chronic eosinophilic leukemia is a clonal neoplasm of eosinophilic precursors that presents with sustained eosinophilia of blood and marrow with 5% to 19% blasts and frequent involvement of other organs (heart, lung, CNS, skin, or gastrointestinal [GI] tract), with absence of Philadelphia chromosome, and *PDGFR* and *FGFR* rearrangements. Release of toxic cationic granular proteins by the infiltrating eosinophils often leads to tissue damage. The term **idiopathic hypereosinophilic syndrome** is applied to similar cases in which, despite the lack of evidence of a secondary cause (parasite or drug) for the eosinophilia, there is no clear evidence of eosinophilic clonality (<5% blasts).

A separate category of clonal neoplastic diseases associated with **eosinophilia** and abnormalities of *PDGFRα, PDGFRβ,* or *FGFR1* genes has been described. These genes encode for receptor tyrosine kinase growth factor receptors that transmit proliferative signals to cells. In most cases, the presentation is that of CMML, with some cases presenting as acute myelogenous leukemia or lymphoblastic leukemia/lymphoma.

Mastocytosis is a clonal neoplastic disorder characterized by proliferation of abnormal mast cells that accumulate in a variety of organs, including the skin, spleen, lymph nodes, liver, and GI tract. Whereas disease confined to the skin is referred to as *cutaneous mastocytosis*, mastocytosis involving extracutaneous sites is termed *systemic mastocytosis*. Whereas cutaneous mastocytosis is most common in young children, systemic mastocytosis is most common in young adults. Rarely,

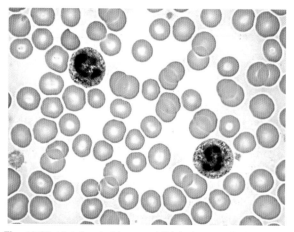

Fig. 13.31 High level of (neutrophilic) leukocyte alkaline phosphatase in leukemoid reaction (peripheral smear).

increased circulating mast cells with significant involvement of marrow are seen, a condition referred to as *mast cell leukemia*. Mast cells can be identified by immunohistochemical staining for mast cell tryptase and stem cell factor (SCF) receptor (CD117). Neoplastic mast cells often abnormally express T-cell markers CD2, CD25, or both.

Polycythemia vera is an MPN marked by erythrocytosis (increased RBC mass) and usually accompanied by neutrophilia, thrombocytosis, and splenomegaly. PV most commonly occurs in older adults (average age, 60 years), who may present with headache, plethora, weakness, dizziness, pruritus, and sweating. Many of these symptoms are related to sluggish blood flow caused by increased blood viscosity (because of the increased hematocrit). Thrombotic complications are common and a major factor in morbidity. Treatment often consists of phlebotomy to reduce the hematocrit and the myelosuppressive agent hydroxyurea to control leukocytosis and thrombocytosis. A significant percentage (15%) of patients with PV progress to end-stage myelofibrosis. In contrast to secondary polycythemia, patients with PV are nonhypoxic (normal PaO_2) with decreased plasma erythropoietin (EPO) levels. *JAK2* mutation is present in nearly all cases of PV.

Secondary polycythemia may be seen in several settings. In patients who inherit a high oxygen affinity hemoglobin variant, inadequate tissue oxygenation induces increased EPO synthesis and EPO-mediated polycythemia. Secondary polycythemia may be seen in patients with chronic hypoxia caused by chronic lung disease, heavy smoking, obesity, sleep apnea, life at high altitude, or cyanotic heart disease. Secondary polycythemia may also be seen in nonhypoxic situations, including solid tumors, benign renal disease, endocrine disorders, and chronic administration of EPO or androgens.

Essential thrombocythemia is an MPN characterized by sustained thrombocytosis, often accompanied by mild anemia, leukocytosis, and mild splenomegaly. ET usually presents in older adults, age 50 to 70 years, with asymptomatic thrombocytosis, often with platelet counts exceeding $1 \times 10^6/\mu L$. The bone marrow is hypercellular, with clusters of giant megakaryocytes that have hyperlobulated nuclei (Fig. 13.32). Because platelet function is often abnormal, patients may experience not only thrombosis but also mucocutaneous bleeding. The prognosis in ET is quite good; the risk of progression to AML is less than 5%. Therefore, ET may be untreated if asymptomatic. Drugs used to reduce the platelet count

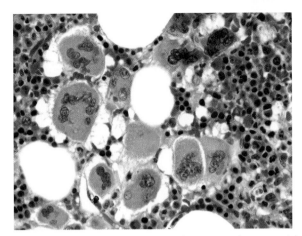

Fig. 13.32 Numerous giant megakaryocytes in essential thrombocythemia.

include hydroxyurea, a myelosuppressive agent, and anagrelide, which blocks megakaryocyte production of platelets.

Because thrombocytosis is common in other subtypes of MPN, it is important to exclude chronic myelogenous leukemia (CML), polycythemia vera (PV), and chronic idiopathic myelofibrosis (CIMF) by demonstrating absence of t(9;22), erythrocytosis, and marrow fibrosis. In addition, it is important to exclude reactive thrombocytosis. Sustained **reactive thrombocytosis** may be seen in a variety of clinical settings, including chronic infection, chronic inflammatory disease, iron deficiency, hemolytic anemia, and cancer.

No mutations in EPO, TPO, or their receptors have been described in PV and ET. Instead, committed hematopoietic elements in each disease are hyperresponsive to their respective growth factors, EPO and TPO. In PV, the increased number of EPO receptor-bearing RBCs leads to negative feedback on renal synthesis of EPO; thus, EPO levels are decreased in PV. In contrast, in ET, the TPO receptor-deficient platelets fail to reduce free TPO levels. Despite reduced TPO binding by megakaryocytes, megakaryocyte growth is increased because of a supra-optimal response to TPO.

Chronic idiopathic myelofibrosis (CIMF) is a chronic MPN usually seen in older adults who present with fatigue, night sweats, weight loss, bone pain, and hepatosplenomegaly, anemia, leukocytosis, thrombocytosis, and massive splenomegaly. The blood count reveals anemia, leukocytosis, and thrombocytosis. The disease is

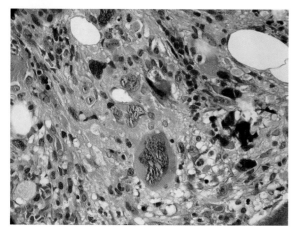

Fig. 13.33 Clusters of bizarre megakaryocytes in chronic idiopathic myelofibrosis.

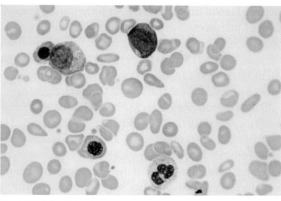

Fig. 13.35 Peripheral smear in myelofibrosis with a nucleated red blood cell (RBC), dacrocytes (teardrop-shaped RBCs), and myeloid left shift (promyelocyte and myelocyte).

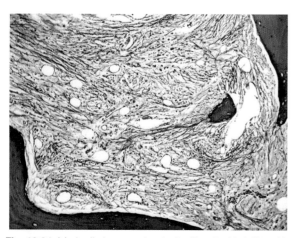

Fig. 13.34 Markedly increased reticulin fibrosis *(dark fibers)* in myelofibrosis (marrow biopsy reticulin stain).

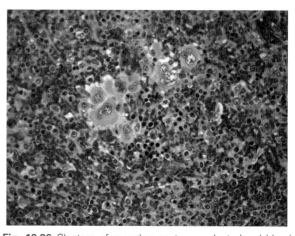

Fig. 13.36 Clusters of megakaryocytes, nucleated red blood cells, and immature myeloid cells in the splenic red pulp (extramedullary hematopoiesis).

marked by slowly progressive marrow fibrosis because of fibroblast proliferation stimulated by **platelet-derived growth factor** released from abnormal (clonal) megakaryocytes (Figs. 13.33 and 13.34). The classic triad of dacrocytes (teardrop-shaped RBCs), nucleated RBCs, and myeloid left shift noted on peripheral blood smears (Fig. 13.35) reflects the infiltrative nature of the myelofibrosis, as normal hematopoiesis is crowded out of the marrow and into the spleen and liver, a process termed **extramedullary hematopoiesis** (Fig. 13.36). Major complications of CIMF include infection (caused by immune deficiency), hemorrhage (caused by dysfunctional platelets), and conversion to AML. A commonly used chemotherapeutic agent in CIMF is hydroxyurea.

A single point mutation in the *JAK2* gene has been described in most cases of PV and about half of all cases of ET and CIMF. The JAK2 protein is a receptor-associated **tyrosine kinase** that is bound to the cytoplasmic domains of cell membrane receptors, including EPO and TPO receptors. Binding of ligand (EPO and TPO) to receptor (EPO receptor and TPO receptor) induces JAK-mediated phosphorylation of several downstream signaling molecules, including **signal transducer and activator of transcription (STAT)**. Phosphorylated STAT migrates to the nucleus, binds to specific gene regulatory sequences, and either activates or represses transcription of specific target genes. The point mutation in *JAK2* is located within the autoinhibitory domain and leads to constitutive (growth factor-independent) JAK2 tyrosine kinase activity and consequential STAT-activated cell proliferation.

Mutations of CALR and MPL genes are also commonly seen in MDS. **CALR** (**calreticulin**) is a calcium-binding protein involved in glycoprotein folding within the endoplasmic reticulum. The **MPL** gene encodes for the megakaryocyte thrombopoietin (TPO) receptor. Binding of TPO to MPL induces megakaryocyte growth and platelet production.

MYELODYSPLASTIC/ MYELOPROLIFERATIVE DISEASES

Some clonal neoplastic marrow neoplasms are characterized by simultaneous ineffective dysplastic hematopoiesis of some lines (MDS-like) and hyperplastic hematopoiesis of other lines (MPN-like). This group of neoplasms includes CMML, JMML, atypical chronic myelogenous leukemia, and MDS/MPN unclassifiable. Patients with these disorders most often present with peripheral blood leukocytosis and a hypercellular myeloid-predominant marrow with dysplastic features.

Chronic myelomonocytic leukemia is a disease of older adults characterized by persistent monocytosis (Fig. 13.37), a hypercellular myeloid-predominant marrow with less than 20% blasts, dysgranulopoiesis, and absence of t(9;22) (BCR-ABL translocation). In most cases, no cytogenetic defect is noted, but a mutation of *ASXL1, TET2, SETBP1,* or *SRSF2* is seen in most cases.

Juvenile myelomonocytic leukemia (JMML) is a disease of young children (younger than 3 years) characterized by monocytosis, left-shifted neutrophilia, a hypercellular myeloid-predominant marrow with less than 20% blasts, and absence of the t(9;22) translocation. As in CMML, no specific cytogenetic defects are present, but *Ras* gene mutations are common. Infiltration of vital organs by the neoplastic myeloid cells is associated with a poor outcome. Hemoglobin F levels are characteristically increased. In vitro studies have demonstrated that the myeloid progenitors in JMML are hypersensitive to the growth-promoting effects of granulocyte–macrophage colony-stimulating factor. JMML is often seen in association with hereditary neurofibromatosis type I.

Atypical chronic myelogenous leukemia is a neoplasm characterized by neutrophilic leukocytosis, thrombocytopenia, a hypercellular myeloid-predominant marrow, myeloid dysplasia, and absence of basophilia, monocytosis, and *BCR-ABL* translocation.

Clonal neoplastic disorders that present with both myelodysplastic and myeloproliferative features but do not meet criteria for CMML, atypical chronic myelogenous leukemia, or JMML are currently classified as **MDS/MPN unclassifiable**.

KEY WORDS AND CONCEPTS

- Accelerated phase
- Acquired Pelger-Huët anomaly
- Acute erythroid leukemia (AML-M6)
- Acute megakaryoblastic leukemia (AML-M7)
- Acute monoblastic/monocytic leukemia (AML-M5)
- Acute myelomonocytic leukemia (AML-M4)
- Acute promyelocytic leukemia (AML-M3)
- Alkylating agents
- Allantoin
- Allogeneic (or autologous) stem cell transplantation
- Allopurinol
- All-*trans* retinoic acid (ATRA)
- AML with 11q23 abnormalities

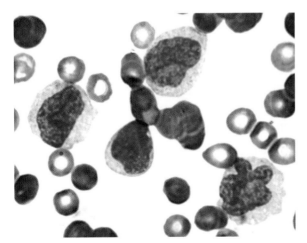

Fig. 13.37 Increased abnormal monocytes in chronic myelomonocytic leukemia (peripheral blood).

- AML with maturation (AML-M2)
- AML with minimal differentiation (AML-M0)
- AML with multilineage dysplasia
- AML without maturation (AML-M1)
- Apoptosis
- Atypical chronic myelogenous leukemia
- B cell lymphoblastic leukemia/lymphoma
- B cell lymphoblastic lymphoma (B-LBL)
- *BCR-ABL*
- Blast crisis
- Bone marrow stem cell transplantation
- *BRAF* kinase gene *(BRAF-V600E)*
- *CALR* (calreticulin)
- Chronic eosinophilic leukemia
- Chronic idiopathic myelofibrosis (CIMF)
- Chronic lymphocytic leukemia (CLL)
- Chronic myelogenous leukemia
- Chronic myeloid leukemia (CML)
- Chronic myelomonocytic leukemia (CMML)
- Chronic neutrophilic leukemia
- Clonal hematopoiesis of indeterminant potential
- Cohesion complex
- Common B-ALL
- Congenital dyserythropoietic anemia
- Consolidation
- Cytotoxic chemotherapeutic drugs
- Disseminated intravascular coagulation (DIC)
- DNA damage response
- Early precursor B-ALL
- Eosinophilia
- Epigenetic modification
- Essential thrombocythemia (ET)
- Extramedullary hematopoiesis
- *FGFR1*
- Hairy cell leukemia
- *HOX*
- Hyperdiploidy
- Idiopathic cytopenia of undetermined significance

- Idiopathic hypereosinophilic syndrome
- Imatinib
- Imatinib mesylate
- Indolent NK cell lymphocytosis
- Induction
- Ineffective hematopoiesis
- Intrathecal chemotherapy
- inv(16), t(16;16)
- *JAK2*
- Juvenile myelomonocytic leukemia (JMML)
- Large granular lymphocytic (LGL) leukemia
- Lamin B receptor gene
- Leukemia
- Leukemoid reaction
- Mastocytosis
- MDS with excess blasts
- MDS with increased ring sideroblasts
- MDS with unilineage or multilineage dysplasia
- MDS/MPN unclassifiable
- MDS/MPN neoplasms
- *MPL*
- Myelodysplastic syndrome (MDS)
- Myeloablative therapy
- NK cell LGL leukemia
- Oncogenes
- Pancytopenia
- ***PDGFRα***
- ***PDGFRβ***
- Philadelphia chromosome
- Platelet-derived growth factor
- Polycythemia vera (PV)
- Pre-B-ALL
- Precursor B cell ALL (B-ALL)
- Primary myelofibrosis
- Prolymphocytic transformation
- *Ras*
- Rasburicase
- Reactive thrombocytosis

- Refractory anemia
- Remission
- Richter transformation
- RNA splicing
- Secondary myelodysplasia
- Secondary polycythemia
- *SF3B1*
- Sideroblastic anemia
- Signal transducer and activator of transcription (STAT)
- t(8;21)

- Tartrate-resistant acid phosphatase (TRAP)
- T-cell ALL (T-ALL)
- T cell LGL leukemia
- Topoisomerase type II inhibitors
- Tumor lysis syndrome
- Transcription factors
- Tyrosine kinase
- Uric acid
- Zeta-associated protein (ZAP-70)

REVIEW QUESTIONS

1. Which of the following is **not** a feature of ET?
   A. Elevated platelet count
   B. Hypercellular marrow with fibrosis
   C. Thrombosis
   D. Mild splenomegaly

2. Which of the following is **not** a characteristic laboratory feature of tumor lysis syndrome?
   A. Hyperkalemia
   B. Hyperphosphatemia
   C. Hyperuricemia
   D. Hypercalcemia

3. Which neoplastic condition below is **not** classified as an MPN?
   A. CML
   B. Chronic idiopathic myelofibrosis
   C. Refractory anemia
   D. PV

4. Causes of secondary polycythemia include all **except**
   A. low-affinity hemoglobin.
   B. mountain life.
   C. sleep apnea,
   D. cyanotic heart disease.

14

Lymphoma and Related Disorders

KEY POINTS

- Lymphomas are malignant clonal neoplasms of lymphocytes.

- Lymphomas are classified by cell of origin (B, T, or natural killer cell), degree of maturation (immature [blastic], or mature), cell size (small or large), mitotic rate (low or high), histologic pattern (nodular, diffuse, or sinusoidal), immunophenotype (e.g., CD10+ Bcl-6+ germinal center B cell, CD5+ B cell, cyclin D1+ mantle B cell), and cytogenetics (e.g., t(8;14), t(14;18), t(11;14), t(2;5)).

- Lymphoma often presents with painless lymphadenopathy or mass lesions in extranodal sites such as the skin and gastrointestinal tract; some lymphomas present with significant blood and marrow involvement (leukemic presentation).

- Hodgkin lymphoma differs from non-Hodgkin lymphoma in several ways: bimodal age distribution; uncommon extranodal disease; common symptoms of malaise, fever, and weight loss; and unique histology with peculiar B cell–derived Reed-Sternberg tumor cells accompanied by a usually prominent reactive cellular background.

- Several chromosome translocations in B-cell lymphoma lead to overexpression of oncoproteins that in turn leads to unregulated proliferation (e.g., c-Myc in Burkitt lymphoma, cyclin D1 in mantle cell

lymphoma, ALK-1 in anaplastic large cell lymphoma) and inhibition of apoptosis (e.g., Bcl-2 in follicular lymphoma and API2-MALT1 in mucosa-associated lymphoid tissue lymphoma).

- Plasma cell neoplasms include plasma cell myeloma, plasmacytoma, and monoclonal gammopathy of undetermined significance.

- Amyloidosis is a disease process caused by deposition of insoluble fibrillar protein in a variety of tissues that leads to tissue damage and organ failure. In some cases, the abnormal protein is derived from immunoglobulin (Ig) light chain produced by plasma cells, and in other cases, the amyloid protein is derived from serum amyloid A, an acute phase reactant produced in chronic inflammatory states, or transthyretin, a thyroxine and retinol transporter.

- Cryoglobulinemia is a clinicopathologic condition caused by intravascular deposition of cold-precipitable Ig protein that leads to necrotizing vasculitis and tissue damage.

- Tumors of histiocytes and dendritic cells include Langerhans cell histiocytosis, histiocytic sarcoma, follicular dendritic cell sarcoma, interdigitating dendritic cell sarcoma, and blastic plasmacytoid dendritic cell neoplasm.

Lymphomas are malignant neoplasms of lymphocytes that arise most often in lymph nodes and other lymphoid organs such as the spleen and thymus. Lymphoid malignancies that arise in the bone marrow are classified as lymphoid leukemias because they present primarily with bone marrow failure and blood involvement rather than lymphadenopathy. Lymphomas are

broadly classified into **Hodgkin lymphoma** and **non-Hodgkin lymphoma**.

Non-Hodgkin lymphoma is far more common than Hodgkin lymphoma. Although both diseases often present with painless lymph node enlargement (lymphadenopathy), Hodgkin lymphoma, more often than non-Hodgkin lymphoma, presents with systemic symptoms of fever, night sweats, and weight loss. Whereas non-Hodgkin lymphoma often presents with widespread (generalized) lymphadenopathy and extranodal disease, Hodgkin lymphoma most often presents with localized nodal disease and only rarely involves extranodal sites. Bone marrow involvement is more common in non-Hodgkin lymphoma. The age distribution of Hodgkin lymphoma is bimodal, with a peak in young adults and a slow rise after the age of 50 years. In contrast, the age distribution of non-Hodgkin lymphoma is unimodal, with a steady rise with advancing age. Some infectious agents, including **Epstein-Barr virus (EBV), human T-cell lymphotrophic virus type 1 (HTLV-1)**, and *Helicobacter pylori*, are implicated as etiologic agents in specific subtypes of lymphoma. Some non-Hodgkin lymphomas are associated with specific chromosome translocations of proto-oncogenes into either the immunoglobulin (Ig) (in B-cell lymphoma) or the T-cell receptor (TCR) (in T-cell lymphoma) gene locus. Translocation into these active sites results in markedly increased oncogene expression. Translocated oncogenes of this sort include *c-Myc* in Burkitt lymphoma, *cyclin D1* in marginal cell lymphoma, *Bcl-2* in **follicular lymphoma (FL)**, and *Bcl-6* in diffuse large B-cell lymphoma. In Hodgkin lymphoma, although no specific gene defects are known, recurrent gains on chromosomes 2, 9, and 12, and amplifications on chromosomes 4 and 9 have been described.

Non-Hodgkin lymphoma represents about 5% of all malignancies. Most (90%) are B-cell lymphomas; the other 10% are T or **natural killer (NK) cell** lymphomas. The most common subtypes of non-Hodgkin lymphoma in the United States are diffuse large B-cell lymphoma (31%) and FL (22%) (Table 14.1). Although the overall median age at presentation of non-Hodgkin lymphoma is 60 to 70 years, some non-Hodgkin lymphoma subtypes (**mediastinal large B-cell lymphoma [MLBCL], anaplastic large cell lymphoma [ALCL]**, and Burkitt lymphoma) present at an earlier age (median age, 30–40 years). Non-Hodgkin lymphoma is generally more common in adults than in children. The most common forms of non-Hodgkin lymphoma in children include Burkitt lymphoma, ALCL, and lymphoblastic lymphoma. There is an overall slight male predominance in non-Hodgkin lymphoma that is marked in **mantle cell lymphoma (MCL)**, and a female predominance is seen with FL and primary MLBCL. Marrow involvement is common in some non-Hodgkin lymphoma subtypes, including small lymphocytic lymphoma (SLL), **lymphoplasmacytic lymphoma (LPL)**, MCL, and FL. In

TABLE 14.1 Frequency of Non-Hodgkin Lymphoma

Subtype	Frequency (%)
Diffuse large B cell	31
Follicular	22
Marginal (MALT)	8
Peripheral T cell	7
Small lymphocytic (SLL/CLL)	7
Mantle cell	6
Others	19

CLL, Chronic lymphocytic leukemia; *MALT,* mucosa-associated lymphoid tissue; *SLL,* small lymphocytic lymphoma.

general, non-Hodgkin lymphomas composed of small lymphocytes more often involve bone marrow than do lymphomas composed of large lymphocytes (Table 14.2).

Although the most common presentation of non-Hodgkin lymphoma is painless lymphadenopathy, extranodal involvement does occur. Common extranodal sites of involvement include the gastrointestinal (GI) tract, skin, bone, brain, and lung. Clinical findings at presentation that are associated with a poor prognosis include symptoms of fever, fatigue, and unexplained weight loss (so-called B symptoms). Other adverse prognostic factors include high pathologic grade (high mitotic rate, cellular anaplasia, and tumor necrosis), widespread disease (high clinical stage), advanced age (older than 60 years), elevated serum (lactate dehydrogenase) (LDH) (indicative of a large tumor burden), poor physical performance status, and extranodal disease. Involvement of the bone marrow may lead to peripheral blood cytopenia, including anemia, neutropenia, and thrombocytopenia, that in turn lead to fatigue, infection, and bleeding, respectively.

Non-Hodgkin lymphomas are classified pathologically based on histology and immunophenotype (by immunohistochemistry, flow cytometry, or both) into low- and high-grade tumors of the B, T, or NK cell type. Whereas low-grade tumors are slow-growing indolent tumors composed of relatively mature small lymphocytes, high-grade tumors are rapidly growing tumors composed of large lymphocytes or lymphoblasts.

The clonal nature of B- and T-cell lymphoma can be confirmed by Ig heavy chain gene or TCR-gamma gene polymerase chain reaction (PCR) analysis of extracted tumor DNA. PCR probes designed to flank regions of DNA that undergo rearrangement and deletion during

TABLE 14.2   **Differences Between Hodgkin and Non-Hodgkin Lymphoma**

	Hodgkin Lymphoma	Non-Hodgkin Lymphoma
Age distribution	Bimodal	Unimodal
Initial presentation	Localized nodal disease (often cervical)	Generalized nodal disease, often extranodal
Fever, night sweats, weight loss	More common	Less common
Nodal disease progression	Often contiguous	Noncontiguous
Cell of origin	Reed-Sternberg B cell	B, T, or natural killer cell
Reactive cell background	Abundant	Usually minimal
Genetic defects	Recurrent chromosome gains and amplifications	Specific oncogene translocations into antigen receptor loci

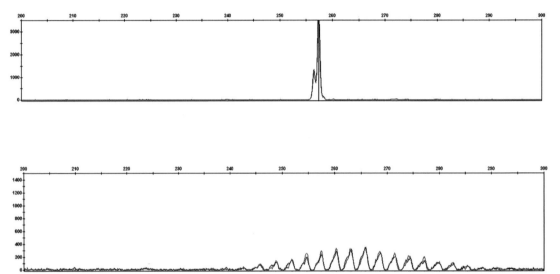

Fig. 14.1 Polymerase chain reaction for immunoglobulin (Ig) heavy chain gene rearrangement. In this example, the single peak noted on the *top chromatogram* indicates the presence in this DNA sample of a single clone of B lymphocytes (i.e., a monoclonal population). This result is most consistent with B-cell lymphoma. In contrast, the multiple small peaks noted in the *bottom chromatogram* are indicative of a polyclonal population of B lymphocytes, a result indicative of a large population of reactive (benign) B lymphocytes, each of which carries a unique Ig heavy chain rearrangement. This same approach, using T-cell receptor gene primers rather than B-cell *Ig* gene primers, can be used to evaluate T-cell lesions for clonality. (Courtesy of Dr. Pei Hui of the Yale University Department of Pathology.)

lymphocyte maturation are used. DNA from nonlymphoid cells does not yield PCR products because the distance between the unrearranged (germline) primer binding sites precludes adequate primer extension during the PCR reaction. In contrast, DNA from lymphoid cells yields amplifiable PCR products because the distance between the primer binding sites is dramatically reduced as a result of splicing out of the intervening DNA. In the case of a clonal lymphocyte infiltrate, the PCR reaction yields a prominent single (or double) product that represents the unique rearrangement or rearrangements carried by the malignant clone (Fig. 14.1). Given that diploid cells contain two copies of each autosomal gene (maternal and paternal alleles), any given clonal B or T cell can harbor either one or two rearrangements of Ig or TCR receptor gene loci, respectively. In most cases, the first attempt at rearrangement at one allele produces a functional gene product. In this case, the clonal cell population carrying the PCR-amplifiable rearranged allele, as well as the non-amplifiable unrearranged (germline) allele, yields a single major PCR product. In contrast, in cases in which the first attempt at rearrangement is unsuccessful (yielding a nonfunctional product), the lymphoid cell rearranges the second allele in hopes of producing a functional product. A tumor that derives from a cell with two rearrangements yields two major PCR products. In the case of a polyclonal (reactive) lymphoid infiltrate, the PCR reaction yields numerous products, each of which varies in length.

After a diagnosis has been established, **clinical staging** is accomplished by physical examination, CBC, bone marrow biopsy, and a variety of radiologic scan procedures that may include standard radiography (for detection of lytic lesions in plasma cell myeloma), **computed tomography (CT)**, **magnetic resonance imaging (MRI)**, and **positron emission tomography (PET)**.

Computed tomography generates a detailed three-dimensional image of the internal physical structure of the body from a large series of two-dimensional x-ray images taken around a single axis of rotation. MRI, like CT, generates a detailed internal anatomic image of the body, but unlike CT, it generates the image with a powerful magnetic field rather than ionizing x-radiation. In MRI, the magnetic field induces the protons (hydrogen atoms) in body water molecules to align with the direction of the magnetic field. Radiofrequency pulses cause the protons to temporarily change their alignment before returning to their original positions relative to the magnetic field. The resonance generated by the repeated change in proton alignment is related to the internal structure of the tissue. Tumors can be detected by MRI because the protons in the tumor tissue return to their equilibrium state at rates different from those of protons in normal surrounding tissues.

Positron emission tomography produces a three-dimensional image of the internal metabolic state of the body by detecting pairs of gamma rays (photons) emitted indirectly by a positron-emitting radionuclide that is incorporated into a nontoxic biologically active molecule that is ingested by the patient. One of the most common molecules used in PET scanning is fludeoxyglucose (FDG), a glucose analog that is taken up by metabolically active tissues. FDG PET scanning provides great detection sensitivity of rapidly growing tumors, such as lymphomas. PET-CT scanning or PET-MRI scanning can now be performed sequentially to provide even greater anatomic detail of PET active sites (Figs. 14.2 and 14.3).

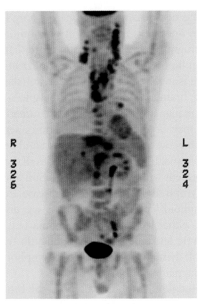

Fig. 14.2 Positron emission tomography/computed tomography scan of the neck, thorax, and abdomen. Note the presence of multiple fludeoxyglucose (FDG)-avid sites *(black)* of metabolically active tumor (lymphoma) in the neck, mediastinum, and abdomen. Note also the normal pooling of FDG in the bladder (urinary excretion).(Provided by Dr. Mehdi Djekidel, Yale University Department of Diagnostic Radiology.)

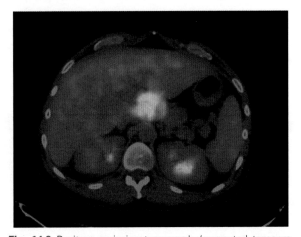

Fig. 14.3 Positron emission tomography/computed tomography scan of the abdomen. Note the fludeoxyglucose (FDG)-avid site *(yellow)* in the porta hepatis (caused by involvement by lymphoma). Whereas the positivity in the kidneys results from normal urinary excretion of FDG. The spleen appears negative *(right)*, the liver is weakly and diffusely positive *(left)*.(Provided by Dr. Mehdi Djekidel, the Yale University Department of Diagnostic Radiology.)

Stage 1 is disease confined to one site only. In stage 2, more than one site is involved but only on one side of the diaphragm. Stage 3 is disease in more than one site present on both sides of the diaphragm. In stage 4 disease, there is involvement of a vital organ (the marrow, liver, lung, brain, or kidney but not the spleen).

When malignant lymphoid cells are numerous in the blood, it may be difficult and sometimes semantic to distinguish between lymphoid leukemia and peripheralized lymphoma. Lymphoid malignancies that characteristically present with involvement of blood and marrow without lymph node or extranodal disease are referred to as lymphoid leukemias. In some cases, disease may present as either leukemia or lymphoma (e.g., **chronic lymphocytic leukemia/small lymphocytic lymphoma [CLL/SLL]**, lymphoblastic leukemia/lymphoma, adult T-cell leukemia/lymphoma).

Non-Hodgkin lymphoma subtypes are broadly classified based on cell of origin (B cell, T cell, or NK cell) and further subdivided into distinct clinicopathologic entities based on clinical presentation, histologic pattern (nodular, diffuse, or sinusoidal), cell maturation (blastic, anaplastic, or mature), cell differentiation (immunophenotype), and tumor cell cytogenetics.

Pathologic classification of non-Hodgkin lymphoma into low- and high-grade forms predicts clinical behavior. Low-grade lymphomas are slow-growing, indolent tumors that may be asymptomatic at presentation. High-grade lymphomas, on the other hand, are rapidly growing tumors often accompanied by fever, fatigue, and weight loss.

B-cell lymphomas are far more common than T-cell lymphomas, representing about 90% of all non-Hodgkin lymphoma cases in North America and Europe. Some subtypes of non-Hodgkin lymphoma occur more commonly in certain geographic regions; examples include **endemic Burkitt lymphoma** in equatorial regions, **adult T-cell leukemia/lymphoma (ATLL)** in southern Japan and the Caribbean basin, and NK/T-cell lymphoma in southern Asia.

B-CELL NON-HODGKIN LYMPHOMA

The most common B-cell lymphoma subtypes include lymphoblastic, CLL/SLL, follicular, mantle, marginal, and diffuse large cell types (Table 14.3). It is worth noting that nearly all these subtypes represent malignancies corresponding to distinct stages of normal B-cell maturation. For example, lymphoblastic lymphoma derives from precursor B lymphoblasts, SLL from naïve B cells, FL from germinal center (GC) B cells, MCL cells from pre-GC mantle zone B cells, and marginal cell lymphoma from post-GC marginal zone B cells (Fig. 14.4). Also, the growth pattern of these lymphomas often recapitulates the microanatomic distribution of their normal counterparts, such as the follicular pattern of FL, the mantle zone pattern of MCL, and the marginal zone pattern of **marginal zone lymphoma (MZL)**.

B lymphoblastic lymphoma is an uncommon high-grade neoplasm of young, often male, adults who present with rapidly growing tumors of lymph nodes, skin, or bone. The tumor cells are precursor B cells (lymphoblasts)

TABLE 14.3 Major B-Cell Lymphoma Types

Lymphoma Type	Cell of Origin	Genetic Defects	Functional Consequence
Lymphoblastic	CD19+ TdT+ B-cell progenitor	t(9;22), 11q23, t(12;21), hyperdiploidy	Poor prognosis: t(9;22), 11q23 Good prognosis: t(12;21), hyperdiploidy
Small lymphocytic	CD5+ post-GC B cells	del 13q	Deletion of regulatory microRNA
Follicular	GC B cells	*Bcl-2* translocation	Apoptosis inhibition
Mantle cell	CD5+ pre-GC mantle zone B cells	*Cyclin D1* translocation	Cell cycle progression
Marginal zone	Post-GC marginal zone B cells	*API2-MALT1* translocation	Apoptosis inhibition and cell cycle progression
Large cell	GC and postgerminal center B cells	*Bcl-6* mutations	Prevention of germinal center B-cell maturation

GC, germinal center.

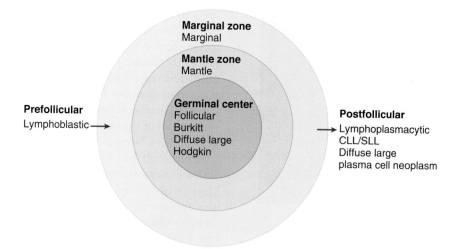

Fig. 14.4 Cellular origin of B-cell lymphoma. *CLL,* Chronic lymphocytic leukemia; *SLL,* small lymphocytic lymphoma.

that express the B cell–specific membrane protein CD19 and the lymphoblast-specific intranuclear enzyme terminal deoxynucleotidyl transferase (TdT). Although the immature cells typically do not express surface Ig, in some cases, they may express cytoplasmic mu heavy chain, a finding characteristic of late-stage precursor B cells. Many features of this disease are shared with that of B lymphoblastic leukemia, so much so that the most widely used disease classification scheme combines these two diseases together as **B lymphoblastic leukemia/ lymphoma.** However, in contrast to B lymphoblastic lymphoma, B lymphoblastic leukemia is a relatively common disease of young children who present with signs of bone marrow failure (i.e., anemia, neutropenia, thrombocytopenia, or a combination of these) along with bone pain and arthralgia. Somewhat surprisingly, the two most common cytogenetic abnormalities detected in B lymphoblastic leukemia/lymphoma, hyperdiploidy with more than 50 chromosomes per cell and translocation t(12;21) producing a ***TEL-AML1* fusion gene** of uncertain function, are associated with a favorable prognosis. Other abnormalities including hypodiploidy, t(9;22) producing a ***BCR-ABL*** fusion gene with tyrosine kinase activity and t(1;19) producing an ***E2A-PBX1* fusion gene** that may block cell differentiation are all associated with an unfavorable prognosis. More than 80% of children with B lymphoblastic leukemia are cured with multiagent chemotherapy. The most favorable outcomes are seen in children between the ages of 4 and 10 years, with a less favorable prognosis in infants and adults.

Chronic lymphocytic leukemia/small lymphocytic lymphoma is a relatively common low-grade neoplasm of older adults (mean age, 65 years), with a male predominance (male-to female ratio, 2 to 1), which presents with either generalized lymphadenopathy (a lymphomatous [SLL] presentation) or peripheral blood lymphocytosis with marrow involvement (a leukemic [CLL] presentation). In either case, most patients are asymptomatic at presentation. Progressive involvement of the bone marrow may lead to fatigue caused by anemia, pyogenic skin infections caused by neutropenia, mucocutaneous bleeding caused by thrombocytopenia, or a combination of these. Autoantibody production may lead to autoimmune hemolytic anemia, autoimmune thrombocytopenia, or both. The small tumor cells are derived from CD5+ CD23+ B cells, often with autoreactive specificity. CD5+ B cells normally represent a very small subpopulation of B cells of uncertain function located primarily in the abdominal region. The most common cytogenetic abnormalities in CLL are in the **13q14 gene** (50%), associated with indolent disease, and **trisomy 12** (20%), associated with aggressive disease. The small lymphocytic infiltrate in SLL is diffuse, often with vaguely defined aggregates of larger cells called proliferation centers (or pseudofollicles) (Fig. 14.5).

The immunophenotypic diagnosis of CLL/SLL (as well as many other lymphomas and leukemias) can be made by **flow cytometry**. In flow cytometry, single-cell suspensions prepared from fresh tissue are stained with fluorochrome-tagged antibodies specific for cellular

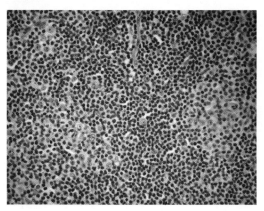

Fig. 14.5 Small lymphocytic lymphoma (lymph node) with a diffuse small lymphocytic infiltrate. Note the two poorly demarcated aggregates of larger cells called proliferation centers (or pseudofollicles).

antigens and run through a flow cytometry instrument. Although most antibodies are designed to detect cell surface antigens, intracellular antigens may also be detected in cells pretreated with permeabilizing agents. Within the instrument, the labeled single-cell suspension is focused into a narrow stream of fluid that allows only single cells to pass through one at a time (hydrodynamic focusing). The stream of cells passes through a tightly focused beam of laser light designed to stimulate fluorescence of cell-bound antibody. A set of electronic detectors instantaneously records the magnitude of the light signals emitted by each cell. These signals include the following:

1. Laser light that is deflected by the cell along the forward angle (180-degree) axis (forward scatter)
2. Laser light that is deflected by the cell along the side angle (90-degree) axis (side scatter)
3. Fluorescent light emitted by the fluorochrome-labeled antibodies bound to the cell

The magnitude of the forward scattered light is directly proportional to the size of the cell, whereas the magnitude of the side scattered light is directly proportional to the cytoplasmic granularity of the cell. After interrogation of approximately 10^4 cells per sample, the data for all three parameters from each cell can be displayed as a dot plot. On the dot plot, each cell can be plotted as a point on a two (or more) dimensional Cartesian plot. Typically, the cells are first displayed on a forward scatter (x-axis)–side scatter (y-axis) dot plot. This plot allows for identification of clusters of cell

types in a complex cell mixture. For example, in blood and marrow, this plot allows for identification of granulocyte, monocyte, and lymphocyte subpopulations (see Fig. 2.4B). By electronically gating on a cell population of interest (e.g., lymphocytes), the fluorescent data for this population can be selectively displayed to determine the precise antigen expression pattern (immunophenotype) of the cells of interest. The number of antigens that can be simultaneously evaluated on each cell is limited only by the number of fluorescent detectors on the instrument and the number of available fluorochrome-labeled antibodies with nonoverlapping emission spectra. New-generation instruments allow for six or more antigens detected per cell. Using this approach, the detailed immunophenotype of lymphomas and leukemias can be determined. For example, in the case of CLL/SLL, flow cytometry easily demonstrates the unique co-expression of CD5 and CD19 on the tumor cells (Fig. 14.6).

Chronic lymphocytic leukemia can be subclassified into two variants based on the presence or absence of somatic hypermutation of the *Ig* heavy chain locus. Under normal physiologic circumstances, naïve B cells with unmutated *Ig* genes encounter antigen within the GC and undergo somatic hypermutation of the *Ig* genes to generate functional high-affinity antibody. CLL cells with evidence of somatic hypermutation (**activated CLL**) presumably derived from mature post-GC cells) are less clinically aggressive than cases without somatic hypermutation (**naïve CLL**) presumably derived from immature pre-GC cells. These two CLL subtypes can be distinguished based on expression of two surrogate cell

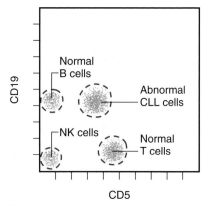

Fig. 14.6 Flow cytometry dot plots. *CLL*, Chronic lymphocytic leukemia.

membrane proteins CD38 and zeta-associated protein (ZAP-70), with positive expression marking naïve CLL (with adverse prognosis). Morphologically, CLL cells are small and "mature," with round nuclei containing irregularly clumped chromatin and indistinct nucleoli. The CD5+ B cells of the closely related (but more aggressive) neoplasm MCL, unlike CLL/SLL, typically do not coexpress the low-affinity IgE receptor protein CD23. With time, some of the small slow-growing CLL tumor cells may acquire additional new mutations that lead to transformation into either large cell lymphoma (**Richter transformation**) or **prolymphocytic leukemia**, both of which are rapidly progressive neoplasms.

Follicular lymphoma is a common, often low-grade disease of middle-aged adults who typically present with asymptomatic generalized lymphadenopathy. This disease is rare in childhood. The tumor cells are derived from CD10+ Bcl-6+ GC B cells, including a variable number of small centrocytes and large centroblasts. **Centrocytes** are small lymphocytes with irregular cleaved nuclei and indistinct nucleoli, and **centroblasts** are larger lymphocytes with non-cleaved nuclei and distinct nucleoli. Most FLs are low-grade tumors composed primarily of centrocytes (grades 1 and 2), but those composed primarily of larger centroblasts are high-grade 3 tumors. Lymph node involvement is marked by effacement (replacement) of normal architecture with abnormal, haphazardly arranged lymphoid follicles (Fig. 14.7). Bone marrow involvement at presentation is common, with a highly characteristic paratrabecular pattern of involvement (Fig. 14.8). FL cells carry the highly specific chromosome translocation **t(14;18)** involving the *Ig* heavy chain gene on chromosome 14 and the **Bcl-2** gene

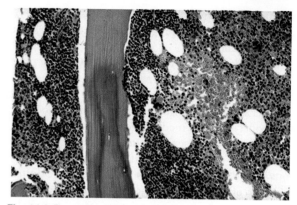

Fig. 14.8 Paratrabecular lymphoid aggregates of follicular lymphoma in bone marrow (alongside both sides of the trabecular bone). Normal marrow is on the *far right*.

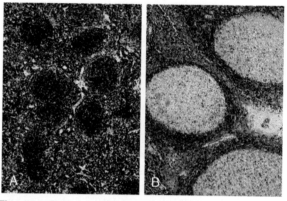

Fig. 14.9 *Bcl-2* immunostain. **A,** Follicular lymphoma, with positive staining *(red)* of the malignant follicles. **B,** Follicular hyperplasia, with negative staining *(clear nodular zones)* of the benign follicles. Note the normal *Bcl-2* positivity of the mantle zones surrounding the benign germinal centers.

on chromosome 18. Insertion of the antiapoptotic *Bcl-2* gene into the highly active Ig region leads to markedly increased production of Bcl-2 protein, which inhibits apoptotic cell death. The increased *Bcl-2* expression of FL is a powerful clue to the diagnosis because normal GC B cells do not express detectable amounts of *Bcl-2* by immunohistochemistry (Fig. 14.9). The immortalized centrocytes and centroblasts undergo slow but inexorable proliferation with progressive enlargement of affected lymph nodes. The course of the disease is indolent (5-year survival rate, >70%) but is incurable with chemotherapy alone. However, combination chemotherapy supplemented with monoclonal anti-CD20 antibody (rituximab) has led to long-term remission. In a

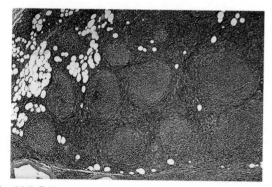

Fig. 14.7 Follicular lymphoma. Note the multiple irregular nodules (10–11) of tumor involving perinodal fat tissue.

significant minority of cases (25%–35%), further cytogenetic defects lead to progression to high-grade large B-cell lymphoma.

Diffuse large B-cell lymphoma (DLBCL), the most common lymphoma subtype in adults (also seen in childhood), is an aggressive high-grade disease that presents as a rapidly growing tumor of lymph nodes or extranodal sites. The median age of DLBCL is 64 years, with a nearly equal gender ratio. Common extranodal sites include the skin, bone, GI tract, and central nervous system (CNS). The tumor is composed of a diffuse infiltrate of large morphologically diverse lymphoid cells with numerous mitotic figures (Fig. 14.10). The most common molecular defects in DLBCL are activating translocations of *Bcl-6, Bcl-2,* and *c-Myc* genes into the Ig heavy chain gene locus. **Bcl-6** is a transcription factor that induces growth and differentiation of GC-derived B cells. Bcl-2 is an antiapoptotic protein. **c-Myc** is a transcription factor that promotes cyclin-mediated G0 to G1 cell cycle entry. Translocation of these genes into the highly active Ig heavy chain locus leads to excessive production of these three growth-promoting proteins. Two prognostic subtypes of diffuse large B-cell lymphoma, the GC type and the nongerminal (activated) type, are based on differential tumor cell expression patterns of three proteins: CD10, Bcl-6, and MUM1/IRF4. Whereas the GC type (CD10+, or Bcl-6+ and MUM1/IRF4−) is associated with a favorable prognosis, the non-GC B-cell type (CD10−, Bcl-6+/−, and

MUM1/IRF4+/−) is associated with a poor prognosis. Although aggressive, some diffuse large B-cell lymphomas are curable with combination chemotherapy, often supplemented with anti-CD20 immunotherapy. In addition to the non-GC phenotype, poor prognostic factors for diffuse large B-cell lymphoma include advanced age (older than 60 years), high serum LDH (related to large tumor burden), low physical performance status, and advanced stage with more than one extranodal site of involvement.

Burkitt lymphoma is a high-grade B-cell lymphoma with features distinct from diffuse large B-cell lymphoma. Morphologically, Burkitt lymphoma is composed of medium-sized post-GC B cells with deeply basophilic cytoplasm containing numerous small lipid vacuoles. The mitotic rate is high and apoptosis is prominent, with numerous debris-laden macrophages giving a "starry sky" appearance (Fig. 14.11). The tumor cells invariably contain one of three translocations— *t(8;14), t(2;8), or t(8;22)*—all involving the *c-Myc* gene on chromosome 8 and the Ig heavy chain, kappa light chain, or lambda light chain loci, all leading to c-Myc protein overexpression and continuous cell cycling. Burkitt lymphoma occurs sporadically throughout the world as well as specifically in two highly characteristic settings: in young children (often a jaw tumor) in malarial endemic regions of equatorial Africa and New Guinea (**endemic Burkitt lymphoma**) and in patients with immune deficiency (immunodeficiency-associated

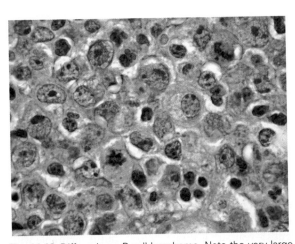

Fig. 14.10 Diffuse large B-cell lymphoma. Note the very large size of the numerous tumor cells in contrast to the small aggregate of four small lymphocytes in the *lower center* of the field. Also note the two mitotic figures.

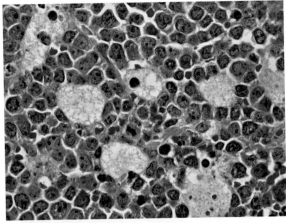

Fig. 14.11 Burkitt lymphoma with numerous blastic lymphoid cells and several (seven) large clear spaces inhabited by foamy macrophages (i.e., the starry sky pattern).

Burkitt lymphoma). In the developed world, Burkitt lymphoma typically presents in older children as an abdominal (ileocecal) mass, a disease referred to as **sporadic Burkitt lymphoma**. Two other differences between endemic and sporadic Burkitt lymphoma are as follows:

1. Epstein-Barr virus (EBV) positivity is much more common in endemic (90%) than sporadic (<30%) tumors. EBV likely contributes to Burkitt tumor cell growth via constitutive CD40-like tyrosine kinase-based proliferative signaling induced by the **EBV latent membrane protein 1 (LMP-1)**.

2. Molecular sites of *c-Myc* chromosome translocation breakpoints are different.

Burkitt tumors are highly chemosensitive, and patients with large tumor burden are at increased risk of treatment-related tumor lysis syndrome.

Mantle cell lymphoma is a high-grade B lymphoma, seen primarily in men, derived from CD5+ mantle zone B cells that carry a specific translocation *t(11;14)* involving the **cyclin D1** and Ig heavy chain genes. Increased expression of cyclin D1 protein induces mantle cell B-cell proliferation by driving the cells through the cyclin D1–dependent G1 cell cycle checkpoint. without cyclin D1 translocation carry a *SOX-11 gene* mutation. SOX-11 encodes for a transcription factor protein. Although MCL (like CLL/SLL) is derived from CD5+ B cells (as in CLL/SLL), the small centrocyte-like cells express a memory (mantle cell) B-cell phenotype and do not coexpress the low-affinity IgE receptor CD23. Lymph node involvement is often marked by a vaguely nodular infiltrate of cyclin D1–positive mantle zone cells that surround small atrophic GCs (Figs. 14.12 and 14.13). Although the most common presentation is generalized lymphadenopathy, some patients may present with abdominal complaints (pain, diarrhea, constipation, or rectal bleeding) caused by GI involvement in the form of multiple lymphomatous polyps known as **lymphomatous polyposis**.

The characteristic chromosome translocation seen in MCL, *t(11;14)*, can be directly detected in individual tumor cells by fluorescence in situ hybridization. In this technique, two DNA probes, each specific for one chromosome (11 or 14) and each labeled with a specific fluorochrome (red or green), are hybridized to fixed cells either on cell smears or in tissue sections and viewed under a fluorescence microscope. Normal cells are marked by two red signals (normal chromosomes 11)

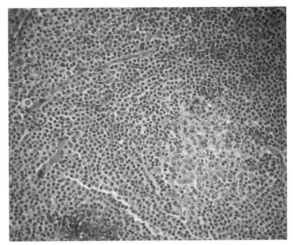

Fig. 14.12 Mantle cell lymphoma. A monotonous expanse of small lymphocytes surrounds the atrophic germinal center (*pink area* in the *right center* of the field).

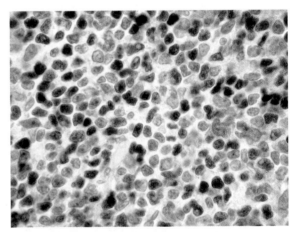

Fig. 14.13 Cyclin D1 immunostain in mantle cell lymphoma. Note the numerous tumor cells with nuclear expression (*brown stain)* of cyclin D1.

and two green signals (normal chromosomes 14). Tumor cells are marked by at least one overlapping red-green signal that appears yellow (Fig. 14.14). This same technique can be applied to a variety of other translocations in lymphoma and leukemia, including *t(9;22)* in CML, *t(8;14)* in Burkitt lymphoma, and *t(14;18)* in FL.

Marginal zone lymphoma is a low-grade lymphoma derived from post-GC B cells that presents most often as an **extranodal mucosa-associated lymphoid tissue (MALT) lymphoma** and less often as a node or spleen-based

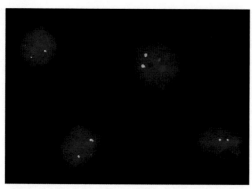

Fig. 14.14 Fluorescence in situ hybridization of the t(11;14) translocation in mantle cell lymphoma. Four nuclei are shown in blue. Each cell should contain four separate signals—two green signals for chromosome 11 and two red signals for chromosome 14. Instead, in each cell shown here there are three distinct signals, one green signal (normal chromosome 11), one red signal (normal chromosome 14), and one hybrid signal (green and red, yielding yellow) that represents a translocation between chromosomes 11 and 14, that is, t(11;14).(Provided by Dr. Pei Hui, Yale University Department of Pathology.)

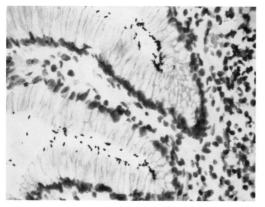

Fig. 14.15 *Helicobacter pylori* (*red-stained* bacilli) attached to the gastric mucosa in extranodal marginal zone (mucosa-associated lymphoid tissue) lymphoma of the stomach (*H. pylori* immunostain).

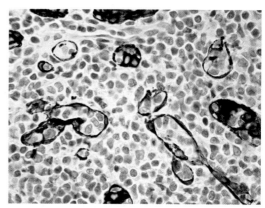

Fig. 14.16 Cytokeratin immunostaining of gastric mucosa-associated lymphoid tissue lymphoma. Note the disruption of the cytokeratin-positive (*brown stain*) glands by numerous cytokeratin-negative (unstained) lymphoid tumor cells.

disease. MALT lymphomas are most often seen in association with a variety of chronic persistent infections and autoimmune conditions. Examples of MALT lymphoma include gastric lymphoma (Fig. 14.15) with *H. pylori* infection, intestinal lymphoma with *Campylobacter jejuni* infection, thyroid lymphoma with **Hashimoto thyroiditis**, and parotid lymphoma with **Sjögren syndrome**. A characteristic biopsy finding in MALT lymphoma is the presence of lymphoepithelial lesions formed by lymphocytic infiltration of cytokeratin-positive glandular epithelium (Fig. 14.16). These lymphomas apparently arise from neoplastic marginal B-cell clones that develop from of the intense chronic inflammation triggered by chronic infection. Early in the disease, these tumors may undergo complete remission with antibiotic therapy alone, begging the question of true malignancy. Clonal evolution with acquisition of mutations, including the *t(11;18)* translocation involving the **apoptosis inhibitor 2 (API2)** and **MALT1 genes** leads to higher grade disease for which antibiotic therapy is ineffective and conventional chemotherapy is required. MZL may also present as primary node-based disease, one-third of which occurs in association with a MALT lymphoma. Marginal cell lymphoma may also arise in the spleen as a **primary splenic marginal cell lymphoma** with marked expansion of the splenic marginal zone (Fig. 14.17), often accompanied by circulating tumor cells with irregular cytoplasmic projections called *villous lymphocytes*.

Plasma cell myeloma (multiple myeloma) is the most common lymphoid malignancy in African Americans and the second most common lymphoid malignancy in European Americans. The disease is most often seen in older adults. The risk of myeloma is increased in cosmetologists, farmers, laxative takers, and those with exposure to pesticides, petroleum products, asbestos, rubber, and wood products, strongly suggesting a role for environmental exposure to toxins in development of the disease. Plasma cell myeloma is

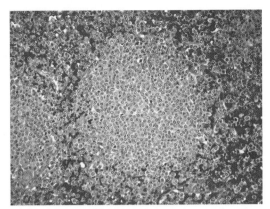

Fig. 14.17 Primary splenic marginal zone lymphoma. Note the characteristic nodular expansion of the white pulp by the lymphoid infiltrate *(center of the field)*. The red pulp is uninvolved.

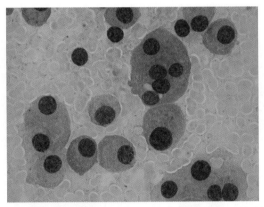

Fig. 14.18 Plasma cell myeloma (bone marrow aspirate). Note the numerous markedly enlarged plasma cells with oval nuclei and abundant blue cytoplasm.

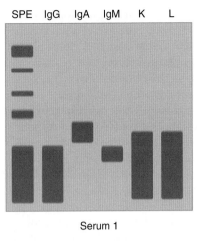

Serum 1

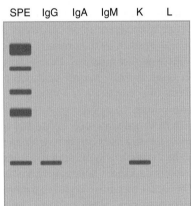

Serum 2

Fig. 14.19 Immunofixation electrophoresis of human serum. Two gels are shown. The *upper gel* (serum 1) depicts normal results. After electrophoresis normal serum proteins separate into five discrete bands (shown in the serum protein electrophoresis [SPE] lane from *top* to *bottom*—albumin, alpha 1 globulins, alpha 2 globulins, beta globulins, and gamma globulins). Immunofixation of immunoglobulin (Ig) heavy chains IgG, IgA, and IgM, and Ig light chains kappa and lambda reveals a normal polyclonal distribution of IgG, IgA, IgM, kappa, and lambda. In contrast, the *lower gel* (serum 2) reveals an abnormal pattern, with a prominent discrete gamma globulin band on SPE caused by the presence of a monoclonal IgG kappa protein. Note that in the presence of a monoclonal protein the levels of nonclonal Ig are markedly suppressed.

a tumor composed of malignant (monoclonal) plasma cells that most often arises in the bone marrow, causing painful lytic bone lesions, pathologic fractures, and hypercalcemia. Although usually more than 10% of the plasma cells in the bone marrow are abnormal, no minimal number of marrow plasma cells is required for diagnosis (Fig. 14.18). Instead, the diagnosis is based on three criteria: the presence of a monoclonal serum or urine protein (Fig. 14.19), monoclonal plasma cells in tissue, and related organ or tissue impairment (hypercalcemia, renal insufficiency, anemia, or bone lesions). Neoplastic plasma cells express the plasma cell markers CD138, MUM1, and either kappa or lambda light chain protein. Production of large quantities of

monoclonal Ig (**paraprotein**) leads to renal tubular deposition of free light chains, known as **Bence-Jones protein**, and development of renal failure; to polyclonal hypogammaglobulinemia leading to recurrent bacterial infections; and in some cases, to deposition of free light chains in soft tissues throughout the body (amyloidosis). **Smoldering myeloma** is defined as asymptomatic disease marked by a monoclonal serum or urine protein and at least 10% clonal plasma cells. **Extraosseous plasmacytoma** is a plasma cell neoplasm presenting in an extramedullary site, most often the upper respiratory tract, with disease only rarely progressing to involve bone marrow. **Osseous plasmacytoma** presents as a solitary tumor in bone (not bone marrow). Many patients progress to involve marrow or other bone sites. Patients with localized plasma cell disease may be effectively treated by radiation therapy, but those with extensive disease (including myeloma) are treated with combination chemotherapy. The overall median survival period is 3 years. A common related condition, termed **monoclonal gammopathy of undetermined significance**, is a chronic asymptomatic condition of older adults (seen in 3% of adults older than 70 years of age) marked by the presence of monoclonal Ig in serum and accompanied by a slight increase (<10%) in bone marrow plasma cells. Up to 25% of patients with this condition eventually progress to plasma cell myeloma.

Amyloidosis is a disease process caused by deposition of insoluble fibrillary protein with beta-pleated sheet secondary structure in numerous tissues that may lead to heart failure, kidney failure, peripheral neuropathy, and abnormal bleeding. **Light chain amyloidosis** results from deposition of monoclonal light chain Ig produced by a clonal plasma cell disorder that in some cases meets the diagnostic criteria for plasma cell myeloma. Amyloid appears in biopsy material (often subcutaneous fat) as an eosinophilic extracellular material within the walls of small blood vessels (Fig. 14.20) that can be confirmed by Congo red staining. Amyloidosis A is caused by tissue deposition of **serum amyloid A (SAA)** in chronic infectious and inflammatory states. SAA is an insoluble protein by-product derived from the circulating precursor protein apo-SAA that normally serves as an acute phase reactant.

Lymphoplasmacytic lymphoma is a rare low-grade neoplasm of older adults that is most often associated with a monoclonal serum IgM paraprotein and a *MyD-88* gene mutation. The MyD-88 protein is involved in lymphocyte signal activation. The lymphoma is composed of plasmacytoid lymphocytes, small ovoid IgM+ lymphocytes with slightly eccentric nuclei, moderately abundant cytoplasm, and a prominent perinuclear Golgi region (Fig. 14.21). The IgM paraprotein may in

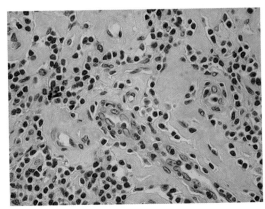

Fig. 14.20 Amyloidosis (soft tissue biopsy). Note the homogenous eosinophilic *(pink)* extracellular material (amyloid) deposited within the walls of blood vessels. To confirm that this material is amyloid, the tissue can be stained with Congo red (not shown). Also present in this section are numerous scattered reactive lymphocytes.

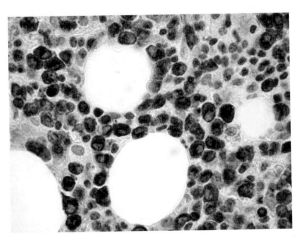

Fig. 14.21 Immunoglobulin (Ig) M immunostain (bone marrow) in lymphoplasmacytic lymphoma. Note the marked increase in IgM+ plasmacytoid lymphocytes (brown stain).

some cases lead to **hyperviscosity syndrome** (increased blood viscosity, fatigue, weakness, anorexia, and weight loss), cryoglobulinemia, and autoimmune phenomena such as peripheral neuropathy and coagulopathy caused by factor antibodies. Most patients who present with the clinical syndrome known as **Waldenstrom macroglobulinemia** (monoclonal serum IgM protein and symptoms of hyperviscosity) have LPL.

Cryoglobulinemia is a clinicopathologic condition caused by increased production of Igs that reversibly precipitate at temperatures below body temperature

(37°C). Intravascular deposition of cryoprecipitate leads to necrotizing vasculitis and tissue damage. End organs that may be damaged include the skin, joints, peripheral nerves, kidneys, liver, CNS, and intestines. The most common symptoms include purpura, arthralgia, and weakness. There are three types of cryoglobulins:

1. **Type I (monoclonal) cryoglobulin** is composed entirely of monoclonal Ig, most often IgM (as in LPL).
2. **Type II (mixed monoclonal–polyclonal) cryoglobulin** is composed of a mixture of monoclonal and polyclonal Igs. The monoclonal component (most often IgM) has rheumatoid factor–like antibody specificity, and the polyclonal component is IgG. Type II cryoglobulinemia is often seen in hepatitis C infection and lymphoproliferative disorders.
3. **Type III (polyclonal) cryoglobulin** is composed entirely of polyclonal Ig. In most cases, some polyclonal Ig has rheumatoid factor–like anti-IgG activity such that much of the precipitate is composed of Ig–anti-Ig complexes. Type III cryoglobulinemia is seen in association with various infections and autoimmune diseases.

Mediastinal large B-cell lymphoma most often presents as a mediastinal mass in young women (Fig. 14.22). Because Hodgkin lymphoma often presents as a mediastinal mass in young women and shares some histologic features with MLBCL, distinction from Hodgkin lymphoma in some cases may be difficult. In contrast to the **Reed-Sternberg (RS) cells** of Hodgkin lymphoma, the large cells of MLBCL are positive for CD45 and CD20, negative for CD15, and only weakly positive for CD30.

Lymphomatoid granulomatosis is a rare, often aggressive T cell–rich EBV+ B-cell lymphoma of middle-aged adults that presents as a necrotizing angiodestructive process in extranodal sites, most commonly the lung, kidney, or CNS. Clinical symptoms may include fever, cough, weight loss, and neurologic defects.

Primary effusion lymphoma (PEL) is a rare high-grade B-cell lymphoma most often seen in patients with human immunodeficiency virus/acquired immunodeficiency syndrome who present with a rapidly enlarging pleural, pericardial, or peritoneal serous effusion. The large tumor cells usually express a null (non-B, non-T) immunophenotype and are positive for **human herpesvirus 8** and sometimes EBV. The B-cell origin of this tumor can be demonstrated by detection of clonal *Ig* gene rearrangements.

T-CELL AND NATURAL KILLER CELL LYMPHOMA

T-cell and NK cell lymphomas, at least in North America and Europe, are much less common than B-cell lymphomas, accounting for only about 10% of all non-Hodgkin lymphoma cases. The many subtypes include T-cell lymphoblastic lymphoma, **peripheral T-cell lymphoma (PTCL)**, angioimmunoblastic T-cell lymphoma, ALCL, **enteropathy-associated T-cell lymphoma (EATL)**, primary cutaneous T-cell lymphoma (mycosis fungoides), ATLL, subcutaneous panniculitis-like T-cell lymphoma, hepatosplenic T-cell lymphoma, primary cutaneous anaplastic T-cell lymphoma, and extranodal T/NK cell lymphoma (Table 14.4). The correspondence of the T-cell lymphomas to normal T-cell subsets is not as well understood as in B-cell lymphoma. This may be because our knowledge of normal T-cell subsets is incomplete, and most T-cell subsets do not populate distinctive histologically recognizable microanatomic compartments, the exceptions being the anterior mediastinal origin of T lymphoblastic lymphoma (thymic T cells) and mediastinal large B-cell lymphoma (thymic B cells).

Although most T-cell lymphomas derive from CD3+ CD4+ helper/inducer T cells, there are many exceptions. Some T-cell lymphomas derive from CD8+ cytotoxic T cells (ALCL, subcutaneous panniculitis-like T-cell lymphoma), others from dual CD4/

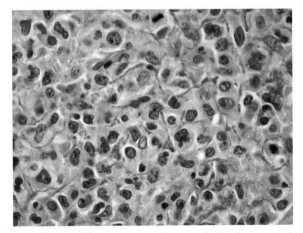

Fig. 14.22 Mediastinal large B-cell lymphoma. Characteristic delicate fibrosis separates the infiltrate into small nests of large tumor cells.

TABLE 14.4 Major T-Cell and Natural Killer Cell Lymphoma Types

Lymphoma Type	Cell of Origin	Genetic Defects	Functional Consequence
Lymphoblastic	CD7+ TdT+ T cell progenitor or thymocyte	*HOX11* translocations, *CDKN2A* loss, *NOTCH1* mutations	Transcription control defect (HOX), loss of cell cycle control (CDK), Myc activation (NOTCH)
Peripheral T cell	CD3+ CD4+ central memory T cell	Complex defects	Unknown
Angioimmunoblastic	CD3+ CD4+ CD10+ T follicular helper cell	Trisomy 3, trisomy 5, +X	Unknown
Extranodal T/NK	CD2+ CD56+ EBV+ NK cell	Complex defects	Unknown
Mycosis fungoides	CD3+ CD4+ skin-homing T cell	Complex defects	Unknown

CDK, cyclin dependent kinase; *EBV*, Epstein-Barr virus.

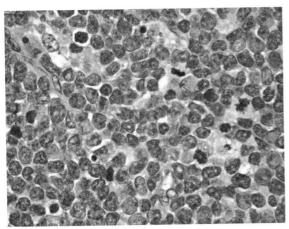

Fig. 14.23 Lymphoblastic lymphoma (mediastinal mass). Note the immature blastic chromatin pattern (salt and pepper chromatin), the two mitotic figures, and the two or three small apoptotic cells.

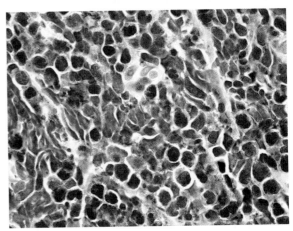

Fig. 14.24 Terminal deoxynucleotidyl transferase immunostain in lymphoblastic lymphoma. Note the brown intranuclear staining pattern in the tumor cells.

CD8 negative cytotoxic T cells (enteropathy-associated T-cell lymphoma), gamma-delta T cells (hepatosplenic lymphoma), NK cells (T/NK lymphoma, nasal type), and precursor T lymphoblasts (lymphoblastic lymphoma).

T lymphoblastic lymphoma is a high-grade disease often seen in male adolescents who present with a rapidly growing anterior mediastinal mass, often with pleural effusion (Fig. 14.23). Compression of soft tissues in the neck by a large mediastinal tumor may cause superior vena cava syndrome, with dyspnea, cough, headache, and facial edema. The tumor is derived from precursor (thymic) T lymphoblasts that most often express CD3 (cytoplasmic), CD7, and TdT (Fig. 14.24). The most common

cytogenetic defects are translocations of a variety of transcription factor and tyrosine kinase genes into the transcriptionally active TCR loci (alpha, beta, gamma, and delta), leading to autonomous cell growth. When presenting with blood and marrow involvement rather than a solid tumor, this disease is referred to as precursor T-cell acute lymphoblastic leukemia. The demographic, phenotypic, and genotypic features of these two closely related conditions are identical.

Peripheral T-cell lymphoma is the most common subtype of T-cell lymphoma. This disease is most often seen in older adults who often present with generalized lymphadenopathy, fever, weight loss, pruritus, and eosinophilia (caused by interleukin (IL)-5 production by malignant T cells). Patients with PTCL sometimes develop profound cytopenia characteristic of **hemophagocytic syndrome (HPS)**. In HPS, hyperactive macrophages ingest marrow cells and produce excessive quantities of proinflammatory cytokines interferon-γ (IFN-γ), tumor necrosis factor α, and transforming growth factor β that suppress normal hematopoiesis. Macrophage activation is induced by proinflammatory cytokines (IFN-γ) released by the malignant T cells. The tumor cells in peripheral T-cell lymphoma are CD3+ CD4+ T cells that may exhibit aberrant lack of expression of pan–T cell antigens. The pathology is marked by a diffuse polymorphous infiltrate of lymphocytes, histiocytes, and eosinophils (Fig. 14.25).

Anaplastic large cell lymphoma is a high-grade tumor of children and adults composed of large pleomorphic cells of null or T-cell immunophenotype (Fig. 14.26). The tumor cells, derived from cytotoxic T cells, usually express the cytotoxic granule proteins perforin and granzyme. Characteristic large cells with kidney-shaped nuclei and abundant cytoplasm are known as *hallmark cells*. Most tumors are marked by a **t(2;5)** translocation involving the **anaplastic lymphoma kinase 1** *(ALK-1)* gene on chromosome 2 and the **nucleophosmin** gene on chromosome 5. Interestingly, nucleophosmin mutations are quite common in AML. Several alternative translocations all involving the *ALK-1* gene are seen in 20% to 30% of cases. Overexpression of ALK-1 protein can be detected in the tumor cells by immunohistochemistry. Primary

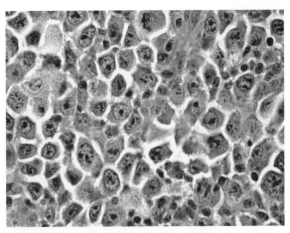

Fig. 14.26 Anaplastic large cell lymphoma. Note the very large tumor cells, many with prominent nucleoli and amphophilic *(red-blue)* cytoplasm.

cutaneous anaplastic large cell lymphoma is a low-grade ALK1− CD30+ tumor seen most often in adults that may spontaneously regress.

Mycosis fungoides is the most common T-cell lymphoma of skin. It is seen in older adults who present with pruritic erythematous patches and plaques on the trunk that progress to form large skin tumors (Fig. 14.27). The malignant T cells characteristically infiltrate the epidermis to form **Pautrier microabscesses** (Fig. 14.28). The CD4+ T cells often lack CD7 coexpression. Disease progression marked by generalized skin involvement (erythroderma) and involvement of the blood and local lymph nodes is known as **Sezary syndrome**. Patients with mycosis fungoides are immunocompromised, and the most common cause of death is bacterial septicemia or pneumonia from cutaneous infection.

Adult T cell leukemia/lymphoma is an HTLV-1+ CD4+ T-cell neoplasm seen in areas of world endemic for HTLV-1 infection (i.e., Japan, the Caribbean region, and Africa). Patients with acute disease present with marked lymphocytosis, generalized lymphadenopathy, skin rash, and hypercalcemia (Fig. 14.29). Patients with chronic disease present with lymphocytosis and skin rash only. Patients are often immunocompromised and have opportunistic infections, including *Pneumocystis carinii* pneumonia and cryptococcal meningitis. The pathogenesis of the disease results from excessive **HTLV-1 *tax* gene**–mediated production of IL-2, leading to cell proliferation followed by acquisition of mutations that result in neoplastic transformation. The

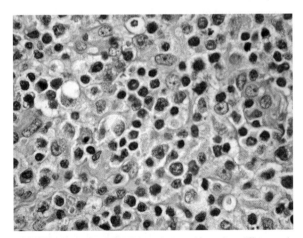

Fig. 14.25 Peripheral T-cell lymphoma. Note the diffuse polymorphous infiltrate composed of small and large lymphocytes, histiocytes, and eosinophils.

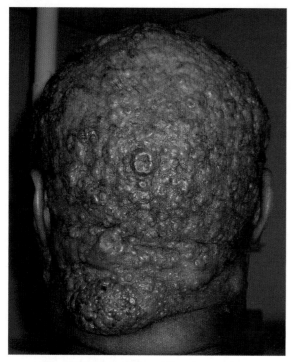

Fig. 14.27 Mycosis fungoides—tumor stage.

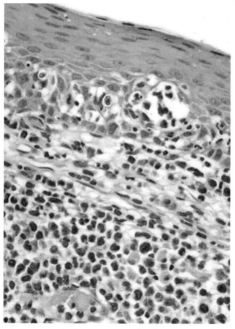

Fig. 14.28 Mycosis fungoides (skin biopsy). Note the epidermal involvement by the abnormal T-cell infiltrate with formation of Pautrier microabscesses (clear spaces in the epidermis filled with lymphoid cells).

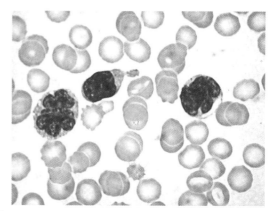

Fig. 14.29 Adult T-cell leukemia/lymphoma (peripheral blood). Abnormal T cells with highly irregular convoluted nuclei ("flower cells").

CD4+ tumor cells characteristically express high levels of the IL-2 receptor protein CD25.

Angioimmunoblastic T-cell lymphoma often presents in middle-aged and older adults with generalized lymphadenopathy, hepatosplenomegaly, pruritic skin rash, and several autoimmune manifestations, including arthritis, serous effusions, positive rheumatoid factor, and polyclonal hypergammaglobulinemia. The lymphoid infiltrate is diffuse, with numerous malignant CD4+ T cells, scattered large EBV+ B cells, increased follicular dendritic cells, and prominent high endothelial venules. Although no specific gene translocation has been identified, the malignant T cells tumor often carry major cytogenetic defects, including *trisomy 3, trisomy 5, and +X*. The clinical course is aggressive and often complicated by systemic infection.

Extranodal T/NK cell lymphoma, nasal type, is an aggressive tumor seen primarily in Asia, Mexico, and Central and South America. Patients typically present with necrotic, angiodestructive, locally aggressive lesions of the nasal region. The tumor cells are most often EBV+ NK cells that express cytotoxic granule proteins granzyme B, T-cell intracellular antigen 1 (TIA-1), and perforin. In most cases, the *TCR* genes are not rearranged, that is, in a germline configuration. The tumor may rapidly disseminate to distant sites and be complicated by HPS, a complex of fever, pancytopenia, hepatosplenomegaly, and proliferation of hemophagocytic histiocytes in the marrow and spleen.

Subcutaneous panniculitis-like T-cell lymphoma is a rare disease of young adults who present with subcutaneous nodules of the extremities and trunk (Fig. 14.30).

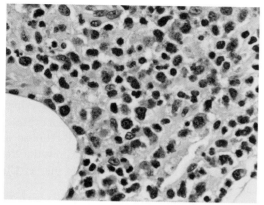

Fig. 14.30 Subcutaneous panniculitis-like T-cell lymphoma (biopsy of subcutaneous tissue—lower extremity). Note the infiltrate of abnormal lymphoid cells with characteristic rimming of fat spaces (*clear space* on the *left* of the field).

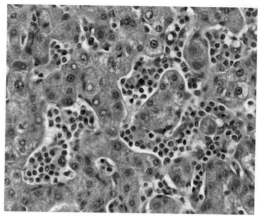

Fig. 14.31 Hepatosplenic T-cell lymphoma (liver biopsy). Note the highly characteristic involvement of the hepatic sinusoids by the T-cell infiltrate.

The tumor derives from clonal CD3+ CD8+ cytotoxic T cells that express cytotoxic granule proteins granzyme B, TIA-1, and perforin. Some cases are complicated by HPS. The clinical course is aggressive, but combination chemotherapy is often effective at controlling disease manifestations.

Enteropathy-associated T-cell lymphoma, although uncommon, is seen most frequently in patients with **celiac disease**, an autoimmune disease of the small intestine associated with gluten hypersensitivity. Patients with long-standing refractory celiac disease are at greatest risk for tumor development. The typical clinical presentation is sudden onset of severe abdominal pain caused by intestinal perforation. The tumor arises from CD3-positive (alpha-beta) dual CD4/CD8-negative intraepithelial cytotoxic T cells that invade the jejunum and ileum. The poor prognosis largely results from the rapid development of bacterial peritonitis and sepsis following bowel perforation.

Hepatosplenic T-cell lymphoma is a rare neoplasm of male adolescents and young men who present with hepatosplenomegaly and marked thrombocytopenia caused by marrow involvement. Lymphadenopathy is characteristically absent. The tumor cells are clonal CD3-positive dual CD4/CD8-negative gamma-delta T cells that infiltrate the sinusoids of the spleen, liver, and bone marrow (Fig. 14.31). Rare cases of hepatosplenic T-cell lymphoma with alpha-beta TCRs have been described in females. The course is aggressive, and the prognosis is poor.

HODGKIN LYMPHOMA

Hodgkin lymphoma is a peculiar B cell–derived malignancy with several highly distinctive features that justify separate classification from B-cell non-Hodgkin lymphoma. Hodgkin lymphoma is less common than non-Hodgkin lymphoma and, unlike non-Hodgkin lymphoma, has a bimodal age distribution in adults, with one peak in young adults and another in older adults (older than 50 years). Unlike non-Hodgkin lymphoma, Hodgkin lymphoma often presents with disease limited to a lymph node or nodes in one anatomic site and only rarely involves extranodal tissues. The treatment and prognosis of Hodgkin lymphoma are determined primarily by clinical staging, with a minor role played by pathologic grading.

Unlike non-Hodgkin lymphoma, Hodgkin lymphoma tumors are usually composed of relatively few scattered malignant cells surrounded by numerous inflammatory cells. The malignant cells in **classic Hodgkin lymphoma (CHL)** are large pleomorphic cells with multinucleated or multilobated nuclei and large prominent nucleoli—**classical Reed-Sternberg (RS) cells** (Fig. 14.32). Classic RS cells exhibit a unique immunophenotype—they are CD30 positive (Fig. 14.33) and (usually) CD15 positive, and even though RS cells are derived from B lymphocytes, they are usually negative for the pan-lymphocyte marker CD45 and the B cell marker CD20. RS cells are hypertetraploid with numerous cytogenetic defects, none of which have so far been shown to be

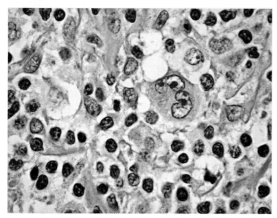

Fig. 14.32 Classic Hodgkin lymphoma. Note the large classic Reed-Sternberg cell (multinucleated with prominent nucleoli) to the *right of center* of the field, as well as the numerous reactive lymphocytes and histiocytes.

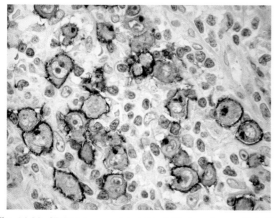

Fig. 14.33 CD30 immunostain in Hodgkin lymphoma. Note the numerous large CD30+ Reed-Sternberg cells (brown membrane and Golgi staining pattern).

In contrast to the multi-nucleated Reed-Sternberg (RS) cells of classical HL, the LP cells of **nodular lymphocyte predominant HL (NLPHL)** contain single multi-lobulated popcorn-shaped nuclei. Despite their morphologic dissimilarity, both **RS cells** and **LP cells** are clonal neoplastic cells derived from B lymphocytes. However, RS cells, unlike LP cells, carry crippling mutations in immunoglobulin genes, do not express immunoglobulin protein, do not express B cell-associated proteins CD45 and CD20, aberrantly express the granulocyte marker CD15 and the activation marker CD30, and are often EBV positive.

The two major types of Hodgkin lymphoma have different clinical and pathologic features. The more common classical Hodgkin lymphoma is seen in children and adults with dual peak incidence, in adolescents or young adults, and in older adults, with a nearly equal gender ratio. In contrast, NLPHL occurs primarily in men between 30 and 50 years of age. Although patients with both forms of Hodgkin lymphoma most often present with peripheral lymphadenopathy, patients with NLPHL are more likely to present with disease confined to one lymph node region (stage 1). Patients with CHL are more likely to present with widespread disease and with symptoms of fever, night sweats, and weight loss (so-called B symptoms). As previously discussed, although the malignant cells of CHL and NLPHL (classic RS cells and LP cells, respectively) both derive from GC B cells, they are morphologically and phenotypically distinctive (Fig. 14.34). Whereas the reactive infiltrate of CHL

specific for Hodgkin lymphoma. The clonal B-cell origin of RS cells has been demonstrated by detection of clonal rearrangements of the Ig heavy chain genes. The presence of numerous crippling mutations of *Ig* genes that interfere with expression of Ig proteins suggests that RS cells represent preapoptotic GC B cells rescued from apoptosis by some unrecognized transforming event. In many cases, classic RS cells are latently infected by EBV and express large amounts of the EBV protein LMP-1. LMP-1 likely contributes to uncontrolled RS cell growth by providing a constitutive CD40-like activation signal. CD40 is a B cell growth factor receptor that upon binding of CD40 ligand triggers nuclear factor κB–mediated transcriptional activation.

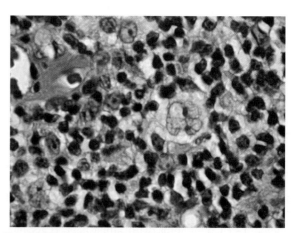

Fig. 14.34 A small lymphocyte background with scattered large neoplastic cells called LP (or popcorn) cells is characteristic of nodular lymphocyte-predominant Hodgkin lymphoma (the large multilobated cell just to right of *center*).

contains numerous T cells, histiocytes, and eosinophils, the reactive infiltrate of NLPHL contains numerous B cells. Disease progression in CHL is often characterized by progressive fibrosis with lymphocyte depletion and increased RS cells. In contrast, disease progression in NLPHL is characterized by transformation to DLBCL.

CLASSIC HODGKIN LYMPHOMA

Classic Hodgkin lymphoma is subclassified into four histopathologic subtypes: nodular sclerosis, mixed cellularity, lymphocyte-rich, and lymphocyte-depleted Hodgkin lymphoma (Table 14.5).

Nodular sclerosis Hodgkin lymphoma, the most common Hodgkin lymphoma subtype (70% of cases), is often seen in young adults (median age, 28 years) who commonly present with an anterior mediastinal mass. The lymphoid infiltrate is nodular and intersected by broad bands of collagenous fibrosis. Within the nodules are classic RS cells admixed with numerous reactive T cells and relatively few histiocytes, eosinophils, granulocytes, and/or plasma cells. The RS cells are often surrounded by clear spaces (lacuna); these RS cells are referred to as lacunar RS cells. The RS cells are EBV positive in up to 40% of cases.

Mixed cellularity Hodgkin lymphoma, representing 20% of CHL cases, is most often seen in middle-aged adults (median age, 37 years) with a male predominance. The lymphoid infiltrate is diffuse and nonfibrotic and composed of relatively numerous scattered classic RS cells within a heterogeneous (mixed) population of T cells, histiocytes, eosinophils, neutrophils, and plasma cells. EBV-positive RS cells are detected in up to 75% of cases.

Lymphocyte-rich Hodgkin lymphoma is an uncommon CHL subtype (5% of cases) that is usually seen in older adults with a male predominance. Like NLPHL, this subtype usually presents with limited localized disease, rarely accompanied by B symptoms. The lymphoid infiltrate is usually nodular, with regressed GCs and greatly expanded B cell–rich mantle zones containing scattered classic RS cells. The reactive infiltrate is composed entirely of T cells without neutrophils and eosinophils. EBV-positive RS cells are seen in about 50% of cases. The course of the disease is indolent, and the prognosis is quite good.

Lymphocyte-depleted Hodgkin lymphoma is the least common (<5% of cases) and most aggressive form of CHL. It is most often seen in middle-aged men. This is the most common Hodgkin lymphoma subtype seen in HIV-positive men and is more common in people from developing countries. The lymphoid infiltrate is diffuse, with an abundance of classic, often highly pleomorphic, RS cells, sometimes associated

TABLE 14.5 Hodgkin Lymphoma Subtypes					
Type	**Frequency (%)**	**Malignant Cell**	**Reactive Cells**	**Pattern**	**EBV**
Nodular lymphocyte predominant	5	CD20+ lymphocyte predominant	Small B lymphocytes	Nodular without fibrosis	Negative
Nodular sclerosis	70	CD30(CD15)+ lacunar Reed-Sternberg	Small T lymphocytes, eosinophils, histiocytes	Nodular with fibrosis	10%–40% positive
Mixed cellularity	20	CD30(CD15)+ classic Reed-Sternberg	Small T lymphocytes, eosinophils, histiocytes	Diffuse	75% positive
Lymphocyte rich	5	CD30(CD15)+ classic Reed-Sternberg	Small B lymphocytes (nodular form); small T lymphocytes (diffuse form)	Nodular (most common) or diffuse	40%–60% positive
Lymphocyte depleted	<1	CD30(CD15)+ pleomorphic Reed-Sternberg	Fibroblasts, histiocytes	Diffuse	75%–100% positive

EBV, Epstein-Barr virus.

with diffuse fibrosis. EBV-positive RS cells are detected in nearly all cases.

HISTIOCYTIC AND DENDRITIC CELL NEOPLASMS

This group of disorders is rare, accounting for fewer than 1% of all lymph node tumors. These tumors derive either from myelomonocytic bone marrow precursors that differentiate within tissues into histiocytes (macrophages) and dendritic cells (including Langerhans cells), or from mesenchymal cells that differentiate into **follicular dendritic cells (FDCs)**. **Langerhans cell histiocytosis** is the most common tumor in this group. These tumors are most common in young boys who present either with isolated lytic bone disease or with disseminated disease, often involving skin, bone, liver, spleen, and marrow. Langerhans cells are oval cells with longitudinally grooved nuclei that express the markers CD1a and S100 (Fig. 14.35). By electron microscopy, these cells can be identified by **Birbeck granules**, tennis racket–shaped cytoplasmic inclusions. **Interdigitating dendritic cell (IDC) sarcomas** and FDC sarcomas are rare spindle cell tumors of lymph nodes. IDC tumors express S100 but not CD1a, and FDC tumors express the markers CD21 and CD35. **Histiocytic sarcomas** are rare tumors that most often involve extranodal sites, including the intestine, skin, and soft tissues, and express histiocyte markers CD68, CD163, and lysozyme.

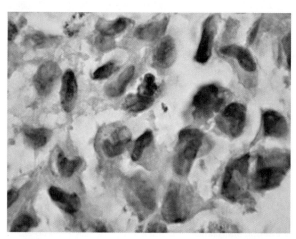

Fig. 14.35 Langerhans cell histiocytosis. Note the large irregular-shaped cells with delicately grooved nuclei (Langerhans cells) and the eosinophils.

Blastic plasmacytoid dendritic cell neoplasms are rare tumors that most often present as nodular skin lesions with marrow involvement and are sometimes accompanied by lymphadenopathy. The tumor is derived from immature plasmacytoid dendritic cells that are positive for CD4, CD56, and CD123 but negative for CD3 and MPO and with nonrearranged (germline) *TCR* genes. The clinical course is highly aggressive. Although the tumor cells are precursors of plasmacytoid dendritic cells, this tumor is currently classified as a myeloid leukemia–related neoplasm rather than a lymphoma-related neoplasm for treatment purposes.

KEY WORDS AND CONCEPTS

- 13q14 gene
- Activated CLL
- Adult T-cell leukemia/lymphoma (ATLL)
- Amyloidosis
- Anaplastic large cell lymphoma
- Anaplastic lymphoma kinase (ALK-1)
- Angioimmunoblastic T-cell lymphoma
- Apoptosis inhibitor 2 (API2)
- B lymphoblastic leukemia/lymphoma
- *Bcl-2*
- Bcl-6
- BCR-ABL
- Bence-Jones protein
- Birbeck granule
- Blastic plasmacytoid dendritic cell neoplasm
- Celiac disease
- Centroblasts
- Centrocytes
- Chronic lymphocytic leukemia (CLL)
- Classic Hodgkin lymphoma (CHL)
- Clinical staging
- c-Myc
- Computed tomography (CT)
- Cryoglobulinemia
- Cyclin D1
- Diffuse large B-cell lymphoma (DLBCL)

- E2A-PBX1 fusion gene
- EBV latent membrane protein 1 (LMP-1)
- Endemic Burkitt lymphoma
- Enteropathy-associated T-cell lymphoma
- Epstein-Barr virus (EBV)
- Extranodal mucosa-associated lymphoid tissue (MALT) lymphoma
- Extranodal T/NK cell lymphoma, nasal type
- Extraosseous plasmacytoma
- Flow cytometry
- Follicular dendritic cells (FDCs)
- Follicular lymphoma (FL)
- Helicobacter pylori
- Hashimoto thyroiditis
- Hemophagocytic syndrome (HPS)
- Hepatosplenic T-cell lymphoma
- Histiocytic sarcoma
- Hodgkin lymphoma
- HTLV-1
- Human herpesvirus 8
- Human T-cell lymphotropic virus type 1 (HTLV-1)
- Hyperviscosity syndrome
- Interdigitating dendritic cell (IDC) sarcomas
- Langerhans cell histiocytosis
- Light chain amyloidosis
- Lymphocyte-depleted Hodgkin lymphoma
- Lymphocyte-rich Hodgkin lymphoma
- Lymphomatoid granulomatosis
- Lymphomatous polyposis
- Lymphoplasmacytic lymphoma (LPL)
- Magnetic resonance imaging (MRI)
- MALT1 gene
- Mantle cell lymphoma (MCL)
- Marginal zone B-cell lymphoma
- Mediastinal large B-cell lymphoma
- Mixed cellularity Hodgkin lymphoma
- Monoclonal gammopathy of undetermined significance
- Mucosa-associated B-cell lymphoma (MALT lymphoma)
- Mycosis fungoides
- Naïve CLL
- Natural killer (NK) cells
- Neoplasm mantle cell lymphoma
- Nodular lymphocyte-predominant Hodgkin lymphoma (NLPHL)
- Nodular sclerosis Hodgkin lymphoma (NSHL)
- Non-Hodgkin lymphoma
- Nucleophosmin
- Osseous plasmacytoma
- Paraprotein
- Pautrier microabscesses
- Peripheral T-cell lymphoma
- Plasma cell myeloma (multiple myeloma)
- Plasmacytoma
- Positron emission tomography (PET)
- Primary effusion lymphoma (PEL)
- Primary splenic marginal cell lymphoma
- Prolymphocytic leukemia
- Reed-Sternberg (RS) cell
- Richter transformation)
- Serum amyloid A (SAA)
- Sezary syndrome
- Sjögren syndrome
- Small lymphocytic lymphoma (SLL)
- Smoldering myeloma
- SOX-11 gene
- Sporadic Burkitt lymphoma
- Subcutaneous panniculitis-like T-cell lymphoma
- T lymphoblastic lymphoma
- t(2;5)
- t(2;8)
- t(8;14)
- t(8;22)
- t(11;18)
- t(14;18)
- tax gene
- TEL-AML1 fusion gene
- Trisomy 12

- Type I (monoclonal) cryoglobulinemia
- Type II (mixed monoclonal–polyclonal) cryoglobulinemia
- Type III (polyclonal) cryoglobulinemia
- Waldenstrom macroglobulinemia

REVIEW QUESTIONS

1. All of the following are often seen in hyperviscosity syndrome secondary to lymphoplasmacytic lymphoma **except**
   A. peripheral neuropathy.
   B. monoclonal IgG paraprotein.
   C. coagulopathy.
   D. *MyD88* mutation.

2. Marginal zone lymphoma occurs in all the following settings **except**
   A. *H. pylori* gastritis.
   B. Hashimoto thyroiditis.
   C. Sjögren syndrome.
   D. lymphomatous polyposis.

3. The BCL-2 translocation in follicular lymphoma has what oncogenic effect on tumor cells?
   A. Blocks apoptosis
   B. Increases growth rate
   C. Blocks tumor immunity
   D. Increases metastasis

4. Which of the following T-cell lymphomas is associated with celiac disease?
   A. Anaplastic large cell lymphoma
   B. Mycosis fungoides
   C. Enteropathy-type T-cell lymphoma
   D. Hepatosplenic T-cell lymphoma

5. RS cells in which subtype of Hodgkin lymphoma are most often positive for EBV?
   A. Nodular lymphocyte predominant
   B. Nodular sclerosis
   C. Mixed cellularity
   D. Lymphocyte depleted

15

Blood Coagulation

KEY POINTS

- Liver-derived coagulation factors circulate in an inactive state and are activated in a cascading fashion, leading to thrombin-mediated fibrin formation.

- Thrombosis is triggered in most cases by vessel wall damage and exposure of blood to tissue factor, collagen, and von Willebrand factor (VWF).

- Tissue factor leads to factor VIIa–mediated activation of the coagulation cascade.

- Exposure of blood to subendothelial collagen and VWF leads to platelet activation.

- Activated platelets provide a phospholipid-rich surface for activation of factors IX and X.

- Thrombin converts fibrinogen to fibrin and plasminogen to plasmin.

- A mature clot is composed of a meshwork of platelets and fibrin.

- Plasmin induces clot dissolution by cleaving fibrin into fibrin degradation products.

- Coagulation factors II, VII, IX, and X require vitamin K–mediated gamma-glutamyl carboxylation for activity.

- The anticoagulant effect of coumarin drugs (vitamin K reductase inhibitors) results from reduced synthesis of functional vitamin K–dependent factors.

- The anticoagulant effect of heparin results from enhancement of antithrombin III–mediated inhibition of factor Xa and thrombin.

- Von Willebrand disease, the most common inherited bleeding disorder, results from deficiency (quantitative or qualitative) of VWF.

- Hemophilia A and B are X-linked bleeding disorders caused by deficiency of factors VIII and IX, respectively.

- Disseminated intravascular coagulation is an acquired bleeding disorder often triggered by sepsis that results from consumption of platelets and coagulation factors by systemic intravascular microthrombosis.

- Hereditary thrombophilia is a group of thrombotic disorders caused by mutations in a variety of coagulation factors, the most common being factor V, that lead to recurrent venous and arterial thrombosis.

Blood is a slightly viscous fluid suspension composed of approximately equal volumes of plasma and cells. If anticoagulated blood in a tube is spun at low speed in a centrifuge, the erythrocytes collect in a layer at the bottom of the tube, and the leukocytes and platelets form a pale layer known as the **buffy coat** on top of the erythrocyte layer, leaving a layer of cell-free plasma above. Under normal circumstances, blood is a fluid suspension that freely circulates through myriad blood vessels throughout the body. However, breaches in or damage to the blood vessel wall initiates a process designed to minimize blood loss, known as blood coagulation or thrombosis. The result of blood coagulation is formation of a semisolid clot composed of fibrin and platelets that acts as a sealant at the site of the blood vessel breach or injury. In the process, platelet-derived growth factor released by clotted platelets stimulate vascular repair. Vascular repair is followed by dissolution of the clot by plasmin-mediated **fibrinolysis**.

The classic coagulation factors are designated by Roman numerals I to XIII. In their active form, factors are referred to by the numeral followed by the letter *a*, as in factor Va. Some factors are referred to more often by their common names than by their Roman numerals, such as fibrinogen (factor I), prothrombin (factor II), tissue factor (factor III), calcium (factor IV). Factor VI is now known as factor Va. The coagulation factors can be functionally classified, with many falling into one of three groups: the zymogens, the cofactors, and the regulators (Table 15.1).

Most coagulation factors are **zymogens**, proteins synthesized by hepatocytes that circulate in plasma as inactive precursors. After limited proteolytic cleavage, zymogens are converted to **serine proteases** (so named for the serine-binding site located within the proteolytic domain) that activate other coagulation zymogens. Two key coagulation reactions take place on the phospholipid-rich cell surface of platelets and endothelial cells with the help of anchoring cofactors V and VIII, both of which are produced by endothelial cells. After thrombin-mediated activation, factors Va and VIIIa stabilize the **"tenase" complex (IXa–VIIIa complex)** and **prothrombinase complex (Xa–Va complex)** on the surfaces of activated platelets and endothelial cells. The platelet proaggregatory factor **von Willebrand factor (VWF)** does not directly contribute to the coagulation cascade; instead, it indirectly contributes by binding to and stabilizing factor VIII. VWF, unlike the other factors, is secreted by endothelial cells and megakaryocytes as high-molecular-weight multimers and quickly converted into smaller multimers by the circulating metalloproteinase **VWF-cleaving enzyme (ADAMTS13)**.

TABLE 15.1 Functional Classification of Coagulation Factors

Group	Factors
Zymogens	II (prothrombin), VII, IX, X, XI, XII
Cofactors	III (tissue factor), V, VIII, HMWK, prekallikrein
Regulators	ATIII, protein C(S), thrombomodulin
Transglutaminase	XIII
Other essential factors	I (fibrinogen), IV (calcium), phospholipid (platelets)

ATIII, Antithrombin III; *HMWK*, high-molecular-weight kininogen.

BLOOD COAGULATION

The coagulation process begins with vessel wall injury, leading to **tissue factor** expression by activated endothelial cells and adhesion of platelets to subendothelial collagen and VWF (Figs. 15.1 and 15.2). Circulating **factor VII** binds to tissue factor and is converted to factor VIIa to form the tissue factor–VIIa complex. Free tissue factor–VIIa complexes are rapidly inactivated in blood by **tissue factor pathway inhibitor**, whereas complexes that bind to endothelial cell and platelet membranes trigger calcium- and phospholipid-dependent surface activation of factors IX and X with help from cofactors VIII and V, respectively. A small amount of factor X is converted to factor Xa on the endothelial cell surface by the tissue factor–VIIa complex, and a small amount of factor V is converted to factor Va by factor Xa, cellular proteases, or both. Factor Va binds to tissue factor-bearing cell membranes and recruits factor Xa to form the stable, membrane-bound Xa–Va prothrombinase complex. Cell-bound factor Xa converts prothrombin to thrombin 300,000 times faster than free factor Xa because free factor Xa is rapidly inactivated in plasma by tissue factor pathway inhibitor. The Xa–Va prothrombinase complex formed on the endothelial cell surface converts a small amount of prothrombin (factor II) to thrombin that, although insufficient for fibrin clot formation, converts factors VIII and IX to VIIIa and IXa, respectively. Unlike factor Xa, free factor IXa is not inactivated by plasma tissue factor pathway inhibitor and can diffuse and bind to activated platelets to form the factor IXa–VIIIa ("tenase") complex that enhances the conversion of factor X to Xa, generating a large amount of **Xa–Va prothrombinase complex** on the surface of activated platelets and yielding enough thrombin to form a fibrin clot. The thrombotic process is further enhanced by thrombin-mediated conversion of factor XI to XIa, thereby further boosting factor IXa production. **Thrombin**, a highly potent serine protease, rapidly converts plasma fibrinogen to **fibrin** monomer and factor XIII to **factor XIIIa**, a transglutaminase that covalently cross-links fibrin monomer to yield stable fibrin polymer. When bound to thrombomodulin on the surface of endothelial cells, thrombin also activates protein C, which, in concert with protein S, inactivates factors Va and VIIIa. Factor Va and VIIIa inactivation prevents generation of factor Xa and thrombin by the "tenase" and prothrombinase complexes, respectively. Thrombin

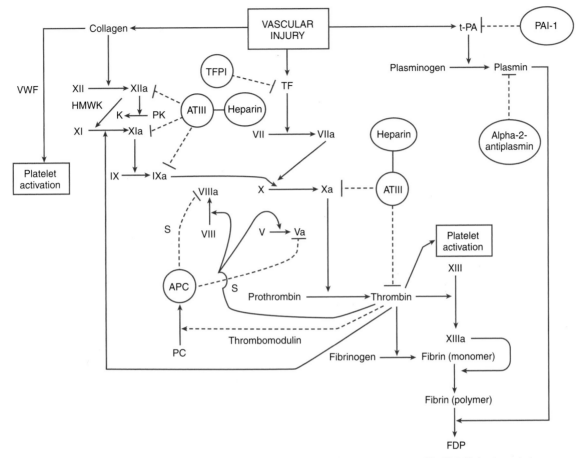

Fig. 15.1 The coagulation cascade. *APC*, Activated protein C; *ATIII*, antithrombin III; *FDP*, fibrin degradation product; *HMWK*, high-molecular-weight kininogen; *K*, kallikrein; *PAI-1*, plasminogen activator inhibitor-1; *PC*, protein C; *PK*, pre-kallikrein; *TFPI*, tissue factor pathway inhibitor; *t-PA*, tissue plasminogen activator.

also plays a role in conversion of plasminogen into plasmin and thus contributes not only to clot formation but to clot dissolution as well. Thrombin plays a central role in coagulation not only by proteolytic activation of fibrinogen; factors V, VIII, XI, and XIII; plasmin; and protein C but also by activation of platelets (Fig. 15.3).

Much of the excess thrombin generated at the site of vascular injury is rapidly inactivated by **antithrombin III (ATIII)**. ATIII inactivates thrombin by binding irreversibly in a one-to-one complex. This binding reaction is enhanced several thousandfold by the closely related sulfated mucopolysaccharides heparan sulfate and heparin. **Heparan sulfate** is expressed on the luminal surface of vascular endothelium, whereas endogenous **heparin** is produced by mast cells and basophils. After

thrombin binding to ATIII, heparan sulfate and heparin are released from the complex, again making them available for binding to free ATIII. The thrombogenic action of thrombin is also controlled by binding of free thrombin to **thrombomodulin**, a membrane protein expressed by endothelial cells. Thrombomodulin-bound thrombin activates protein C, which, when complexed with protein S, inhibits clotting by inactivating coagulation cofactors VIIIa and Va.

Although the preceding model of tissue factor-initiated activation, known as the **extrinsic pathway**, is the predominant pathway operative in the in vivo setting, a second activation pathway known as the **intrinsic pathway** exists. In this pathway, coagulation is initiated by negative-charged surface activation of plasma **factor**

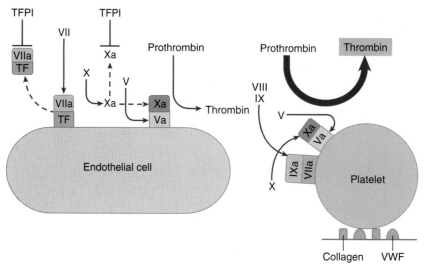

Fig. 15.2 Endothelial cells and platelets in coagulation activation. *TF*, tissue factor; *TFPI*, tissue factor pathway inhibitor; *VWF*, von Willebrand factor.

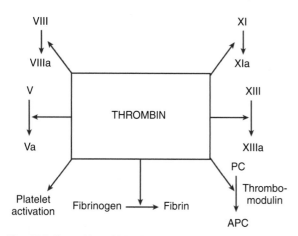

Fig. 15.3 Thrombin, which plays a central role in coagulation. *APC*, activated protein C; *PC*, protein C.

XII (Hageman factor) in the presence of plasma protein cofactors **prekallikrein** and **high-molecular-weight kininogen (HMWK)**. This pathway was discovered during investigations of the in vitro phenomenon of spontaneous (intrinsic) clot formation in uncoated, negatively charged glass tubes. Although factor XIIa can contribute to clotting via activation of the zymogen factor XI, the role of the intrinsic pathway in initiation of the clotting cascade in vivo appears to be minimal because deficiencies of factor XII, prekallikrein, and HMWK are not associated with increased bleeding. In contrast, factor XI deficiency is associated with bleeding, indicating that thrombin-mediated (rather than factor XIIa–mediated) activation of factor XI is critical for normal hemostasis.

FIBRINOLYSIS

The combination of platelet adhesion, fibrin formation, and platelet aggregation at the site of endothelial injury leads to formation of the stable fibrin-platelet clot. Dissolution of the fibrin clot is initiated by the fibrinolytic enzyme **plasmin**, formed by proteolytic cleavage of the plasma precursor plasminogen by thrombin and **tissue plasminogen activator (t-PA)**, released by damaged endothelial cells. The proteolytic byproducts of fibrinolysis, low-molecular-weight fibrinopeptide fragments known collectively as **fibrin degradation products (FDPs)**, including **D-dimer**, interfere with thrombin-mediated fibrin formation by competitive inhibition.

BLEEDING DISORDERS

Deficiencies of fibrinogen; prothrombin; VWF; and factors V, VII, VIII, IX, X, XI, and XIII are all associated with abnormal bleeding, whereas deficiencies of factor XII, prekallikrein, and HMWK (members of the contact factor group) are not associated with increased bleeding.

Hemophilia A (factor VIII deficiency) and **hemophilia B** (factor IX deficiency) are X-linked recessive disorders seen almost exclusively in males. In rare cases, hemophilia in a female is seen if the father has hemophilia and the mother is a carrier. Female carriers themselves are sometimes at risk of excess bleeding secondary to injury or surgery. The clinical severity of these disorders is related to the levels of functional coagulation factor in plasma. Severe spontaneous bleeding is seen in patients with less than 1% functional protein, whereas patients with factor levels higher than 5% experience bleeding only when provoked by trauma or surgery. The bleeding in hemophilia takes the form of bleeding into deep tissues (hemarthrosis, hematomas, and excessive surgical bleeding). In contrast, the bleeding seen with deficiency of VWF (von **Willebrand disease [VWD]**), like that seen with platelet disorders, is more often more superficial cutaneous and mucosal bleeding (**petechiae** and **ecchymosis**). Because VWF is important in platelet adhesion and aggregation, it is not surprising that its deficiency leads to this form of platelet-type bleeding. Other forms of bleeding (easy bruising, **epistaxis**, and **menorrhagia**) may be seen with both types of bleeding disorders.

In factor VIII (hemophilia A), IX (hemophilia B), and XI (hemophilia C) deficiency, the **activated partial thromboplastin time (aPTT)** is prolonged, whereas the **prothrombin time (PT)** and platelet count are normal. Functional assays for factors VIII, IX, and XI confirm a specific factor deficiency. The functional assay is an aPTT performed on a mix of patient plasma with a single factor-deficient plasma (VIII, IX, or XI). Lack of correction of the aPTT by specific factor-deficient plasma identifies the deficient factor. For example, an aPTT that is corrected by factor VIII– and factor XI–deficient plasma but not by factor IX–deficient plasma is indicative of factor IX deficiency. Because VWF acts as a plasma carrier protein for factor VIII, the levels of factor VIII are typically decreased in VWD. Thus, in cases of bleeding in which the factor VIII levels are low, an assay for VWF is performed to clearly differentiate hemophilia A from VWD.

In contrast to deficiencies of factors VIII, IX, and IX that are marked by a prolonged aPTT and a normal PT, deficiencies of factors V, X, and prothrombin are marked by prolongation of both aPTT and PT. Factor VII deficiency is the only factor deficiency marked by a prolonged PT and normal aPTT. Again, confirmation of the specific factor deficiency is made with a mixing study with single factor-deficient plasma.

Factor XIII deficiency is a rare disorder that leads to delayed bleeding because of the production of unstable fibrin clots. Common forms of bleeding include neonatal umbilical cord bleeding, soft tissue hematoma, and intracranial hemorrhage. The PT and aPTT are normal in factor XIII deficiency. Instead, the diagnosis is made with the **urea clot lysis assay**. In this assay, thrombin is added to patient plasma to form a clot, which then is incubated in 5M urea. Under normal circumstances, a stable clot remains insoluble in urea, whereas a clot from factor XIII–deficient plasma is soluble.

In some cases, coagulation factor deficiencies are acquired as a result of the development of factor inhibitors (antibodies). The most common acquired factor inhibitor is directed against factor VIII, a condition known as **acquired hemophilia A**. Whereas 20% to 40% of patients with congenital hemophilia A treated with factor VIII develop alloantibodies to factor VIII, the development of factor VIII autoantibodies in nonhemophiliac individuals is rare. Although most cases of acquired hemophilia in people without hemophilia are idiopathic, patients with autoimmune disease and cancer are at increased risk. The condition is also seen in women in the postpartum setting. Acquired hemophilia, in contrast to congenital hemophilia, develops most often in adults of either gender. The bleeding in acquired hemophilia usually takes the form of purpura or soft tissue bleeding unlike the deep hemarthroses typical of congenital hemophilia. The quantity of factor VIII inhibitor can be determined by measuring residual factor VIII activity of normal plasma after incubation with serial dilutions of patient plasma. The result is reported in **Bethesda units**, with Bethesda units defined as the reciprocal of the dilution of patient plasma that yields 50% inhibition of factor VIII activity of normal plasma. For example, if a 1:64 dilution of patient plasma induces 50% factor VIII inhibition of normal plasma, then the titer of factor VIII antibody is 64 Bethesda units. During treatment, the titer of the inhibitor as measured in Bethesda units can be followed as a measure of treatment efficacy. Methods of treatment include those designed to increase factor VIII levels (with factor VIII concentrates or **DDAVP** [1-deamino-8-D-arginine vasopressin]), bypass factor VIII (with recombinant factor VIIa or activated prothrombin complex concentrate), or suppress production of factor VIII antibody (by plasmapheresis, intravenous immunoglobulin (Ig), and/or drug-induced immunosuppression). The vasopressin derivative DDAVP acts by stimulating release of factor VIII by vascular endothelial cells.

Von Willebrand factor, the only coagulation factor not made by hepatocytes, is produced by endothelial cells and megakaryocytes and released as a high-molecular-weight multimer that acts as a platelet "glue" by forming molecular bridges between activated platelets in a process known as **platelet aggregation** and between platelets and subendothelial collagen in a process known as **platelet adhesion**. VWF can bind to platelets via two cell surface receptors, glycoprotein (GP) Ib/IX and GPIIb/IIIa. Given the importance of platelet adhesion and aggregation to clot formation, it should come as no surprise that deficiency or defects in VWF leads to abnormal bleeding. These conditions are collectively known as VWD, which is not only the most common inherited bleeding disorder but is also seen as an acquired condition. VWD is characterized by so-called platelet-type mucosal bleeding, that is, bleeding into the skin (petechiae), nasal mucosa (epistaxis), mouth (gingival bleeding), soft tissues (hematoma), and endometrium (menorrhagia). Because factor VIII is stabilized in a plasma complex with VWF, factor VIII levels are often reduced in VWD (as indicated by a prolonged aPTT), which in some cases contributes to the bleeding disorder.

There are several subtypes of VWD that differ in bleeding severity. The most common type, **type 1 VWD**, is an autosomal dominant disease characterized by quantitatively reduced plasma levels of VWF antigen. Because VWF does not participate in the coagulation cascade leading to fibrin clot formation, VWF function cannot be measured by clotting assays (PT and aPTT). Instead, VWF is best measured by a platelet aggregation assay known as the ristocetin cofactor activity assay. **Ristocetin cofactor activity** is determined by measuring platelet aggregation induced by patient plasma (as a source of VWF) in the presence of the compound ristocetin. **Ristocetin** is a synthetic molecule that induces platelet aggregation by forming molecular bridges between VWF molecules bound to adjacent platelets.

The second most common type of VWD, **type 2A VWD**, is a usually autosomal dominant disease characterized by qualitative defects of VWF leading to greater loss in functional ristocetin cofactor activity than in VWF antigen concentration. The characteristic loss of high and intermediate molecular weight VWF multimers in type 2A VWD can be measured by **agarose gel protein electrophoresis**. The third most common VWD variant, **type 2B VWD**, is an autosomal dominant condition characterized by selective loss of only high-molecular-weight VWF multimers, leading to ristocetin cofactor activity that ranges from normal to mildly decreased. Type 2B VWD can be identified by performing **ristocetin-induced platelet aggregation (RIPA)**, an assay performed by adding ristocetin directly to patient platelet-rich plasma and monitoring platelet aggregation with an optical device called a platelet aggregometer. After platelet aggregation, an optically dense suspension of platelet-rich plasma (low light transmittance) is converted to more optically clear plasma with large platelet aggregates (high light transmittance). In contrast to the ristocetin cofactor activity assay, RIPA uses the patient's own platelets coated in vivo with VWF. Curiously, type 2B VWD is characterized by increased RIPA to low concentrations of ristocetin, a result shared with a rare von Willebrand–like autosomal dominant disease known as **pseudo-VWD** that results from a mutation in the platelet GPIb VWF receptor. **Type 2N VWD** is an uncommon autosomal recessive disease characterized by factor VIII deficiency that is caused by a VWF defect, leading to poor factor VIII binding. **Type 3 VWD** is an uncommon but severe, usually autosomal recessive form of VWD characterized by virtual absence of VWF protein.

Under some clinical circumstances, such as massive tissue damage (trauma or burns) and septic shock, release of tissue factor or tissue factor–like substances into the bloodstream triggers a pathologic hypercoagulable process known as **disseminated intravascular coagulation (DIC)**. This process leads initially to small vessel thrombosis, rapid depletion of coagulation factors and platelets, and extensive fibrinolysis with production of increased amounts of fibrin split products and ultimately to generalized bleeding and vascular collapse. Laboratory diagnosis of DIC is best established by documenting prolonged PT and aPTT, thrombocytopenia, and elevated fibrin degradation products, including D-dimers. D-dimers are plasmin-mediated FDPs that are composed of two cross-linked D fragments. D-dimers, in contrast to generic FDP, are formed only from fibrin (not fibrinogen) degradation. Thus, D-dimers are increased in fibrinolytic conditions such as DIC and not increased in fibrinogenolytic conditions such as primary fibrinogenolysis (see later discussion). Treatment of patients with DIC is best directed at treatment of the underlying cause (trauma, cancer, or sepsis), supplemented in some cases with heparin to inhibit clotting and plasma or platelet transfusions to replace consumed coagulation factors and platelets.

Primary fibrinogenolysis is a rare DIC-like bleeding condition caused by plasmin-mediated fibrinogenolysis. Conversion of plasminogen to plasmin is initiated by the plasminogen activators tissue plasminogen activator t-PA and **urokinase (u-PA)**. Under normal circumstances, plasmin activity is limited to fibrinolysis, with free plasmin rapidly inactivated by plasmin inhibitors. However, in some circumstances, such as severe liver disease and disseminated cancer, excess free plasmin leads to fibrinogenolysis. The source of most of the released t-PA is endothelial cells and u-PA is released primarily by malignant, often urothelial, tumors. Although similar to DIC, D-dimers are not increased and the platelet count is normal in primary fibrinogenolysis. The **euglobulin clot lysis test** is abnormally shortened in both DIC and primary fibrinogenolysis.

Thrombotic thrombocytopenic purpura (TTP)–hemolytic uremic syndrome (HUS) is a DIC-like disorder most commonly seen in females and classically characterized by thrombocytopenia, microangiopathic hemolytic anemia, fever, neurologic symptoms, and acute renal failure. The disease is most often caused by an inherited or acquired autoantibody-induced deficiency in ADAMTS13 that leads to increased levels of thrombogenic high-molecular-weight multimers of VWF, spontaneous platelet aggregation, deposition of platelet microthrombi in small vessels, red blood cell fragmentation, and thrombocytopenia. Unlike DIC, TTP-HUS is characterized by relatively normal coagulation test results (PT, aPTT, and D-dimer). The distinction from DIC is important because current treatment of patients with TTP-HUS is immediate plasma exchange, presumably effective because of removal of thrombogenic high-molecular-weight VWF multimers and autoantibodies and repletion of the VWF-cleaving enzyme. syndrome HUS is an acquired TTP-like condition that primarily affects young children who present with *Escherichia coli* diarrhea followed by renal microthrombosis and renal failure.

Another DIC-like condition is **HELLP syndrome** (acronym for *hemolytic* anemia, *elevated liver* enzymes, and *low platelet* count), which occurs in pregnant women with severe **preeclampsia** (hypertension, proteinuria, and edema developing during pregnancy) who further develop microangiopathic hemolytic anemia, elevated liver enzymes, and thrombocytopenia in the third trimester or postpartum period.

Loss of normal hepatocyte function in **liver disease** leads to decreased factor synthesis and ultimately to multiple factor deficiencies and increased bleeding. Synthesis of the vitamin K–dependent factors II, VII, IX, and X is suppressed in liver disease because gamma-carboxyl modification of the precursors takes place within hepatocytes. Because factor VII (labile factor) has the shortest plasma half-life of all coagulation factors, it is the first to drop below normal levels in liver disease, thus explaining why the factor VII–dependent PT is a more sensitive indicator of liver disease than the aPTT. On the other hand, because factor V (a stable factor) has the longest plasma half-life of the coagulation factors, reduced levels of factor V in patients with liver disease indicate a severe reduction in hepatic function. Other contributing factors to the abnormal bleeding seen in liver disease include **hypofibrinogenemia**, synthesis of abnormal fibrinogen (dysfibrinogenemia), and reduced hepatic clearance of plasma fibrin or fibrinogen split products that interfere with normal clotting.

Vitamin K deficiency leads to increased bleeding from functional deficiencies of the vitamin K–dependent factors II, VII, IX, and X. Under normal circumstances, vitamin K converts the inactive precursors of these factors in hepatocytes to active precursors by carboxylation of gamma-glutamyl residues. In vitamin K deficiency, the inactive precursors, known as **proteins induced by vitamin K antagonism or absence (PIVKA)**, accumulate in the circulation. The anticoagulant coumadin, a vitamin K antagonist, also leads to accumulation of PIVKA. Gamma-glutamyl carboxylation allows coagulation factors to efficiently bind to phospholipid-rich endothelial cell and platelet surfaces via divalent calcium bridges. Although proteins C and S are also vitamin K–dependent factors, deficiency does not lead to increased bleeding.

HEREDITARY THROMBOPHILIA

Thrombophilia refers to any clinical condition marked by an increased risk of thrombosis. Inheritance of several coagulation factor mutations and polymorphisms (factor V, prothrombin, fibrinogen, protein C, protein S, and ATIII) leads to recurrent venous (often deep vein), arterial, or both types of thrombosis in some patients. Disease may be seen not only in the homozygous condition but also in the heterozygous condition. Disease severity is often modified by a variety of contributing factors. Acquired deficiencies of protein C, protein S, and ATIII that result from liver disease or autoantibody formation may also lead to thrombophilia.

Antiphospholipid syndrome is an acquired autoimmune thrombophilic condition resulting from development of antibodies to phospholipids and associated proteins, most commonly the phospholipid **cardiolipin** (diphosphatidylglycerol) and the associated apolipoprotein beta-glycoprotein 1. These antibodies are often referred to as lupus anticoagulants because they are often seen in patients with systemic lupus erythematosus and interfere with in vitro phospholipid-dependent clotting assays such as the **dilute Russell viper venom test (dRVVT**; see the discussion of coagulation testing). Despite their anticoagulant effects in vitro, these antibodies are associated with venous and arterial thrombosis in vivo.

Activated protein C resistance (also known as resistance to activated protein C), the most common hereditary thrombophilia and seen in up to 12% of whites, is associated with recurrent venous thrombosis. The disease results from inheritance of an abnormal factor V gene with a specific point mutation (**factor V Leiden**) that resists inactivation by activated protein C, thus leading to poorly controlled factor Va activity. The heterozygous conditions increases the thrombotic risk four- to eightfold, whereas it is estimated that half of all those with homozygosity will experience significant thrombosis. The risk of thrombosis in heterozygotes is markedly increased in combination with protein C deficiency, physical inactivity, and oral contraceptive use. The risk of arterial thrombosis is increased in smokers.

Protein C deficiency typically presents as an autosomal dominant condition, with most heterozygotes being asymptomatic. Recurrent venous thrombosis results from inadequate protein C- or S-dependent inhibition of thrombin-activated procoagulant cofactors Va and VIIIa. Newborns with severe deficiency may present with **neonatal purpura fulminans**, a serious condition characterized by arterial and venous thrombosis that leads to widespread ecchymosis and hemorrhagic necrosis of subcutaneous tissues. Protein C deficiency is a risk factor for **coumarin skin necrosis**, a purpura fulminans–like condition seen in patients treated with coumarin (warfarin). In this case, inherited deficiency of protein C is exacerbated by coumarin-mediated inhibition of protein C.

Protein S deficiency is an autosomal dominant condition with features similar to protein C deficiency. Recurrent venous thrombosis results from inadequate inhibition of procoagulant cofactors Va and VIIIa by the protein C–protein S complex. Protein S deficiency may also be seen as an acquired condition.

ATIII in conjunction with heparin or heparan is a potent inhibitor of factors IXa, Xa, XIa, and IIa (thrombin). **ATIII deficiency** leads to increased risk of venous thrombosis in older children and young adults. A 10- to 20-fold increased risk of thrombosis—venous more than arterial—peaks in the second decade of life. Heparin resistance is not a strong indicator of ATIII-deficient reduced levels with liver disease and heparin use.

Some patients with hereditary **dysfibrinogenemia**, defined by hepatic production of dysfunctional fibrinogen caused by a variety of fibrinogen point mutations, are susceptible to venous thrombosis in young adulthood. Many patients with dysfibrinogenemia present with a bleeding disorder rather than thrombophilia. In young women, the defect may present as spontaneous abortion, stillbirth, or postpartum hemorrhage. Coagulation testing most often demonstrates a prolonged thrombin time, reptilase time, or both. An acquired form of dysfibrinogenemia is seen in chronic liver disease. In chronic liver disease, a hypersialated form of fibrinogen that functions poorly in fibrin polymerization is produced.

Thrombophilia is also seen in patients with elevated plasma prothrombin (caused by a specific prothrombin gene polymorphism), elevated factor VIII levels, and elevated homocysteine levels (**hyperhomocysteinemia**). Elevated blood homocysteine is associated with both accelerated arteriosclerosis and thrombosis, likely as a result of toxic effects on endothelial cells. Causes of hyperhomocysteinemia include mutations in enzymes involved in homocysteine metabolism and deficiencies of vitamin B_6, vitamin B_{12}, and folate.

ANTICOAGULATION

Warfarin, and other coumarin drugs (including coumadin), are oral anticoagulants that act by inhibiting vitamin K reductase, thus blocking vitamin K–dependent gamma-glutamyl carboxylation of **vitamin K–dependent factors** II, VII, IX, X, protein C, and protein S. The coagulation factor proteins that are produced by the liver in the presence of warfarin are functionally inactive. The anticoagulant effect of warfarin is rapidly reversed by vitamin K administration. Because common pathway factors II, IX, and X are inhibited by warfarin, it could be predicted that the intrinsic pathway as measured by the aPTT would be inhibited. However, because factor VII has the shortest half-life of these coagulation factors, its inhibition by warfarin leads to a more rapid and dramatic inhibition of the PT. Major complications of warfarin therapy include bleeding, often gastrointestinal, and skin necrosis. The skin necrosis may be caused by a hypercoagulable state as a result of severe warfarin-mediated protein C and S deficiency that develops in some patients. Other oral anticoagulants act by direct inhibition of thrombin or factor Xa.

The other major anticoagulant, heparin, is a high-molecular-weight sulfated glycosaminoglycan that binds to ATIII, greatly enhancing its inhibitory effect (more than 1000-fold), primarily upon thrombin and factor Xa. In contrast to warfarin, heparin must be administered parenterally. Because the anticoagulant effect of warfarin is delayed until vitamin K–dependent factors are depleted (3–4 days), patients requiring long-term anticoagulation are typically initially treated with both intravenous heparin and oral warfarin, with heparin withdrawn after the warfarin effect is optimal. There are three major types of pharmacologic heparin: **unfractionated heparin (UFH)**; low-molecular-weight heparin; and a synthetic pentasaccharide, fondaparinux, that specifically blocks factor Xa. UFH is a complex mixture of polysulfated glycosaminoglycans of various molecular weights whose anticoagulant effect is not entirely predictable, requiring periodic monitoring with the aPTT. **Low-molecular-weight heparin (LMWH)** is a more purified preparation whose anticoagulant effect is more predictable than UFH. Unlike UFH, LMWH has a more dramatic inhibitory effect on factor Xa than thrombin and is more accurately monitored with an **anti-Xa** test. In some patients, heparin therapy yields a poor anticoagulant effect. This phenomenon, termed **heparin resistance**, most often results from high levels of factor VIII produced in response to inflammation. In some cases, heparin resistance is caused by ATIII deficiency. In this situation, heparin is ineffective because it cannot form a functional ATIII–heparin complex.

Endogenous heparin is produced by and stored in the secretory granules of tissue mast cells. Heparin released by mast cells located near small blood vessels likely maintains the patency of the microvascular system. The endogenous glycosaminoglycan heparan sulfate also possesses anticoagulant properties, albeit to a lesser extent than heparin. Unlike heparin, heparan sulfate is a ubiquitous compound produced by many

cell types and found throughout the extracellular matrix. Heparan sulfate produced by endothelial cells plays an important role in maintaining normal intravascular blood flow. The anticoagulant potency of both heparin and heparan sulfate is directly related to the presence of a specific polysulfated pentasaccharide that binds the circulating protein ATIII with high affinity. Heparan sulfate expresses this pentasaccharide moiety at a lower frequency than heparin. ATIII inhibits coagulation by binding to and inhibiting the activity of several activated coagulation factors, most importantly factors Xa and thrombin.

Adverse side effects of UFH include excessive bleeding, **heparin-induced thrombocytopenia (HIT)** with thrombosis, and heparin-induced osteoporosis. Several anticoagulants that act as specific thrombin inhibitors have recently been developed. These newer agents, as well as low-molecular-weight heparin, are useful in patients who cannot tolerate UFH therapy.

Heparin-induced thrombocytopenia results from development of IgG antibodies to heparin–platelet factor 4 (PF4) complexes. PF4, a procoagulant chemokine also known as CXCL4, is released from platelet alpha granules and binds strongly to heparinlike substances. Heparin–PF4 immune complexes bind to platelets via platelet Fc receptors, inducing intravascular platelet aggregation and thrombosis. HIT is less often seen in patients treated with LMWH. The mechanism of heparin-induced osteoporosis has not been clearly determined but likely involves direct effects on metabolic bone formation and resorption.

Other anticoagulants include ADP receptor antagonists and direct inhibitors of factor Xa or thrombin (**hirudin**). Inhibitors of platelet aggregation include aspirin (cyclooxygenase inhibitor), adenosine diphosphate receptor antagonists, and GPIIb/IIIa receptor antagonists.

COAGULATION TESTING

The PT is defined as the time in seconds needed for citrate-anticoagulated plasma to form a clot at 37°C after addition of calcium and tissue factor (provided by rabbit brain extract that also contains a small amount of phospholipid) (Table 15.2). Normally, a clot forms within 12 to 14 seconds. A prolonged PT is seen in patients with abnormalities (mutation, deficiency, or inhibitor) of factor VII, X, or V; prothrombin; fibrinogen;

TABLE 15.2	Coagulation Tests
Test	**Clinical Conditions Detected**
Prothrombin time	Factor VII, X, V, II, and I deficiency; liver disease; warfarin effect
Activated partial thromboplastin time	Factor XI, X, IX, VIII, V, II, and I deficiency; presence of heparin; antiphospholipid syndrome
Thrombin time	Fibrinogen deficiency or dysfunction; presence of heparin; presence of FDP
Reptilase time	Differentiates heparin from FDP effect on thrombin time
Dilute Russell viper venom time	Antiphospholipid syndrome
Plasma mixing study	Factor inhibitors (antibodies)
Urea clot lysis	Factor XIII deficiency
Ristocetin cofactor activity	VWD
Euglobulin clot lysis	Fibrinolysis; fibrinogenolysis

FDP, Fibrin degradation product; *VWD,* von Willebrand disease.

or a combination of these (extrinsic pathway) and in patients treated with the anticoagulant coumadin.

The aPTT is defined as the time needed for citrate-anticoagulated plasma to form a clot at 37°C after addition of calcium, phospholipid (partial thromboplastin), and kaolin, a clay mineral that serves as a surface activator. Normally, a clot forms within 28 to 30 seconds. A prolonged aPTT is seen in patients with abnormalities (mutation, deficiency, or inhibitor) of prekallikrein; HMWK; factors XII, IX, VIII, X, and V; prothrombin; fibrinogen; or a combination of these (intrinsic pathway) and in patients treated with the anticoagulant heparin (see Table 15.1).

The **thrombin time** is defined as the time it takes for citrated plasma to form a clot following addition of calcium and thrombin. Normally, a clot forms within 10 to 12 seconds. A prolonged thrombin time is seen with abnormalities (mutation, deficiency, or inhibitor) of **fibrinogen** or in the presence of **thrombin inhibitors** (FDP or heparin). To differentiate between FDP and heparin as the cause of a prolonged thrombin time, the **reptilase time** may be performed. Reptilase (a snake venom) directly converts plasma fibrinogen to fibrin and unlike thrombin is not inhibited by heparin. Thus, assuming that the thrombin time defect is not caused by fibrinogen deficiency or dysfibrinogenemia, a prolonged reptilase time is strongly suggestive of increased FDP, as seen in DIC. Elevated FDP can be confirmed by direct measurement of FDP (or D-dimer) by immunoassay. On the other hand, confirmation that a prolonged thrombin time associated with a normal reptilase time resulting from heparin contamination can be obtained by repeating the assay following pretreatment of the plasma with heparinase to destroy the heparin or by

first passing the plasma through an anion exchange column to remove the heparin.

Given a prolonged PT or aPTT, screening for the presence of a factor inhibitor (autoantibody) is performed by a **plasma mixing study**. In a mixing study, patient plasma and normal control plasma are mixed in a 1:1 ratio, and a repeat PT or aPTT is performed. If the prolonged PT or aPTT is caused by a factor deficiency (e.g., hemophilia B [factor IX deficiency]), the presence of normal amounts of the deficient factor in the normal plasma will lead to correction of the test result. It is important to recognize that 50% of a normal factor level is more than sufficient to normalize the test result. In contrast to factor deficiency, the mix fails to correct the PT or aPTT in the presence of a factor inhibitor. After a positive mixing study result (one without correction), specific factor assays are performed to identify the specificity of the inhibitor, for example, factor X inhibitor, factor VII inhibitor, and so on.

If an antiphospholipid antibody inhibitor is suspected, a dRVVT is performed. In this test, ethylenediaminetetraacetic acid (EDTA)–anticoagulated patient plasma is recalcified in the presence of a dilute preparation of phospholipid and Russell viper venom, and the time to clot formation is recorded. Russell viper venom converts factor X to factor Xa in the presence of sufficient phospholipid and factor Va. A prolonged result in comparison with the aPTT is suspicious for **antiphospholipid antibody**. A correction in the dilute Russell viper venom test with addition of a large amount of phospholipid (that binds and inactivates the entire antiphospholipid antibody) provides confirmation of antiphospholipid antibody. Patients with antiphospholipid syndrome often develop antibodies to cardiolipin, a lipid with anticoagulant properties found in the inner mitochondrial membrane. **Cardiolipin antibodies** are detected and measured by enzyme-linked immunosorbent assay.

A **urea clot solubility assay** is performed when factor XIII deficiency is suspected. In this assay, a clot formed by adding thrombin to patient plasma is suspended in 5M urea. An unstable clot caused by lack of factor XIII-mediated cross-linking is soluble in urea, whereas a normal clot is insoluble.

In the **euglobulin clot lysis test**, the time for a euglobulin clot to dissolve is measured. Euglobulin, a precipitate of clotting factors formed by the acidification of citrated plasma, is dissolved in buffer and then recalcified to form a euglobulin clot. The rate of clot lysis is proportional to the plasma fibrinolytic activity. The euglobulin clot lysis time is shortened in DIC and primary fibrinogenolysis.

KEY WORDS AND CONCEPTS

- Acquired hemophilia A
- Activated partial thromboplastin time (aPTT)
- Activated protein C resistance
- Agarose gel protein electrophoresis
- Antiphospholipid antibody
- Antiphospholipid syndrome
- Antithrombin III (ATIII)
- Anti-Xa
- ATIII deficiency
- Bethesda units
- Buffy coat
- Cardiolipin
- Cardiolipin antibodies
- Coumarin skin necrosis
- DDAVP
- Dilute Russell viper venom test (dRVVT)
- Disseminated intravascular coagulation (DIC)
- Dysfibrinogenemia
- Ecchymosis
- Epistaxis
- Euglobulin clot lysis test
- Extrinsic pathway
- Factor V Leiden
- Factor VII
- Factor XII (Hageman factor)
- Factor XIII deficiency
- Factor XIIIa
- Fibrin
- Fibrin degradation products (FDP)
- Fibrinogen
- Fibrinolysis
- HELLP syndrome
- Hemolytic uremic syndrome (HUS)
- Hemophilia A
- Hemophilia B
- Heparan sulfate
- Heparin
- Heparin resistance
- Heparin-induced thrombocytopenia (HIT)
- High-molecular-weight kininogen (HMWK)
- Hirudin
- Hyperhomocysteinemia
- Hypofibrinogenemia
- Intrinsic pathway
- Liver disease
- Low-molecular-weight heparin (LMWH)
- Menorrhagia
- Neonatal purpura fulminans
- Petechiae
- Plasma mixing study
- Plasmin
- Platelet adhesion
- Platelet aggregation
- Prekallikrein
- Primary fibrinogenolysis
- Protein C deficiency
- Protein S deficiency
- Proteins induced from vitamin K antagonism or absence (PIVKA)

- Prothrombin time (PT)
- Prothrombinase complex
- Pseudo-VWD
- Reptilase time
- Ristocetin cofactor activity
- Ristocetin
- Ristocetin-induced platelet aggregation (RIPA)
- Serine proteases
- Tenase complex (IXa–VIIIa complex)
- Thrombin
- Thrombin inhibitors
- Thrombin time
- Thrombomodulin
- Thrombophilia
- Thrombotic thrombocytopenic purpura (TTP)
- Tissue factor
- Tissue factor pathway inhibitor
- Tissue plasminogen activator (t-PA)
- Type 1 VWD
- Type 2A VWD
- Type 2B VWD
- Type 2N VWD
- Type 3 VWD
- Unfractionated heparin (UFH)
- Urea clot solubility assay
- Urokinase (u-PA)
- Vitamin K deficiency
- Vitamin K–dependent factors
- von Willebrand disease (VWD)
- von Willebrand factor (VWF)
- VWF-cleaving enzyme (ADAMTS13)
- Warfarin
- Xa–Va prothrombinase complex
- Zymogens

REVIEW QUESTIONS

1. Tissue factor activates which of the following coagulation factors?
   A. Factor XII
   B. VWF
   C. factor X
   D. factor VII

2. The anticoagulant heparin acts by
   A. activating plasmin.
   B. stabilizing ATIII.
   C. inhibiting protein C.
   D. inhibiting vitamin K reductase.

3. Increased thrombosis (thrombophilia) is seen in all of the following conditions below **except**
   A. antiphospholipid antibody.
   B. protein C deficiency.
   C. factor VIII deficiency.
   D. homocysteinemia.

4. All of the following statements about VWD are true **except**
   A. VWD Can be monitored with prothrombin and partial thromboplastin time.
   B. Quantitative and qualitative defects of VWF lead to defective platelet adhesion and aggregation.
   C. VWD presents with mucosal bleeding (petechial, nasal, gingival).
   D. VWD is most often autosomal dominant.

5. Which one of the following statements about DIC is **incorrect**?
   A. Trauma or sepsis induces tissue factor release.
   B. Fibrinogen and platelets are decreased.
   C. Fibrin-platelet microthrombi form in small vessels.
   D. Increased FDPs lead to intravascular thrombosis.

16

Platelets

KEY POINTS

- Megakaryocytes in the bone marrow are stimulated by the liver-derived cytokine thrombopoietin to produce platelets by cytoplasmic budding.

- Platelets are small anucleate cytoplasmic fragments that circulate in the blood with a half-life of 8 to 10 days..

- The normal platelet count ranges from 150,000 to 400,000/μL of blood; one third of all platelets in the vascular pool reside in the spleen (marginal pool).

- Bleeding solely caused by thrombocytopenia seldom occurs above a blood platelet count of 50,000/μL.

- Platelet-type (mucosal) bleeding is characterized by petechiae, ecchymosis, and purpura.

- Subendothelial collagen and von Willebrand factor (VWF) exposed by endothelial damage trigger platelet adhesion to the damaged vessel wall.

- Adherent platelets release the platelet activation factor adenosine diphosphate and bind to circulating platelets (platelet aggregation) via fibrinogen and VWF bridges to form hemostatic platelet plugs at sites of vascular injury.

- Aggregated platelets trigger vasoconstriction (serotonin) and induce vascular repair at the site of vascular injury.

- The mature blood clot is composed of an adherent meshwork of platelets and fibrin.

- Inherited platelet bleeding disorders are caused by mutations in platelet surface receptors for VWF, fibrinogen, or both; granule deficiency; and granule release defects.

- Causes of acquired platelet bleeding disorders include splenomegaly, aplastic anemia, hematopoietic malignancy, drugs, and immune-mediated destruction.

Platelets are small anucleate cells produced by cytoplasmic budding from bone marrow megakaryocytes (Fig. 16.1). Megakaryocyte growth and platelet production are largely controlled by **thrombopoietin (TPO)**, a growth factor produced by the liver. The TPO level is constant and does not vary with platelet count. The **TPO receptor** (*c-mpl* gene) is expressed on both megakaryocytes and platelets. Because under normal conditions the platelet mass greatly exceeds the megakaryocyte mass, the amount of TPO available for binding to megakaryocytes is limited. In situations in which the platelet mass is reduced, such as thrombocytopenia, more TPO is available for binding to megakaryocytes, which stimulates megakaryocyte growth and increased platelet production. Increased platelet production is marked by release into

blood of numerous young platelets that are relatively large with abundant cytoplasmic RNA. These platelets, known as reticulated platelets, have an increased mean platelet volume and can be enumerated by automated complete blood count instruments after staining with the fluorescent RNA-binding dye thiazole orange.

On Wright-stained peripheral smears, platelets appear as small, blue-gray particles with purple-red granules about one-tenth the size of red blood cells (RBCs; Fig. 16.2). The normal platelet count ranges from 150,000 to 400,000/μL, yielding a ratio of platelets to RBCs on a peripheral smear of about 1 to 20. About one-third of all platelets are sequestered in the spleen. Platelets in the **splenic pool** freely exchange with circulating platelets and can be immediately released to the blood in

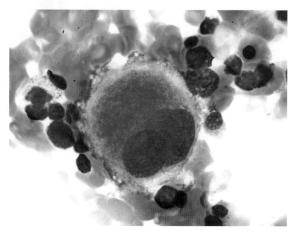

Fig. 16.1 Large megakaryocyte *(center)* with a multilobated nucleus and irregular cytoplasmic borders (marrow aspirate smear and Wright-Giemsa stain).

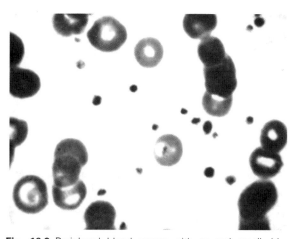

Fig. 16.2 Peripheral blood smear with several small, blue platelets and many larger red blood cells (Wright stain).

Clotting is initiated at the site of vascular injury not only by factor VII surface activation on damaged endothelial cells by tissue factor but also by **platelet activation**. Circulating platelets bind to **subendothelial collagen** and **von Willebrand factor (VWF)** exposed by loss of endothelial cells via platelet surface glycoprotein receptors **GPIa/IIa** and **GPIb/IX**, respectively, in a process termed **platelet adhesion** (Fig. 16.3). Exposure to collagen, **adenosine diphosphate (ADP)**, and thrombin induces shape changes in adherent platelets with release of platelet granule contents and expression of the high-affinity fibrinogen–VWF receptor **GPIIb/IIIa**. The platelet shape change results from calcium-dependent contraction of actin–myosin bundles within the platelet cytoplasm.

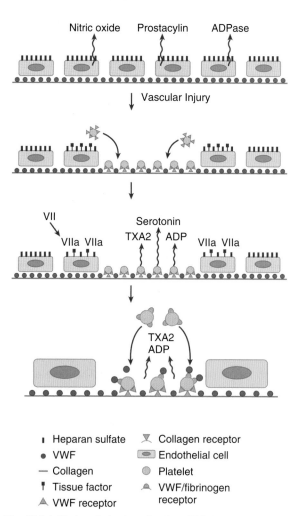

Fig. 16.3 Initiation of platelet adhesion. *ADP,* Adenosine diphosphate; *TXA2,* thromboxane A2; *VWF,* von Willebrand factor.

response to epinephrine (from stress). Splenomegaly of any cause is often accompanied by thrombocytopenia because of increased size of the splenic pool. The normal platelet lifespan is 8 to 10 days. Aged or damaged platelets are removed primarily by the spleen, with contributions by the liver and bone marrow. The age-associated loss of terminal sialic acid residues on platelet surface glycoproteins exposes mannose residues that are recognized by mannose receptor bearing macrophages, leading to phagocytosis. In addition, nonimmune immunoglobulin (Ig) G bound to aged or damaged platelets leads to ingestion by IgG (Fc) receptor-bearing macrophages.

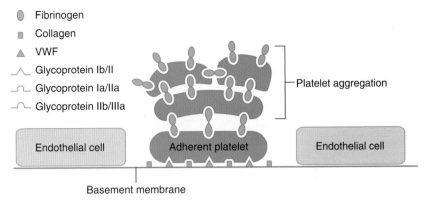

Fig. 16.4 Platelet adhesion and aggregation. *VWF,* Von Willebrand factor.

Nearby platelets bind to adherent platelets via fibrinogen and VWF bridges in a process termed **platelet aggregation** (Fig. 16.4). Phosphatidyl serine residues exposed on the surface of activated platelets serve as sites for calcium-dependent binding of the **vitamin K–dependent coagulation factors** (II, VII, IX, and X). Aggregated platelets at the site of a clot further contribute to thrombosis by binding circulating tissue factor-containing vesicles; releasing ADP, factor V, and fibrinogen; and providing a phospholipid surface receptive to binding of coagulation cofactors Va and VIIIa and subsequent production of factor Xa and thrombin by membrane-bound IXa-VIIIa and Xa-Va complexes, respectively.

Platelets contain several granules that are released upon platelet activation (Fig. 16.5). **Alpha granules** contain procoagulants (factor V, fibrinogen, VWF, and PF4) and growth factors (**platelet-derived growth factor [PDGF]** and transforming growth factor β [TGF-β]). **Platelet factor 4 (PF4)** contributes to clot formation by inactivating endogenous heparan sulfate at the site of endothelial cell injury. (PDGF) enhances vascular repair by stimulating fibroblast and smooth muscle cell growth. Both platelet-derived TGF-β and vascular endothelial growth factor induce vessel wall repair by stimulating endothelial cell and myofibroblast proliferation. **Dense granules** contain ADP, serotonin, and calcium. ADP is important in the recruitment and activation of platelets at the site of platelet adhesion. **Serotonin** minimizes bleeding at sites of injury by inducing vasoconstriction. **Calcium (Ca^{2+})** induces platelet shape change by stimulating contraction of the actin–myosin cytoskeleton. Calcium also serves as an essential co-factor in the coagulation cascade by bridging vitamin K–dependent factors with platelet membrane

phospholipid and as co-factor for **phospholipase C**, leading to the production of platelet **thromboxane A2**, a potent inducer of both platelet aggregation and vasoconstriction. **Arachidonic acid** is formed from platelet membrane phospholipid by phospholipase C. Arachidonic acid is converted to endoperoxides by the platelet enzyme **cyclooxygenase**, which are then converted to thromboxane A2 by thromboxane synthase. **Aspirin (acetylsalicylic acid)** inhibits platelet activation by irreversibly acetylating cyclooxygenase, thus preventing formation of thromboxane A2 by platelets. Endothelial cells inhibit platelet activation (and vasoconstriction) by converting endoperoxides to the potent platelet inhibitor (and vasodilator) **prostacyclin** through the action of the enzyme **prostacyclin synthase**. Endothelial cell prostacyclin activates platelet **adenylate cyclase**, increasing the intracellular concentration of **cyclic adenosine monophosphate (cAMP)**, which, by reducing intracellular calcium, inhibits platelet activation. Similarly, the antiplatelet drug **dipyridamole**, a phosphodiesterase inhibitor, inhibits platelet activation; it increases the level of platelet cAMP by inhibiting the cAMP-degradative action of phosphodiesterase. **Lysosomes** contain several proteolytic enzymes, including acid phosphatase, collagenase, and elastase. **Microperoxisomes** contain **catalase**, an enzyme that neutralizes toxic hydrogen peroxide released by leukocytes.

THROMBOCYTOPENIA AND THROMBOCYTOSIS

Reductions in the blood platelet count (thrombocytopenia) are commonly encountered in a variety of reactive and neoplastic conditions. In most cases, platelet counts

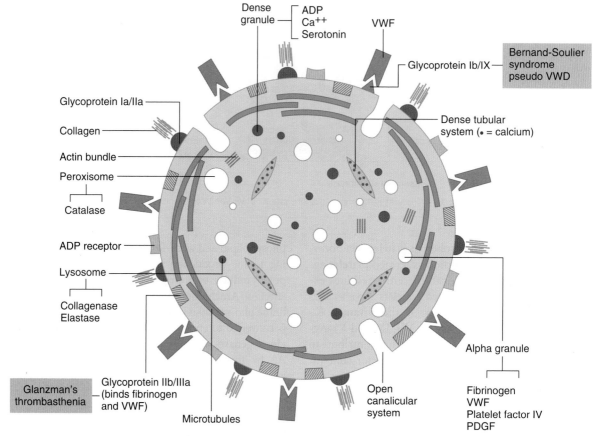

Fig. 16.5 Platelet structure and function. *ADP,* Adenosine diphosphate; *PDGF,* platelet-derived growth factor A2; *VWF,* von Willebrand factor.

greater than 50,000/μL are not associated with bleeding. Assuming normal platelet function, evidence of mucosal bleeding (petechiae, purpura) is seldom encountered with platelet counts greater than 20,000/μL of blood. A reduced blood platelet count may be detected in patients with massive splenomegaly. In this situation, a massive number of platelets are stored within the enlarged spleen (a condition known as pseudothrombocytopenia) (Box 16.1).

PLATELET FUNCTION DEFECTS

Several inherited and acquired defects of platelet function lead to clinical bleeding disorders.

Inherited Platelet Defects

The most common inherited disorder of platelet function, **von Willebrand disease (VWD)**, results not from an intrinsic platelet defect but rather from a deficiency of VWF. Without VWF, platelets are unable to aggregate properly in vivo. Inherited (autosomal recessive) deficiency of the platelet GPIb/IX receptor, known as **Bernard-Soulier syndrome**, is a rare autosomal recessive condition that not surprisingly shares many features with VWD. The disease is characterized by mucocutaneous bleeding (usually present from birth), prolonged bleeding time, decreased platelet count with giant platelets, and absent ristocetin-induced platelet aggregation (RIPA) that, unlike VWD, cannot be overcome by addition of normal plasma (a source of VWF). Inherited (autosomal recessive) deficiency of the platelet GPIIb/IIIa fibrinogen receptor, known as **Glanzmann thrombasthenia**, is a rare autosomal recessive condition characterized by mucocutaneous bleeding (usually present from birth), a normal platelet count, and absent platelet

BOX 16.1 Platelets by the Numbers

Causes of Thrombocytosis
- Chronic infections (tuberculosis, osteomyelitis, subacute bacterial endocarditis)
- Myeloproliferative disorders (extremely high in primary thrombocythemia)
- Malignancy (variety)
- Chronic inflammatory disorders (rheumatologic)
- Iron-deficiency anemia

Causes of Thrombocytopenia
- *Decreased Production*
  - Aplastic anemia
  - Megaloblastic anemia
  - Myelodysplastic syndrome
  - Acute leukemia
  - Cytotoxic chemotherapy and radiotherapy
  - Liver disease (decreased thrombopoietin)
- *Increased Destruction*
  - Autoimmune thrombocytopenia (idiopathic thrombocytopenic purpura)
  - Thrombotic thrombocytopenic purpura
  - Hemolytic uremic syndrome
  - Drug-induced (heparin, quinidine, sulfa drugs, carbamazepine, methyldopa, gold salts, rifampin, oral antidiabetics)
  - Disseminated intravascular coagulation (sepsis, leukemia)
  - Hypersplenism (cirrhosis, infiltrative diseases)
  - Posttransfusion purpura (alloimmune mediated)
  - Human immunodeficiency virus infection

aggregation by all agonists (platelet-aggregating agents ADP, thrombin, collagen, and epinephrine) except for ristocetin. There are a variety of defects in activation-induced secretion of platelet granule contents collectively referred to as *platelet release defects*. These disorders are characterized by easy bruising and mild mucocutaneous bleeding. The most common type of release defect is often referred to as "aspirinlike" because the platelet dysfunction is similar to that induced by aspirin. Aspirin, by inhibiting platelet cyclooxygenase, prevents the secondary wave of platelet aggregation by blocking the production and release of thromboxane A2 in response to the weak platelet agonists ADP and epinephrine. Similarly, in **aspirinlike release defects**, platelet activation by exogenous agents such as ADP and epinephrine fails to stimulate release of platelet granule contents, thus preventing the secondary wave of platelet aggregation. In some cases, the aspirinlike defect has been attributed to mutations in the cyclooxygenase gene. Other platelet release reaction defects, the **storage pool disorders**, result from absence of dense, alpha, or both types of granules. Thus, like aspirinlike defects, there is an absence of the secondary wave of platelet aggregation in response to ADP and epinephrine, not because the granule release mechanism is defective but because there are no granules to be released. Dense granule deficiency is characteristic of a few inherited disorders, most notably **Hermansky-Pudlak syndrome**, a disease commonly seen in northwest Puerto Rico characterized by partial albinism, pulmonary fibrosis, inflammatory bowel disease, and bleeding. Alpha granule deficiency is characteristic of **gray platelet syndrome**, a disease characterized by mild mucocutaneous bleeding; thrombocytopenia; and large, pale platelets on peripheral smears.

Acquired Platelet Defects

Several acquired platelet function defects usually present as easy bruising, mild mucocutaneous bleeding, or both. **Uremia** is associated with a mild bleeding diathesis, presumably because of effects on platelets of elevated nitrogenous waste products that would normally be rapidly eliminated by the kidneys. Platelet function is also impaired in **chronic liver disease** because of a variety of biochemical changes to the platelet membrane. Platelet function defects have also been described with **cardiopulmonary bypass** (caused by platelet trauma), **idiopathic thrombocytopenic purpura (ITP)**, **chronic myeloproliferative disorders**, and drugs (aspirin, other nonsteroidal antiinflammatory drugs, penicillin, and heparin).

In ITP, antibody-coated platelets are cleared from the circulation by splenic macrophages in the red pulp of the spleen, leading to thrombocytopenia, petechiae, purpura, and bleeding. Somewhat curiously, in contrast to **hypersplenism**, splenomegaly is not a feature of ITP. Antibodies formed are often directed against platelet VWF receptors GPIIb/IIIa and GPIb/IX. There are two distinct clinical forms of ITP: the childhood form (peak age, 2–4 years) and the adult form (peak age, 15–40 years). **Childhood ITP**, sometimes seen after a viral infection, is acute and in most cases resolves spontaneously. Treatment, when required, may include intravenous gamma globulin, corticosteroids, splenectomy, or a combination of these. **Adult ITP** is chronic and does not resolve spontaneously. Initial treatment consists of corticosteroids and splenectomy. However, more than one-third of adult-type patients do not respond to initial therapy and may require chemotherapy.

Platelet Aggregation Testing

Platelet-rich plasma is produced from ethylenediaminetetraacetic acid (EDTA)–anticoagulated whole blood by centrifugation. Individual platelet agonists are added to aliquots of platelet-rich plasma in clear tubes, and the change in light transmittance with time is measured in an aggregometer. In the presence of agonists, normal platelets are rapidly activated, change shape, and bind together to form aggregates. Initially, the light transmittance of the dense platelet suspension is very low. Soon after adding an agonist, normal platelets aggregate into progressively larger clumps. Light transmittance increases as aggregation proceeds. Two waves of aggregation are seen with weak agonists (e.g., ADP and epinephrine), the primary wave resulting from reversible agonist-dependent aggregation and the secondary wave resulting from irreversible platelet-dependent aggregation after the release of endogenous platelet-aggregating agents (Fig. 16.6). Only one large wave of aggregation is seen with strong agonists (e.g., collagen and thrombin). Specific platelet function defects can be identified by this approach. For example, in Bernard-Soulier syndrome, platelets do not aggregate in response to the nonphysiologic agonist ristocetin but exhibit normal aggregation with all other agonists. This results from inherited deficiency of the platelet VWF receptor Ib/IX. **Ristocetin** induces platelet aggregation by forming molecular bridges between VWF molecules bound to VWF receptors on adjacent platelets. Without platelet-bound VWF, RIPA cannot occur. Therapeutic inhibitors of platelet function include aspirin, ADP receptor antagonists, and GPIIB/IIIA antagonists.

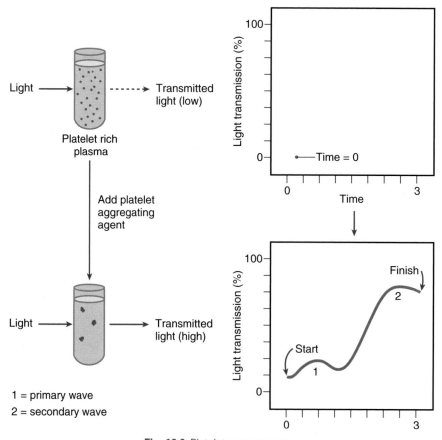

Fig. 16.6 Platelet aggregometry.

KEY WORDS AND CONCEPTS

- Adenylate cyclase
- Adenosine diphosphate (ADP)
- Adult ITP
- Alpha granules
- Arachidonic acid
- Aspirin (acetylsalicylic acid)
- Aspirinlike release defects
- Bernard-Soulier syndrome
- Calcium (Ca^{2+})
- Catalase
- Cardiopulmonary bypass
- Childhood ITP
- Chronic liver disease
- Chronic myeloproliferative disorders
- Cyclic adenosine monophosphate (cAMP)
- Cyclooxygenase
- Dense granules
- Dipyridamole
- Glanzmann thrombasthenia
- GPIa/IIa
- GPIb/IX
- GPIIb/IIIa
- Gray platelet syndrome
- Hermansky-Pudlak syndrome
- Hypersplenism
- Idiopathic thrombocytopenic purpura (ITP)
- Lysosomes
- Microperoxisomes
- Phospholipase C
- Platelet activation
- Platelet adhesion
- Platelet aggregation
- Platelet-derived growth factor (PDGF)
- Platelet factor 4 (PF4)
- Platelet release defects
- Prostacyclin
- Prostacyclin synthase
- Ristocetin
- Serotonin
- Splenic pool
- Storage pool disorders
- Subendothelial collagen
- Thrombopoietin (TPO)
- Thromboxane A2
- TPO receptor (*c-mpl* gene)
- Uremia
- Vitamin K—dependent coagulation factors
- von Willebrand disease (VWD)
- von Willebrand factor (VWF)

REVIEW QUESTIONS

1. Platelets express receptors for all following thrombosis-related molecules **except**
   A. collagen.
   B. thrombomodulin.
   C. VWF.
   D. fibrinogen.
   E. ADP

2. All of the following endothelial cell derived products inhibit thrombosis **except**
   A. ADPase.
   B. prostacyclin.
   C. Tissue factor.
   D. nitric oxide.

3. Which disorder below is due to platelet GPIIB/IX deficiency?
   A. Release defect
   B. Alpha granule deficiency
   C. Glanzmann thrombasthenia
   D. Bernard-Soulier syndrome

4. Which factor-function association is **incorrect**?
   A. ADP–platelet recruitment
   B. VWF–platelet binding
   C. Prostacyclin–platelet aggregation
   D. Serotonin–vasoconstriction

17

Benign Conditions of Lymphoid Organs

KEY POINTS

- Lymph nodes are composed of four major compartments: the cortical B cell–rich follicles, the paracortical T cell–rich interfollicular zone, the medullary region, and the sinusoidal compartment.

- Lymphoid hyperplasia may be classified according to the compartment and major cell type that is affected: B-cell follicular hyperplasia, T-cell paracortical hyperplasia, or histiocytic sinusoidal hyperplasia.

- *Lymphadenopathy* refers to any lymph node enlargement, whether caused by lymphoma, metastatic cancer, lymphoid or histiocytic hyperplasia, granulomatous disease, or infection.

- *Lymphadenitis* often refers to an acute painful form of lymph node enlargement (lymphadenopathy) seen with infection or necrosis.

- Clues as the cause of granulomatous lymphadenitis include the presence or absence of necrosis, the type of necrosis (caseating or noncaseating), the presence or absence of multinucleated giant cells, and the detection of microorganisms by a variety of techniques (including immunohistochemistry, polymerase chain reaction, culture, and serology).

- Benign causes of splenic enlargement (splenomegaly) include chronic passive congestion, infection, chronic hemolytic anemia, storage diseases, and vascular defects.

- *Hypersplenism* refers to any form of peripheral blood cytopenia caused by increased splenic sequestration or destruction of blood cells and is often accompanied by splenomegaly.

- Conditions leading to thymic enlargement include thymic hyperplasia (often seen in myasthenia gravis), hyperthyroidism, thymoma (usually benign tumor of thymic epithelium), and malignant lymphoma.

Lymph nodes constantly respond to antigens arriving from lymph and blood. However, in most instances, the antigen load is small and triggers only minimal transient enlargement of responding lymph nodes. Immune reactions that take place within lymph nodes often lead to follicular, paracortical, or both types of hyperplasia. **Follicular hyperplasia** results from proliferation of **germinal center (GC)** B cells within secondary follicles (Fig. 17.1), whereas **paracortical hyperplasia** results from proliferation of T cells within the interfollicular zone (Fig. 17.2). In some cases, reaction to antigen leads instead to a proliferation of histiocytes that remain confined to **lymphoid** sinuses, a process termed **sinus histiocytosis** (Fig. 17.3).

Significant enlargement of lymph nodes (>1 cm³) is generally considered abnormal and is termed **lymphadenopathy**. The most common causes of lymphadenopathy are infection, cancer (most commonly lymphoma), autoimmune disorders (rheumatoid arthritis and systemic lupus erythematosus [SLE]), and drug hypersensitivity (e.g., Dilantin). Lymphadenopathy may be classified as either localized or generalized.

Painful lymphadenopathy, often referred to as **lymphadenitis**, most often results from acute inflammation related to infection. Lymphadenitis is seen with all types of infection, including viruses (**Epstein-Barr virus** [EBV], cytomegalovirus, and human immunodeficiency virus [HIV]), bacteria (*Mycobacteria*, *Bartonella*, and

170

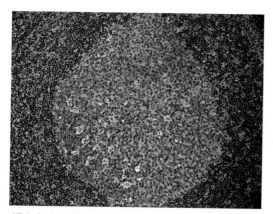

Fig. 17.1 A single large secondary lymphoid follicle with a central germinal center surrounded by an intact peripheral mantle zone (reactive follicular hyperplasia). Most lymphocytes in this field are CD20+ B cells (in both germinal center and mantle zone).

Fig. 17.2 Paracortical (interfollicular) hyperplasia with numerous small T lymphocytes and scattered large pale histiocytes.

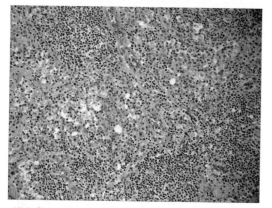

Fig. 17.3 Sinus histiocytosis (center) with numerous light pink histiocytes located within a dilated lymph node sinus. Note the peripheral aggregates of normal lymphoid tissue (top and bottom).

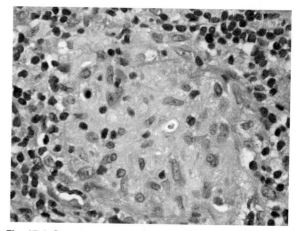

Fig. 17.4 Granulomatous lymphadenitis with a non-necrotizing granuloma (center of the field) composed of large epithelioid histiocytes surrounded by small lymphocytes.

Treponema spp.), fungi (*Histoplasma* and *Cryptococcus* spp.), and protozoa *(Toxoplasma gondii).*

Granulomatous lymphadenitis is characteristic of some infectious diseases; of the idiopathic condition sarcoidosis; and as a reaction to foreign materials such as talc, silica, and nylon suture. Granulomas are collections of activated macrophages (histiocytes) and CD4+ T lymphocytes that form in response to certain microbes, microbial products, foreign material, or keratinaceous debris (Fig. 17.4). The general idea is that granulomas form in response to antigenic material that cannot be effectively cleared from tissues. Granuloma formation has been shown in some experimental models to depend on a Th2 response and a variety of cytokines, including interferon-γ, transforming growth factor β, and tumor necrosis factor α. In many cases, fusion of macrophages leads to the formation of **multinucleated giant cells** (Fig. 17.5). Granulomas are generally classified as either necrotizing (as in tuberculosis and cat scratch disease) or non-necrotizing (as in sarcoidosis and toxoplasmosis). Necrosis can be further defined as either caseous or noncaseous necrosis. **Caseous necrosis** is devoid of identifiable cellular and nuclear debris and is particularly characteristic of **tuberculous lymphadenitis**. In tuberculosis, the caseous necrosis is accompanied by multinucleated giant cells with horseshoe-shaped arrangements of the nuclei known as **Langhans-type giant cells**. In contrast to infection with *Mycobacterium tuberculosis*, infection with atypical mycobacteria such as *Mycobacterium*

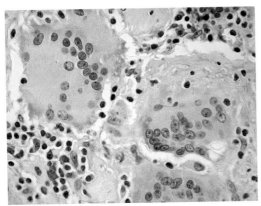

Fig. 17.5 Multinucleated giant cells formed by fusion of numerous mononucleated histiocytes.

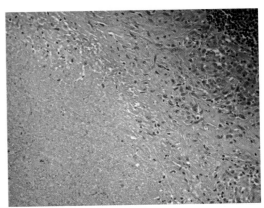

Fig. 17.7 Cat scratch lymphadenitis. Almost the entire field of view of this lymph node is obscured by a large granuloma with central eosinophilic necrosis *(bottom left)* surrounded by a layer of epithelioid histiocytes *(right)*. A small bit of normal lymphoid tissue is also present *(top right)*. Stains for the microorganism *(Bartonella henselae)* are seldom positive.

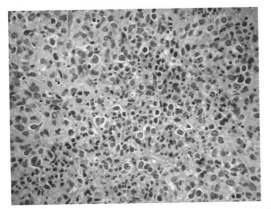

Fig. 17.6 Histiocytic necrotizing lymphadenitis (Kikuchi disease) with cellular nuclear debris (small, dark blue particles in the *center* of the field).

avium-intracellulare is more often characterized by non-necrotizing granulomas devoid of giant cells.

It is important to recognize that **necrotizing lymphadenitis** can also be seen in the absence of granulomas. Examples include bacterial and fungal infection, **SLE lymphadenitis**, and **Kikuchi-Fujimoto disease** (a rare idiopathic condition that is seen most commonly in young females) (Fig. 17.6).

Noncaseous necrosis, on the other hand, contains identifiable cell fragments and nuclear debris, often neutrophilic debris. **Cat scratch disease** presents as fever and painful localized lymphadenitis caused by infection by *Bartonella henselae*, a bacterium carried by healthy domestic cats. The infection is usually acquired by cat scratch or cat bite, with involvement of draining lymph nodes (often axillary). The lymph node contains numerous

large confluent granulomas with noncaseous necrosis and neutrophilic abscesses (Fig. 17.7). Aggregates of bacteria may be detected in tissue sections with the Warthin-Starry silver stain or by immunostaining with specific antibody (Fig. 17.8). In **syphilis** (*Treponema pallidum* infection), the necrosis is usually accompanied by increased plasma cells and capsular fibrosis. Silver staining of tissue sections highlights the characteristic elongated spiral-shaped bacteria.

Sarcoidosis is an idiopathic, often asymptomatic systemic condition commonly associated with hilar and mediastinal lymphadenopathy, as well as lung involvement. Affected lymph nodes contain numerous nonnecrotizing granulomas with multinucleated giant cells (Fig. 17.9). It is important to exclude all other known infectious causes of granulomatous disease before making this diagnosis.

Toxoplasmosis, caused by infection by the protozoan parasite *Toxoplasma gondii*, leads in most cases to nonnecrotizing granulomatous lymphadenitis, particularly involving cervical lymph nodes. *T. gondii* infection is often acquired by contact with infected cats (the definitive host), cat feces, or contaminated soil. The infection may also be acquired from other animals (mammals and birds) or from undercooked meats. *Toxoplasma* infection is widespread, with a seroprevalence rate in the United States of about 22%. The histology of **Toxoplasma lymphadenitis** is marked by follicular (B-cell) lymphoid hyperplasia, monocytoid B-cell aggregates, and clusters

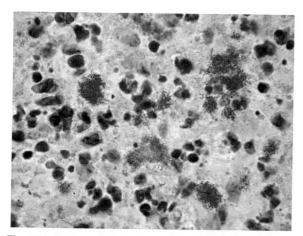

Fig. 17.8 Immunostain for *Bartonella henselae* in cat scratch disease. Note the large clumps of red-staining bacilli. In the first step of the immunostain procedure, the primary anti–*Bartonella* antibody (monoclonal mouse immunoglobulin [Ig] G) binds to the bacilli. In the second step, a secondary antimouse IgG that is covalently coupled to the enzyme horseradish peroxidase binds to the primary antibody. In the third step, a soluble, colorless peroxidase substrate is applied to the tissue section and is converted to an insoluble red-colored product that specifically deposits on the antibody-bound bacilli. In the fourth step, the tissue is counterstained with the nucleophilic dye hematoxylin to provide background staining of the cellular nuclei and nuclear debris. In many cases, a different peroxidase enzyme substrate is used to yield a golden brown (rather than red) color.

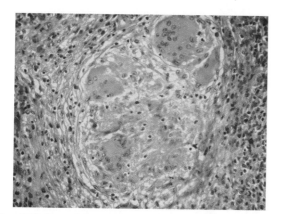

Fig. 17.9 Sarcoidosis with nonnecrotizing granulomas with several multinucleated giant cells.

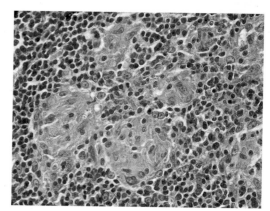

Fig. 17.10 *Toxoplasma* lymphadenitis with small aggregates of epithelioid histiocytes surrounded by small lymphocytes.

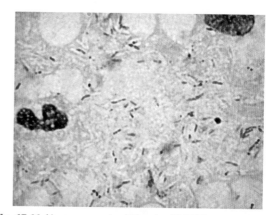

Fig. 17.11 Numerous red acid-fast bacilli (AFB) consistent with atypical mycobacterial infection (AFB stain). In AFB staining, a red dye (carbol fuchsin) that stains all cells (including all bacteria) is applied to the tissue section. This staining is followed by a destaining procedure in acid-alcohol that decolorizes all cells except acid-fast bacilli. A counterstain is applied to stain all other cells (including non–acid-fast bacteria) blue or purple. Mycobacteria do not decolorize because they contain the waxy substance mycolic acid in their cell walls. Acid-fast microorganisms include not only *Mycobacteria* spp. but also *Nocardia* spp. and fungi.

that often cluster together to form granulomas. *Toxoplasma* cysts may rarely be detected in hematoxylin and eosin–stained lymph nodes, and individual organisms can sometimes be detected by immunohistochemistry with *Toxoplasma*-specific antibody.

Acid-fast bacteria (mycobacteria and *Nocardia* spp.), fungi, and non–acid-fast bacteria can be identified in tissue sections by special histochemical stains (acid-fast bacilli stain; silver stain or periodic acid–Schiff; and tissue Gram stain, respectively) (Figs. 17.11 to 17.13).

of epithelioid histiocytes often within or adjacent to GCs (Fig. 17.10). Monocytoid B cells are marginal zone–like B cells with oval nuclei and abundant clear cytoplasm that resemble monocytes. Epithelioid histiocytes are large, activated macrophages with enlarged oval nuclei

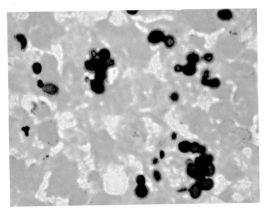

Fig. 17.12 Numerous *(black)* budding yeast forms *(Histoplasma capsulatum)* stained by the Grocott methenamine silver (GMS) stain. In the GMS stain, fungal wall mucopolysaccharides are oxidized and reacted with a methenamine–silver nitrate solution. The silver nitrate is reduced to yield a deposit of metallic silver on fungal walls and enhanced by treatment with gold chloride to allow for additional deposition of metallic gold. After counterstaining with a light green dye, fungi appear as black-colored yeast or filamentous forms.

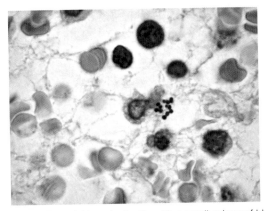

Fig. 17.13 Bacterial lymphadenitis with a small colony of blue, gram-positive cocci in the right center of the field. As with Gram stains applied to smears, gram-positive bacteria stain blue, and gram-negative bacteria stain pink-red.

Other infectious agents can be identified in tissue by immunohistochemical staining with specific antibody. In many cases, however, identification of the infectious agent requires culture and serology. Foreign materials (talc, silica, suture) that induce granuloma formation can often be identified as refractile material with the use of a microscope equipped with a polarizing filter.

Dermatopathic lymphadenitis is a relatively common cause of lymph node enlargement (often axillary or inguinal) that results from proliferation of Langerhans cells and T cells in the lymph node paracortex. Langerhans cells are immature CD1a+ dendritic cells located within the epidermis and mucosal epithelium that, upon encounter with antigen, migrate to regional lymph nodes, where they present antigen to paracortical T cells, leading to paracortical lymphoid hyperplasia (Figs. 17.14 and 17.15). Recent data indicate that Langerhans cells, unlike classic dendritic cells, may not be derived from bone marrow precursors and maintain

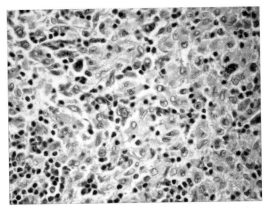

Fig. 17.14 Dermatopathic lymphadenitis. In this section of lymph node, there is a collection of large histiocyte-like dendritic cells with pink cytoplasm and convoluted, delicately folded nuclei (Langerhans cells) associated with melanin pigment-laden macrophages. The melanin-laden macrophages and Langerhans cells have migrated from the skin to the lymph node.

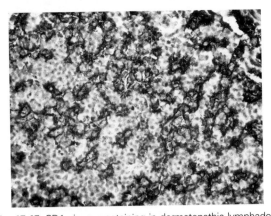

Fig. 17.15 CD1a immunostaining in dermatopathic lymphadenitis. Note the large number of brown-stained CD1a+ Langerhans cells. Langerhans cells are specialized dendritic cells that normally reside in skin and mucosa. Upon activation by antigen, Langerhans cells migrate via lymphatics to draining lymph nodes, enter the paracortical zone, and present antigen to T cells.

their number by local proliferation in the skin and mucosa. Virtually any inflammatory (particularly exfoliative) dermatologic process can lead to dermatopathic lymphadenitis. Dermatopathic lymphadenitis is also seen in cutaneous T-cell lymphoma (mycosis fungoides). The diagnosis of mycosis fungoides can be confirmed by detection of a monoclonal population of T cells with an aberrant CD3+ CD7− immunophenotype. In contrast to mycosis fungoides, the T cells in dermatopathic lymphadenitis are polyclonal, with CD3 and CD7 coexpression.

In **infectious mononucleosis**, cervical lymph nodes are marked by florid follicular and interfollicular B-cell hyperplasia with numerous large, EBV-positive immunoblasts (Fig. 17.16). **Castleman disease** is a rare benign idiopathic condition that in most cases (hyaline vascular variant) is associated with markedly enlarged lymph nodes with many small atretic GCs surrounded by concentric layers of mantle zone B cells (Fig. 17.17). The less common plasma cell variant of Castleman disease, commonly seen in HIV-infected patients, is marked by interfollicular plasmacytosis. **Progressive transformation of germinal centers (PTGC)** is another rare benign idiopathic form of lymphadenopathy marked histologically by significantly enlarged CD20+ lymphoid follicles with infiltration and disruption of GCs by mantle zone B cells (Fig. 17.18). PTGC is sometimes seen in association with nodular lymphocyte–predominant Hodgkin lymphoma. **Kimura disease** is an idiopathic condition marked by

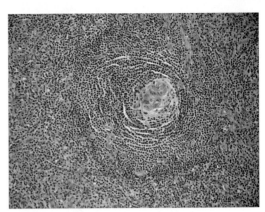

Fig. 17.17 A single abnormal germinal center with regressive features is noted in the *center* of the field. The germinal center displays hyaline vascular change and is surrounded by concentric rings of mantle cells. These changes are consistent with the hyaline vascular variant of the idiopathic condition known as Castleman disease.

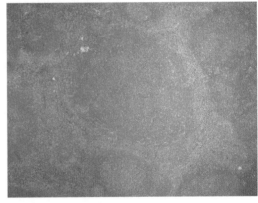

Fig. 17.18 Large irregular lymphoid follicle characteristic of progressive transformation of germinal centers.

large interfollicular aggregates of eosinophils that may sometimes undergo necrosis (Fig. 17.19).

SPLEEN

The spleen is a lymphoid organ located in the left upper quadrant of the abdominal cavity that is composed of two anatomic compartments: the red pulp and the white pulp.

The **red pulp** consists of a branching network of venous structures termed **splenic sinuses** separating cellular zones called **splenic cords**. The splenic cords contain

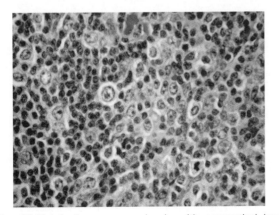

Fig. 17.16 Infectious mononucleosis with paracortical lymphoid hyperplasia. In this field, the large lymphoid cells with prominent nucleoli are activated B cells referred to as *B immunoblasts*. In this case, many of these immunoblasts were positive for Epstein-Barr virus.

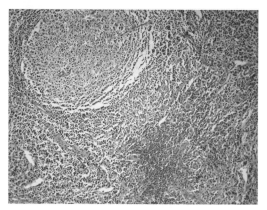

Fig. 17.19 Kimura disease with a large irregular infiltrate of eosinophils within the interfollicular zone *(lower right)*. Also note the reactive lymphoid follicle *(upper left)*.

numerous macrophages, as well as lymphocytes, plasma cells, granulocytes, and red blood cells (RBCs). Blood enters the spleen through the splenic artery; passes through central arteries, central arterioles, and arterial capillaries and then empties into the splenic cords. In the cords, the blood encounters resident phagocytic macrophages that remove debris, microorganisms, immune complexes, and damaged or aged blood cells. After passage through the cords, blood enters the splenic sinuses through specialized gaps (**fenestrations**) between endothelial cells. Blood then passes from the venous sinuses to the splenic vein and out to the inferior vena cava.

The **white pulp** consists of lymphoid tissue that surrounds the central arteries and arterioles. The white pulp is composed of a perivascular T cell–rich zone and an adjacent often prominent B cell–rich lymphoid follicle. Activated lymphoid follicles are composed of a GC, a mantle zone, and a specialized marginal zone that abuts the red pulp at the marginal sinus. Bloodborne antigens captured by marginal zone macrophages are likely presented to marginal zone (memory) B cells. **Marginal zone B cells** are antigen-primed memory B cells capable of rapidly producing immunoglobulin (Ig) G to commonly encountered bloodborne antigens in a T cell–independent fashion. Marginal zone B cells express high levels of the CD21 and CD35 complement receptors that presumably enhance the ability of marginal zone B cells to respond to small amounts of complement-bound (opsonized) antigen.

Pathologic enlargement of the spleen (**splenomegaly**) is seen in several hematologic neoplasms, including myeloproliferative disorders, leukemia, and lymphoma. Benign conditions leading to splenomegaly include **lysosomal storage disease** (e.g., Gaucher disease, Niemann-Pick disease), **infection** (mononucleosis, viral hepatitis, malaria, and tuberculosis), **granulomatous disease** (sarcoidosis), **chronic hemolytic anemia** (hereditary spherocytosis, thalassemia, sickle cell anemia, and pyruvate kinase (PK) deficiency), **chronic venous congestion**, **amyloidosis**, and **autoimmune disease**. Lysosomal storage diseases lead to accumulation of abnormal lipoid material within enlarged hyperplastic Kupffer cells, whereas indigestible amyloid protein is deposited in vascular walls. In hemolytic anemia, the massive RBC destruction in the spleen leads to chronic congestion and hypertrophy of the red pulp. Chronic venous congestion caused by right-sided heart failure, cirrhosis of the liver, or portal or splenic vein obstruction leads to congestive splenomegaly. In myeloproliferative disorders, the splenomegaly results from the compensatory production of blood cells in the spleen, a process termed **extramedullary hematopoiesis** (Fig. 17.20).

Patients with **hyposplenism** caused by asplenia or postsplenectomy are at increased risk of bacterial sepsis because of loss of splenic macrophage function. Common agents include *Staphylococcus pneumoniae*, *Haemophilus influenzae*, and *Neisseria meningitides*. In the

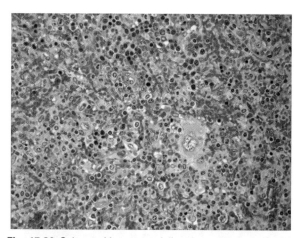

Fig. 17.20 Spleen with extramedullary hematopoiesis. In this field, the red pulp is effaced by scattered megakaryocytes (very large cell *right of center*), erythroid colonies (clusters of small cells with round, dark blue nuclei and pink cytoplasm at the *top* of the field), and scattered myeloid cells (pale-staining medium-sized cells with abundant clear cytoplasm noted throughout the field).

absence of spleen function, RBC inclusions of retained nuclear DNA, or **Howell-Jolly bodies**, are readily seen on Wright-stained peripheral smears. Under normal circumstances, these inclusions would be removed by splenic macrophages.

Hypersplenism is defined as a peripheral cytopenia (anemia, leukopenia, thrombocytopenia, or a combination of these) caused by excessive pooling of blood cells within an enlarged spleen (splenomegaly). The cause of the splenomegaly is almost always a readily identifiable pathologic process, such as chronic venous congestion associated with liver cirrhosis.

In idiopathic thrombocytopenic purpura (ITP), the spleen plays a central role in the removal and destruction of antibody-coated platelets, leading to thrombocytopenia. Although the spleen is typically not enlarged in ITP, microscopic examination reveals white pulp (lymphoid) hyperplasia with prominent GC formation and numerous red pulp macrophages that contain ingested platelets.

THYMUS

The thymus is a lymphoid organ located in the anterior mediastinum that is essential for T-cell selection and maturation. The thymus is composed of two anatomic compartments: the outer cortex and the inner medulla. Major cell types within the thymus include thymocytes (immature T cells), thymic epithelial cells, dendritic cells, and macrophages. **Hassall corpuscles** are distinctive structures in the adult thymic medulla that are composed of concentric whorls of degenerating thymic epithelial cells (Fig. 17.21). Thymic enlargement is seen with thymoma, thymic hyperplasia, and lymphoma. **Thymoma** is a usually benign epithelial tumor composed of varying proportions of cytokeratin-positive thymic epithelial cells and polyclonal CD3+ thymocytes (Fig. 17.22). Interestingly, up to 50% of thymomas are associated with the autoimmune disease myasthenia gravis. The skeletal muscle weakness seen with myasthenia gravis results from the development of autoantibodies to the acetylcholine receptor, a key component of the neuromuscular junction. Most patients with myasthenia gravis who do not develop thymoma develop **thymic hyperplasia**, a process marked by the formation of numerous B cell–rich secondary lymphoid follicles with prominent GCs. **Lymphomas** that arise in the thymic region include T lymphoblastic lymphoma, mediastinal large B-cell lymphoma, and Hodgkin lymphoma.

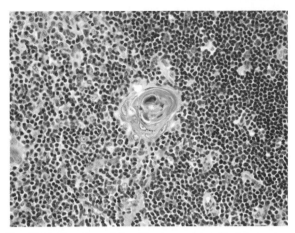

Fig. 17.21 Thymic medulla with a large pink epithelial structure with degenerative change known as a Hassall corpuscle. The Hassall corpuscle is a normal feature of the adult thymus and is derived from thymic epithelial cells. Recent evidence suggests that this structure is responsible for generation of thymus-derived regulatory (suppressor) T cells.

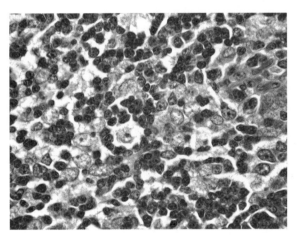

Fig. 17.22 Thymoma, a usually benign tumor of thymic epithelium composed of a variable admixture of small immature lymphoid cells (thymocytes) with basophilic nuclei and larger thymic epithelial cells with pale-staining nuclei. In some cases, it may be difficult to differentiate a lymphocyte-rich thymoma from a thymic lymphoblastic lymphoma.

KEY WORDS AND CONCEPTS

- Amyloidosis
- Autoimmune disease
- Caseous necrosis
- Castleman disease

- Cat scratch disease
- Chronic hemolytic anemia
- Chronic venous congestion
- Dermatopathic lymphadenitis
- Epstein-Barr virus (EBV)
- Extramedullary hematopoiesis
- Fenestrations
- Follicular hyperplasia
- Germinal center (GC)
- Granulomatous disease
- Granulomatous lymphadenitis
- Hassall corpuscles
- Howell-Jolly bodies
- Hypersplenism
- Hyposplenism
- Infection
- Infectious mononucleosis
- Kikuchi-Fujimoto disease
- Kimura disease
- Langhans-type giant cells
- Lymphadenitis
- Lymphadenopathy

- Lymphoid
- Lymphomas
- Lysosomal storage disease
- Marginal zone B cells
- Multinucleated giant cells
- Necrotizing lymphadenitis
- Paracortical hyperplasia
- Progressive transformation of germinal centers (PTGC)
- Red pulp
- Sarcoidosis
- Sinus histiocytosis
- SLE lymphadenitis
- Splenic cords
- Splenic sinuses
- Splenomegaly
- Syphilis
- Thymic hyperplasia
- Thymoma
- *Toxoplasma* lymphadenitis
- Toxoplasmosis
- Tuberculous lymphadenitis
- White pulp

REVIEW QUESTIONS

1. Which of the following benign lymph node conditions is associated with noncaseating granulomas?
   A. Cat scratch disease
   B. Sarcoidosis
   C. Dermatopathic lymphadenitis
   D. Mononucleosis

2. Which of the following pathogens is the causative agent of cat scratch disease?
   A. *Mycobacterium* spp.
   B. *Bartonella* spp.
   C. *Toxoplasma* spp.
   D. EBV

3. Which condition listed below is **not associated** with splenomegaly?
   A. Chronic liver disease
   B. Heart failure
   C. Bacterial sepsis
   D. Gaucher disease

4. Which peripheral blood finding is typically seen in asplenia?
   A. Howell-Jolly bodies
   B. Acanthocytes
   C. Dacrocytes
   D. Thrombocytopenia

18

Blood Transfusion and Stem Cell Transplantation

KEY POINTS

- Donor blood is collected and separated into red blood cell (RBC), platelet, granulocyte, and plasma fractions for transfusion into patients with severe anemia, thrombocytopenia, neutropenia, and bleeding, respectively.

- The ABH blood group antigens (A, B, and O) consist of a family of terminal oligosaccharide residues expressed by a variety of cell types, including RBCs.

- Acute hemolytic transfusion reactions are caused by incompatibility between the ABH blood group type of the blood donor and that of the recipient.

- The Rh blood group antigens (D, C, c, E, and e) derive from a family of integral membrane proteins.

- Hemolytic disease of the newborn results from transplacental migration of maternal anti-Rh(D) immunoglobulin (Ig) G to the Rh(D)-positive fetus, with consequent hemolytic anemia of the fetus.

- Delayed transfusion reactions triggered by recipient antibodies to non-ABO RBC antigens lead to low-grade hemolysis after a delay of 4 to 14 days posttransfusion.

- Febrile transfusion reactions caused by recipient antibodies to platelet or leukocyte antigens lead to a nonhemolytic febrile response that may persist for 12 hours posttransfusion.

- Allergic transfusion reactions result from a hypersensitivity reaction to transfused plasma proteins that leads to a variety of allergic manifestations, including pruritis, urticaria, bronchospasm, angioedema, and anaphylaxis.

- Anaphylactoid transfusion reactions are rare, often serious, conditions caused by transfusion of plasma IgA to patients with IgA deficiency.

- Transfusion-related acute lung injury is a serious condition caused by donor antibodies to leukocyte antigens that trigger neutrophil trapping in the pulmonary circulation with consequent acute respiratory distress.

- Autologous stem cell transplantation, although better tolerated than allogeneic transplantation, is suitable only in cases in which normal stem cells uncontaminated by tumor cells can be harvested from the patient.

- Unlike autologous stem cell transplantation, allogeneic stem cell transplantation may be complicated by graft failure, graft-versus-host disease, infection, and posttransplant lymphoproliferative disease.

- Human leukocyte antigen (HLA) is a large family of highly polymorphic cell surface glycoproteins encoded by a set of genes in the major histocompatibility complex locus.

- HLA class I molecules are expressed on nearly all cell types and normally present endogenous peptide antigens to immune cells.

- HLA class II molecules are normally expressed only on antigen-presenting cells and present exogenous antigen to immune cells.

- In an alloimmune reaction (as in an unmatched allogeneic transplant), recipient (or donor) T cells respond to donor (or recipient) cells.

- HLA matching of the donor and recipient is performed to maximize the odds of engraftment success, the best matches being identical twins or 100% HLA-matched siblings.

BLOOD TRANSFUSION

Blood obtained from healthy adult donors is collected and separated into several components for transfusion, including red blood cells (RBCs), platelets, plasma, and rarely, leukocytes (granulocytes). Laboratory tests performed on donor blood include blood typing (ABO and Rh), RBC antibody detection, hepatitis screening, and screening for the infectious agents hepatitis B virus, hepatitis C virus, human immunodeficiency virus, human T-cell lymphotropic virus, and syphilis. Cell fractions are usually stored in citrate phosphate dextrose adenine (**CPDA**) preservative, a solution containing citrate (anticoagulant), phosphate (buffer), dextrose (energy supply), and adenine (to maintain intracellular adenosine triphosphate). Citrate acts as an anticoagulant by binding to calcium, an essential cofactor in the coagulation cascade.

Preserved RBC concentrates maintain viability for up to 35 days, whereas stored platelet concentrates maintain viability for only about 5 days. Cold storage of plasma leads to depletion of coagulation factors V, VIII, and IX within 48 hours, and granulocyte function begins to decline 24 hours after granulocyte concentrate collection. Frozen storage of **packed RBCs**, platelet concentrates, and plasma significantly extends the shelf life of these blood products. Frozen storage of RBCs and platelets requires the addition of cryoprotective agents to prevent freeze-thaw–mediated cytolysis (glycerol for RBCs and dimethyl sulfoxide for platelets). Frozen storage of granulocytes is not routinely performed because post-thaw recovery of granulocytes rarely exceeds 25%.

The primary indications for transfusion of packed RBCs include severe anemia (hemoglobin >7 g/dL) and significant blood loss. In special circumstances, RBCs can be washed to remove plasma or filtered to remove leukocytes. **Washed RBCs** are used to minimize exposure of patients with hypersensitivity to plasma proteins to plasma protein and to minimize exposure of neonates to the effects of transfused anticoagulant, potassium, or both. **Leukocyte-poor RBCs** are provided to multitransfused patients to prevent febrile reactions in those who may have developed anti–**human leukocyte antigen (HLA)** antibodies to leukocytes and platelets and to immunocompromised patients to reduce the risk of transmission of bloodborne viruses.

Indications for **platelet transfusion** include severe thrombocytopenia (platelet count <5,000–10,000/μL) caused by marrow failure (aplastic anemia or after myelosuppressive therapy), and bleeding caused by idiopathic thrombocytopenic purpura, massive RBC transfusion, cardiopulmonary bypass, and inherited platelet function disorders.

Granulocyte transfusions are generally limited to patients with all of the following: (1) an absolute granulocyte count below 500/μL, (2) fever, (3) an identified responsible infectious agent, and (4) no fever reduction after 48 hours of appropriate antibiotic therapy. Leukocyte antigen matching is useful in minimizing febrile transfusion reactions and maximizing leukocyte half-life. To prevent serious cytomegalovirus (CMV) infection in immunosuppressed patients, granulocyte transfusions from CMV-negative donors are provided. **Graft-versus-host disease** induced by donor lymphocytes can be prevented by irradiation of granulocyte concentrates before administration to immunocompromised patients.

Citrated donor plasma is often frozen immediately after collection (**fresh-frozen plasma**) to preserve labile coagulation factors V and VIII, significantly extending the shelf life of this blood product. Indications for plasma transfusion include coagulation factor deficiencies (excluding factors VIII and IX), rapid reversal of warfarin-induced anticoagulation, plasma exchange for thrombotic thrombocytopenic purpura, bleeding with massive blood transfusion, bleeding caused by liver disease-related coagulopathy, and bleeding caused by disseminated intravascular coagulation (DIC).

Frozen plasma that is slowly thawed at 4°C forms a small amount of precipitated material termed **cryoprecipitate**. Cryoprecipitate is enriched in several procoagulant substances, including factor VIII, von Willebrand factor (VWF), fibrinogen, and factor XIII. Although cryoprecipitate can be used to treat deficiencies of any of these factors, its most common use is in treatment of hypofibrinogenemia. First-line therapies for hemophilia A and VWD are recombinant factor VIII and desmopressin (DDAVP), respectively. DDAVP, an analog of vasopressin, acts by enhancing the release of VWF from endothelial cells.

BLOOD GROUPS

Red blood cells (as well as other cell types) express a variety of highly variable cell surface glycoproteins and glycolipids, termed *blood group antigens*, that are capable of eliciting hemolytic immune reactions in patients transfused with unmatched allogeneic blood and in

Rh-positive fetuses carried by Rh-negative women exposed in a previous pregnancy to Rh-positive fetal blood at delivery. The two major blood group families include the ABO glycolipid antigens and the Rh glycoprotein antigens. ABO blood group includes types O, A, B, and AB, in that order of frequency. The **ABH blood group antigens** consist of a family of specific terminal oligosaccharides expressed by a variety of unrelated cell membrane proteins on a variety of cell types, including RBCs, glandular epithelium, and vascular endothelium. The ABH genetic locus encodes for two codominant alleles for glycosyltransferases A and B, and the O allele encodes for a nonfunctional gene. Thus, genotypes AA and AO yield blood type A, genotypes BB and BO yield blood type B, genotype AB yields blood type AB, and genotype OO yields blood type O. Blood type O individuals express the nonglycosylated base oligosaccharide antigen H.

Early in life, exposure to A- and B-like substances produced by bacteria in the gastrointestinal tract provoke the development of anti-A antibody in those with blood type B, anti-B antibody in those with blood type A, and both anti-A and anti-B antibody in those with blood type O. These antibodies are IgM in type and efficiently fix complement. Individuals of blood type AB produce neither anti-A nor anti-B antibody.

Because their RBCs express no A or B blood group antigens, individuals with blood type O (so-called universal donors) can safely donate packed RBCs to people of any other ABO blood because the H antigen is not recognized as a foreign antigen. However, people with blood type O can be transfused only with type O RBCs because they produce both anti-A and anti-B antibodies. Although individuals with blood type AB can donate RBCs only to people of blood type AB, they can receive RBCs of any other ABO blood type. Patients of blood type A can safely be given either type A or type O RBCs, and patients of blood type B can safely be given either type B or type O RBCs.

Transfusion of ABO-incompatible blood can trigger a life-threatening acute hemolytic process in the recipient. This event, called an **acute hemolytic transfusion reaction**, is triggered by binding of recipient ABO antibody and complement to donor RBCs with rapid intravascular hemolysis, DIC, and shock. Symptoms may include fever, hypotension, low back pain, chest tightness, nausea, and vomiting. Treatment consists of immediate termination of the transfusion, hydration, control of bleeding, and maintenance of renal function.

The second most important blood group system is the Rh system. Rh antigens are expressed on two proteins encoded by two closely related genes, one protein expressing the D antigen and the other expressing CcEe antigens.

The five **Rh blood group antigens** (D, C, E, c, and e) are expressed by two closely linked non-glycosylated integral membrane proteins, RhD and RhCE. Rh-positive individuals express both D (genotype DD or Dd) and CcEe antigens, whereas Rh-negative individuals (genotype dd) express only CcEe antigens. Most whites (85%) are RhD positive, with the three most common genetic haplotypes being CDe, cde, and cDE. Exposure of an RhD-negative individual to RhD-positive blood by transfusion or during pregnancy in most cases provokes formation of anti-D antibody of the IgG type. Similarly, IgG antibodies to RhC(c) and RhE(e) antigens may also form in C(c)- and E(e)-negative people, respectively.

The major clinical problem caused by Rh incompatibility, **hemolytic disease of the newborn**, is a hemolytic condition seen in Rh-positive newborns of Rh-negative mothers who have been previously sensitized to the D antigen by exposure to Rh-positive fetal blood in a previous pregnancy or to Rh-positive transfused blood. Asymptomatic transplacental passage of fetal blood occurs in most pregnancies, and as little as 0.5 mL of blood is sufficient to induce maternal sensitization. Maternal anti-D antibody crosses the placenta and causes hemolysis of fetal RBCs, leading to anemia, jaundice, and hepatosplenomegaly caused by extramedullary hematopoiesis. In severe cases, hepatosplenomegaly is accompanied by portal and umbilical vein hypertension, ascites, placental dysfunction, hypoproteinemia, generalized edema, and cardiac failure, a condition referred to as hydrops fetalis. Rh hemolytic disease of the newborn can be effectively prevented by administering Rh immune globulin (RhIg) shortly after delivery to the nonsensitized Rh-negative mother who gives birth to an Rh-positive infant. Although the mechanism of RhIg action is not known, the two most prevalent hypotheses are that RhIg binds to and inhibits immune reactivity to the D antigen on fetal RBCs and that RhIg induces D antigen-specific T-cell suppression. Transfusion-mediated exposure of Rh-negative people to Rh-positive blood also usually leads to production of anti-D antibody that can be associated with acute hemolytic transfusion reactions.

Although **ABO-associated hemolytic disease of the newborn** (type A or B offspring of type O mothers) is more common than Rh disease, it is generally a milder disease. This is because ABO antibodies are usually of the IgM type and do not cross the placenta, whereas IgG Rh antibodies do cross the placenta. Both ABO and Rh antibodies are non–complement fixing antibodies that bind to RBCs and lead to their removal from the circulation via phagocytosis by Fc receptor–bearing splenic macrophages, a process termed *extravascular hemolysis*. In contrast, binding of RBCs by complement-fixing antibody leads to complement-mediated intravascular hemolysis. In contrast to extravascular hemolysis, intravascular hemolysis leads to hemoglobinemia and indirect hyperbilirubinemia.

TRANSFUSION REACTIONS

Delayed hemolytic transfusion reactions, occurring 4 to 14 days after transfusion, are also seen in response to the RBC antigens Kell, Kidd, and Duffy, which like Rh are usually provoked by prior transfusion or pregnancy. Clinical findings may include falling hemoglobin and jaundice. Diagnosis can often be confirmed with a positive **direct (Coombs) antiglobulin test** result, in which antibody-coated RBCs agglutinate in the presence of anti-IgG. In contrast to the direct antiglobulin test, the **indirect (Coombs) antiglobulin test** is used to detect antibodies to RBCs in patient serum. The incidence of delayed transfusion reactions in recipients who require multiple transfusions can be minimized by transfusing blood matched not only for ABO but also for major non-ABO antigens, as noted earlier.

A common type of transfusion reaction is the non-hemolytic **febrile transfusion reaction** caused by recipient antibodies to donor leukocyte or platelet alloantigens elicited by prior transfusions. Fever may persist for 12 hours after transfusion. Most of these reactions can be prevented by transfusion of (filtered) leukocyte-poor blood. In some cases, it may be necessary to type platelet or leukocyte alloantigens of donors to maximize the effectiveness of transfused platelets or leukocytes in previously sensitized recipients.

Some of the most commonly encountered platelet alloantigens are polymorphic determinants expressed by the fibrinogen–VWF receptor glycoprotein (GP) IIb/IIIa (CD41/CD61).

The leukocyte alloantigens most important in transfusion (and transplantation) medicine are the highly polymorphic **HLA class I molecules** (A, B, and C), which are expressed on nearly all cell and tissue types. The HLA I molecules are membrane glycoproteins composed of heterodimers of polymorphic alpha heavy chains and the invariant beta light chain, β_2-microglobulin. HLA I molecules bind and present endogenous peptide antigens to CD8+ T cells and are critically important in initiation of an immune response to foreign antigens and altered self. During an alloimmune response, immune cells recognize and respond to the non–self-HLA I molecule as if it were a self-HLA bound to a foreign (or abnormal self) peptide.

In contrast to the near-ubiquitous expression of HLA I molecules, **HLA class II molecules** (DP, DQ, and DR) are normally expressed only on B cells, monocytes (macrophages and dendritic cells), endothelial cells, and activated T cells. HLA II molecules are heterodimeric membrane glycoproteins composed of alpha heavy chains and beta light chains, both of which are polymorphic in HLA-DP and HLA-DQ (the alpha chain in HLA-DR is invariant). The function of HLA II molecules is in presentation of exogenous peptide antigens (derived from ingested material) to CD4+ T cells. During an alloimmune reaction, immune cells recognize and respond to a non–self-HLA II molecule as if it were a self-HLA bound to an exogenous peptide.

Allergic transfusion reactions caused by transfused plasma proteins are also fairly common. Although the usual symptoms of generalized pruritus and urticaria respond to oral antihistamines, more serious symptoms (i.e., bronchospasm, angioedema, and anaphylaxis) require parenteral epinephrine.

A rare but often serious **anaphylactoid transfusion reaction** may be seen in patients with **IgA deficiency**. The anaphylactoid reaction, characterized by chills, dyspnea, abdominal cramps, nausea, vomiting, and hypotension, results from formation of immune complexes of recipient anti-IgA with donor IgA. Patients with IgA deficiency who require blood transfusion can safely be given washed or frozen RBCs that are rendered free of donor plasma.

Transfusion-related acute lung injury (TRALI) is the most common cause of transfusion-related fatality. TRALI is characterized by acute respiratory distress with pulmonary edema and hypoxemia occurring within 6 hours of blood transfusion that is unrelated to volume overload or cardiac failure.

The pathogenesis of TRALI involves binding of activated neutrophils to activated alveolar capillary endothelial cells, leading to neutrophil trapping in the pulmonary

TABLE 18.1 Transfusion Reactions

Type	Antigen	Symptoms
Acute hemolytic	ABO blood group	Fever, shock, DIC
Delayed hemolytic	Non-ABO blood group	Anemia, jaundice
Febrile	Leukocyte or platelet	Fever
Allergic	Plasma protein	Pruritus, urticaria
Anaphylactoid	IgA	Chills, hypotension, dyspnea, abdominal distress
TRALI	Leukocyte or endothelial	Acute respiratory distress

DIC, Disseminated intravascular coagulation; *Ig,* immunoglobulin; *TRALI,* transfusion-related acute lung injury.

circulation, release of toxic neutrophil oxidants, and acute alveolar injury. The substances that trigger TRALI include donor-derived leukocyte antibodies and bioactive lipids. Leukocyte antibodies associated with TRALI may be directed against neutrophil-specific alloantigens or HLAs expressed by both neutrophils and endothelial cells. Bioactive lipids, which activate neutrophils, are formed as a result of breakdown of leukocytes and platelets in stored blood. Patients most at risk for TRALI include those with recent surgery, active infection, cardiovascular disease, and leukemia, presumably caused by preactivated neutrophils, endothelial cells, or both. Donor blood obtained from multiparous women (exposed multiple times to paternal leukocyte antigens by the fetus) is most often implicated in TRALI. Given the higher leukocyte antibody content of plasma in comparison with cell concentrates, transfused fresh-frozen plasma from multiparous women is particularly troublesome. Therefore, many blood banks produce fresh-frozen plasma from male donors whenever possible (Table 18.1).

STEM CELL TRANSPLANTATION

Stem cell transplantation is a potentially curative treatment for hematolymphoid malignancies. Stem cell transplantation is highly effective because it allows for delivery of very-high-dose marrow-toxic (myeloablative) therapy to eradicate tumor followed by stem cell rescue. Myeloablation often consists of high-dose chemotherapy with alkylating agents (e.g., cyclophosphamide or busulfan) with or without total-body irradiation.

Sources of stem cells for transplantation include bone marrow, growth factor–mobilized peripheral blood, and umbilical cord blood. Peripheral blood stem cell donors are pretreated with growth factors (granulocyte- or macrophage colony-stimulating factor, interleukin-3, thrombopoietin [TPO], or C-X-C chemokine receptor type 4 antagonist) that induce proliferation and release of marrow stem cells into the peripheral circulation. Umbilical cord blood, like marrow, normally contains stem cells. In any case, stem cells represent a small proportion of the nucleated cells from these sources. Stem cells express several specific cell surface proteins, including CD34, which mediates adhesion to marrow stroma; c-kit receptor, which induces stem cell proliferation; CD133, which induces development of cell membrane protrusions; and c-mpl, the TPO receptor, which promotes stem cell growth. The number of stem cells can be quantified by flow cytometry using fluorescent antibodies to CD34. In some cases, stem cells can be further enriched by flow sorting or with anti-CD34 immunomagnetic beads. Successful marrow transplantation typically requires approximately 5 to 10 million CD34+ stem cells per kilogram of body weight.

In **allogeneic transplantation** for leukemia, protection against residual tumor recurrence is provided by the **graft-versus-leukemia effect**. This effect is a result of a low-grade, T cell–mediated immune response of allogeneic T cells to minor histocompatibility antigens expressed by residual tumor cells that survive high-dose myeloablative chemotherapy.

Autologous stem cell transplantation is better tolerated than allogeneic stem cell transplantation because it does not require posttransplant immunosuppression for prevention of rejection and is not subject to graft-versus-host disease. However, for patients with primary marrow disorders, including aplastic anemia, leukemia, myelodysplastic syndromes, and myeloproliferative disorders, autologous transplantation is inappropriate because normal stem cells are abnormal or markedly reduced in number. In contrast, for patients with lymphoma in which marrow stem cells are normal, autologous transplantation is preferred. Because residual tumor cells may be present in autologous stem cell collections, techniques have been developed for purging of tumor cells by antibody- or complement-mediated removal of tumor cells and enrichment of CD34+ stem cells.

COMPLICATIONS OF ALLOGENEIC STEM CELL TRANSPLANTATION

Acute graft-versus-host disease (aGVHD) occurs less than 100 days posttransplant and is characterized by immune-mediated damage to skin, gastrointestinal tract, and liver by donor T cells reacting to unmatched histocompatibility antigens. aGVHD prophylaxis consists of an immunosuppressant (e.g., cyclosporine or tacrolimus) with the folate antagonist methotrexate. **Chronic graft-versus-host disease (cGVHD)** occurs more than 100 days posttransplant and presents with autoimmune-like symptoms similar to those of the connective tissue disorders scleroderma and dermatomyositis. Treatment consists of immunosuppressive drugs. Patients with cGVHD are also at risk of infection, often by gram-positive bacteria, presumably as a result of immune deficiency.

Bacterial infections occur during periods of severe neutropenia and most often result from gram-positive bacteria. For prophylaxis, broad-spectrum antibiotics are administered to febrile neutropenic patients. Because life-threatening **fungal infections** with *Candida* and *Aspergillus* spp. are also seen in the neutropenic posttransplant setting, antifungal prophylaxis is used in some cases. **Viral infections** are common in the posttransplant setting. One of the most serious viral illnesses in the posttransplant setting is CMV-associated interstitial pneumonitis. Other viral illnesses include those caused by herpes simplex virus, varicella-zoster virus, and Epstein-Barr virus (EBV).

The **posttransplant lymphoproliferative disorders (PTLDs)** are a group of disorders characterized by an abnormal, often clonal proliferation of activated, usually EBV-infected lymphoid cells (B cells > T cells) leading to fever, generalized lymphadenopathy, and damage to vital organs. Factors associated with increased risk of PTLD include pretransplant EBV seronegativity of the recipient and use of high-dose posttransplant immunosuppression.

Other complications of stem cell transplantation include mucositis, bleeding caused by thrombocytopenia, and veno-occlusive disease of the liver.

HUMAN LEUKOCYTE ANTIGENS

The HLAs are a family of highly polymorphic cell surface glycoproteins encoded for by a set of related genes on chromosome 6, collectively referred to as the **major histocompatibility complex (MHC)** locus. There are two major classes of HLAs: class I and class II. There are three classic types of HLA I molecules (A, B, and C) and three types of HLA II molecules (DP, DQ, and DR). Everyone inherits two co-dominant alleles at each locus. Currently, there are more than 100 recognized classic HLA molecules.

The ideal allogeneic stem cell donor is an identical twin or an HLA-matched sibling. The chance of a complete (haploidentical) match between two siblings is 25%. However, in most cases, identical twin or haploidentical sibling donors are not available. In these cases, an HLA-matched unrelated donor is sought.

In addition to the three classic types of HLA I molecule (HLA-A, HLA-B, HLA-C), there are three non-classic HLA types (**HLA-E, HLA-F, and HLA-G molecules**). These antigens are less polymorphic and more restricted in tissue distribution than the classic types (A, B, C) and thus play a minor role in transplantation.

The HLA I phenotype of donors and recipients is determined by a serologic assay known as the microcytotoxicity assay. In this assay, small aliquots of donor (or recipient lymphocytes) are placed in wells with a large panel of HLA-specific antibodies and complement. The pattern of lymphocyte cytotoxicity (cell death) induced by the antibodies defines the HLA phenotype of the cells. The HLA II phenotype of donors and recipients is determined by the mixed lymphocyte reaction assay. In this assay, viable donor or recipient lymphocytes are cocultured with a panel of homozygous typing cells (of known HLA II phenotype) rendered incapable of cell division. Lymphocytes sharing the same HLA type with the typing cells do not proliferate, whereas lymphocytes that differ in HLA type do proliferate. These serologic and cellular assays are quickly becoming supplanted by more rapid and refined flow cytometric and molecular approaches to HLA typing.

A stem donor–recipient pair is a complete match if all 12 MHC alleles are identical. In this case, it is likely that the allogeneic stem cell transplant will not initiate graft-versus-host disease or be subject to rejection.

KEY WORDS AND CONCEPTS

- ABH blood group antigens
- ABO-associated hemolytic disease of the newborn

- Acute graft-versus-host disease (aGVHD)
- Acute hemolytic transfusion reaction
- Allergic transfusion reactions
- Allogeneic transplantation
- Anaphylactoid transfusion reaction
- Autologous stem cell transplantation
- Bacterial infections
- Chronic graft-versus-host disease (cGVHD)
- CPDA
- Cryoprecipitate
- Delayed hemolytic transfusion reactions
- Direct (Coombs) antiglobulin test
- Febrile transfusion reaction
- Fresh-frozen plasma
- Fungal infections
- Graft-versus-host disease
- Graft-versus-leukemia effect

- Granulocyte transfusions
- Hemolytic disease of the newborn
- HLA class I molecules
- HLA class II molecules
- HLA class E, F, and G molecules
- Human leukocyte antigens (HLAs)
- IgA deficiency
- Indirect (Coombs) antiglobulin test
- Leukocyte-poor RBCs
- Major histocompatibility complex (MHC)
- Packed RBCs
- Platelet transfusion
- Post-transplant lymphoproliferative disorders (PTLDs)
- Rh blood group antigens
- Transfusion-related acute lung injury (TRALI)
- Viral infections
- Washed RBCs

REVIEW QUESTIONS

1. Patients with which blood type are considered universal donors?
   A. A positive
   B. Rh positive
   C. AB positive
   D. O positive

2. Which donor antigen source induces febrile transfusion reactions?
   A. RBCs
   B. Leukocytes or platelets
   C. Plasma proteins
   D. IgA

3. Which of the following statements about TRALI is **false**?
   A. TRALI is triggered by leukocyte and platelet antibodies in donor plasma.

   B. TRALI presents with acute pulmonary thrombosis.
   C. TRALI is often seen with use of fresh-frozen plasma from multiparous women.
   D. TRALI is triggered by bioactive lipids in donor blood.

4. Graft-versus-host disease seen after stem cell transplantation is characterized by all of the following **except**
   A. dermatomyositis-like skin changes.
   B. mucositis.
   C. gram-negative bacterial infection.
   D. CMV-positive interstitial pneumonitis.
   E. veno-occlusive disease of the liver.

19

Hematologic Cancer Therapy

KEY POINTS

- Many forms of cancer chemotherapy are designed to inhibit tumor cell proliferation by interfering with DNA synthesis.

- Cancer chemotherapeutic agents can be classified as cell-cycle active agents and non–cell-cycle active agents; cell-cycle agents target actively proliferating cells, whereas non–cell-cycle agents target tumor cells, regardless of their proliferative status.

- Combination chemotherapy is designed both to simultaneously target cycling and noncycling tumor cells and to minimize the risk of emergence of a

- tumor clone that may be refractory to treatment with a single agent alone.

- Chemotherapy-related toxicity is common; cell-cycle active agents in particular are associated with damage to highly proliferative normal tissues such as bone marrow and gastrointestinal tract.

- Newer agents with less toxic side effects include therapeutic monoclonal antibodies targeted to tumor cell–specific antigens, small molecule inhibitors to oncoproteins, and immune checkpoint inhibitors.

Most traditional forms of cancer chemotherapy are designed to interfere with DNA replication and thus prevent cell proliferation. Although use of these agents is complicated by toxic effects on normal tissues, the relative resistance of normal cells, including marrow stem cells, to toxicity perhaps results from a very low proliferation rate and unimpaired ability to detect and repair drug-induced DNA damage. Rapidly dividing normal tissues, such as mucosal epithelium and bone marrow, are particularly susceptible to damage by antineoplastic agents. Toxic effects of chemotherapy on normal tissues, including mucositis and leukopenia, often limit maximum dosage. Combination chemotherapy is designed to reduce the probability of successful clonal selection by using different mechanisms of action, with nonoverlapping mechanisms of resistance and toxic effects. Many agents require dose reduction in patients with preexisting hepatic or renal dysfunction. Drug metabolism is impaired in patients with liver disease, and urinary excretion of drugs and metabolites is reduced in those with renal disease.

Chemotherapeutic agents can be broadly classified into cell-cycle active agents and non–cell-cycle active agents (Fig. 19.1). Cell-cycle active agents kill actively proliferating cells, whereas non–cell-cycle active agents kill both proliferating and resting cells. One approach to combination chemotherapy is to treat patients with a combination of a cell-cycle active agent and a non–cell-cycle active agent.

CELL-CYCLE ACTIVE AGENTS

The folic acid analog methotrexate is a **dihydrofolate reductase inhibitor** that interferes with DNA synthesis by blocking the conversion of deoxyuridine monophosphate to deoxythymidine monophosphate. **Purine and pyrimidine analogs** (cytosine arabinoside and 6-mercaptopurine) interfere with normal DNA synthesis by incorporation of abnormal nucleotides into DNA. The **adenosine deaminase inhibitor** pentostatin leads to toxic accumulation of deoxyadenosine triphosphate, negative feedback on ribonucleotide reductase, and

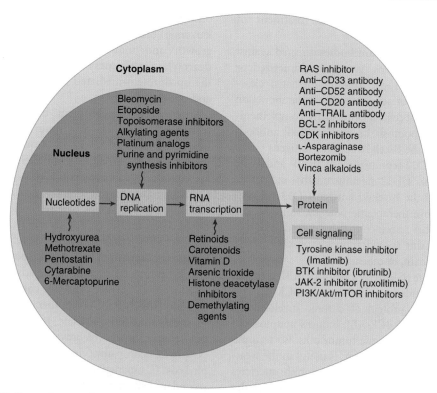

Fig. 19.1 Chemotherapeutic agents: Cellular sites of action. *BTK*, Bruton tyrosine kinase; *CDK*, cyclin-dependent kinase; *JAK*, Janus kinase; *mTOR*, mammalian target of rapamycin; *PI3K*, phosphoinositide 3-kinase.

interference with DNA synthesis. The direct **ribonucleotide reductase inhibitor** hydroxyurea blocks DNA synthesis by reducing the supply of deoxynucleotides. Compounds that bind tubulin (the vinca alkaloids vincristine and vinblastine, as well as taxanes) block cell division by inhibiting **mitotic spindle formation**. Topoisomerases are enzymes that normally allow for unwinding of supercoiled DNA during DNA replication. By interfering with DNA unwinding, **topoisomerase inhibitors** (campothecins, epipodophyllotoxins, and anthracyclines) prevent repair of DNA strand breaks. **Bleomycin** kills tumor cells by inducing multiple DNA strand breaks via oxidative damage. **L-Asparaginase** kills rapidly growing tumor cells by depleting their stores of asparagine, an essential amino acid.

NON–CELL-CYCLE ACTIVE AGENTS

Alkylating agents, including nitrogen mustards (e.g., cyclophosphamide), nitrosoureas (e.g., bischloroethyl nitrosourea), and methylating agents (e.g., dacarbazine),

interfere with DNA function by cross-linking or methylating DNA. **Platinum analogs** (cisplatin and carboplatin) kill tumor cells by forming metal adducts with DNA. **Cell maturational agents** (retinoids, carotenoids, vitamin D, and arsenic trioxide) act by inducing differentiation and cell death of neoplastic cells. In particular, tretinoin (all-*trans* retinoic acid [ATRA]) induces differentiation of neoplastic promyelocytes in acute promyelocytic leukemia.

The cytidine analogs (5-azacytidine and 5-azadeoxycytidine) are **demethylating agents** that act by inhibiting DNA methyltransferase and unblocking gene expression of hypermethylated (presumably antioncogenic) genes in cancer cells. These agents have been useful in the treatment of patients with myelodysplastic syndromes.

Interferon-α (IFN-α) kills tumors by directly inhibiting tumor cell growth, boosting the immune response, and inhibiting angiogenesis. Corticosteroids are **lymphocytotoxic agents** useful in the treatment of patients with lymphoid malignancies. **Thalidomide**, presumably because of inhibition of angiogenesis and

T-cell activation, is effective in the treatment of patients with myeloma.

Therapeutic monoclonal antibodies directed against hematologic tumor antigens have been chimerized or humanized to prevent rapid immune-mediated clearance. The mechanism of action appears to be induction of antibody-dependent cellular cytotoxicity, complement-mediated lysis, and apoptosis. Examples include antibodies directed against the B-cell lymphoma antigens CD20 (rituximab) and CD22 (epratuzumab), the B- and T-cell lymphoma antigens CD52 (alemtuzumab) and CD25 (daclizumab), and the myeloid antigen CD33 (gemtuzumab). To improve therapeutic potency, some monoclonal antibodies have been conjugated to radioisotopes (^{131}I or ^{90}Y) or toxins (pseudomonas exotoxin, ricin A chain, diphtheria toxin, or calicheamicin).

Imatinib mesylate (Gleevec), a synthetic **ABL tyrosine kinase inhibitor**, binds to and inhibits the BCR-ABL tyrosine kinase fusion protein of chronic myelogenous leukemia. Inhibition of BCR-ABL induces apoptosis of chronic myelogenous leukemia tumor cells. Bortezomib (Velcade), a **proteasome inhibitor**, is useful in the treatment of patients with myeloma. Bortezomib interferes with proteasome-mediated degradation of intracellular ubiquitinated proteins. Proteasome inhibition leads to increased levels of the cell-cycle inhibitor p53 and the nuclear factor (NF) κB inhibitor IκB. p53 leads to tumor cell growth arrest, and IκB blocks NFκB-mediated tumor cell growth stimulation and resistance to apoptosis.

Newer, promising antitumor strategies include antisense oligonucleotides or small molecule inhibitors to the apoptosis inhibitor Bcl-2, antibodies to the **tumor necrosis factor–related apoptosis-inducing ligand (TRAIL) death receptor** (inducing tumor cell death), inhibitors to promitotic cyclin-dependent kinases, **farnesyltransferase (*Ras* oncogene) inhibitors**, heat shock protein inhibitors, and histone deacetylase inhibitors.

Heat shock proteins are "molecular chaperones" produced in response to cell injury that repair and protect cell proteins from irreversible damage. Heat shock protein inhibitors sensitize tumor cells to the damaging effects of cytotoxic chemotherapy. Chromosomal DNA that is tightly bound to nonacetylated histone proteins is unavailable for transcription (closed chromatin). Focal histone acetylation by histone acetyltransferases loosens the bound DNA and allows for transcription (open chromatin). Histone deacetylase blocks transcription by reversing histone acetylation and closing the chromatin. By recruiting histone deacetylase, some oncoproteins (e.g., PML-RARα in acute promyelocytic leukemia) block transcription of genes that inhibit cell growth and induce differentiation. Thus, **histone deacetylase inhibitors** block cancer growth by undoing the oncoprotein-mediated block on growth inhibition and cell differentiation.

One recent development in personalized cancer treatment is the use of **chimeric antigen receptor-bearing T cells (CAR-T)** to provoke strong tumor-specific T cell-mediated cytotoxicity. Patient T cells are collected, genetically modified to express chimeric tumor-specific antigen receptor, expanded ex-vivo, and re-infused in the patient. The chimeric receptor is composed of an immunoglobulin antigen-specific binding domain (VH-VL) linked to a T cell transmembrane activation domain. The CAR-T specifically recognize and kill tumor cells, without the adverse side effects so often seen with classic cytotoxic chemotherapy.

Major toxicities of chemotherapy include myelosuppression, mucositis, cardiac toxicity (anthracyclines), pulmonary fibrosis (bleomycin and alkylating agents), peripheral neuropathy (vinca alkaloids and taxanes), anaphylaxis (L-asparaginase), tumor lysis syndrome, and secondary leukemia (alkylating agents, hydroxyurea, and etoposide). ATRA therapy of acute promyelocytic leukemia is sometimes complicated by the **retinoic acid syndrome**, a disorder characterized by fever, altered mental status, respiratory failure, and hyperleukocytosis (Table 19.1 and Box 19.1).

Chemotherapy of large bulky tumors often leads to hyperuricemia, caused by large amounts of uric acid derived from nucleic acids released from dying tumor cells. To prevent uric acid–induced renal failure, the drug **allopurinol**, a **xanthine oxidase** inhibitor, is administered. Xanthine oxidase catalyzes the conversion of hypoxanthine to uric acid. Hypoxanthine is more soluble than uric acid and does not form renal tubular precipitates. **Rasburicase**, a recombinant form of uricase, is also effective in preventing uric acid nephropathy by catalyzing the oxidation of uric acid to the more soluble metabolite allantoin which is freely excreted in the urine. **Leucovorin** (5-formyltetrahydrofolate) is a reduced form of folic acid that is administered shortly after high-dose methotrexate to minimize methotrexate-mediated damage to normal tissues. Leucovorin is effective in this setting because it does not require reduction by dihydrofolate reductase, the enzyme inhibited by methotrexate.

Tumor lysis syndrome is a potentially lethal side effect of massive chemotherapy-induced tumor cell death.

TABLE 19.1 Chemotherapeutic Agents for Nonlymphoid Heme Malignancy

Mechanism	Agents	Effect
Folic acid antagonist	Methotrexate	Inhibits DNA synthesis
Nucleoside analog	6-Mercaptopurine	Inhibit DNA synthesis
	Cytosine arabinoside	
Adenosine deaminase inhibitor	Pentostatin	Inhibits DNA synthesis
Ribonucleotide reductase inhibitor	Hydroxyurea	Inhibits DNA synthesis
Tubulin inhibitor	Vinca alkaloids	Inhibit mitotic spindle formation
Topoisomerase inhibitors	Campothecins	Prevent DNA strand break repair
	Epipodophyllotoxins	
	Anthracyclines	
DNA complex formation	Bleomycin	Induce DNA strand breaks
Topo-2 inhibition	Doxorubicin	
Asparagine depletion	L-Asparaginase	Cell growth inhibition
DNA alkylation	Cyclophosphamide	DNA cross-linking
DNA intercalation	Carboplatin	Formation of metallic adducts
Cell maturation agents	Retinoids	Maturation-induced cell death
	Carotenoids	
	Vitamin D	
	Arsenic trioxide	
Immune response activator	Interferon	Inhibits tumor growth
Lymphocytotoxicity	Corticosteroids	Induce tumor cell death
Antiangiogenic agent	Thalidomide	Inhibits tumor growth
Tumor antigen binding	Gemtuzumab	Antibody-mediated cytotoxicity
Tyrosine kinase inhibitor	Imatinib	Blocks BCR-ABL oncoprotein
Proteasome inhibitor	Bortezomib	p53- and IκB-mediated tumor cell growth arrest
Topoisomerase-2 (TOPO-2) inhibitor	Etoposide	DNA strand breakage
	Daunorubicin	
Inhibition of DNA repair	Etoposide	Tumor cell DNA damage
Histone deacetylase inhibitor	Vorinostat	DNA strand breakage
Histone methyltransferase inhibitor		EZH2 inhibition
DNA demethylation	Decitabine	Suppressor oncogene inhibition

BCR-ABL; EZH2; TOPO-2, Topoisomerase-2.

BOX 19.1 Chemotherapeutic Agents for Lymphoid Heme Malignancy

B-cell receptor signaling (SYK, BTK) inhibitors
BCL2 inhibitors
Immune checkpoint inhibitors (PD-1, CTLA-4)
PI3K/AKT/mTOR inhibitors
JAK–STAT pathway inhibitors
Immune modulators (lenalidomide)
Chimeric antigen receptor T cells (CAR-T)
Epigenetic modifiers (HDAC, DNA demethylase)
Combination chemotherapy (e.g., ABVD)
Antibody–drug conjugates

ABVD, Adriamycin, bleomycin, vinblastine, and dacarbazine; BTK, Bruton tyrosine kinase; CTLA-4, cytotoxic T lymphocyte–associated protein 4; HDAC, histone deacetylase; JAK, Janus kinase; mTOR, mammalian target of rapamycin; PD-1, programmed cell death protein 1; PI3K, phosphoinositide 3-kinase; STAT, signal transducer and activator of transcription.

Tumor cell lysis is accompanied by release of cell constituents, including potassium, phosphate, and nucleic acids into the bloodstream, leading to hyperuricemia, hyperkalemia, hyperphosphatemia, and hypocalcemia, followed in some cases by acute renal failure.

KEY WORDS AND CONCEPTS

- ABL tyrosine kinase inhibitor
- Adenosine deaminase inhibitor
- Allopurinol
- L-Asparaginase
- Bleomycin
- Cell maturational agents
- Demethylating agents
- Dihydrofolate reductase inhibitor

- Farnesyltransferase (*Ras* oncogene) inhibitors
- Heat shock proteins
- Histone deacetylase inhibitors
- Interferon-α (IFN-α)
- Leucovorin
- Lymphocytotoxic agents
- Mitotic spindle formation
- Platinum analogs
- Proteasome inhibitor
- Purine and pyrimidine analogs
- Rasburicase
- Retinoic acid syndrome
- Ribonucleotide reductase inhibitor
- Thalidomide
- Therapeutic monoclonal antibodies
- Topoisomerase inhibitors
- Tumor necrosis factor–related apoptosis-inducing ligand (TRAIL) death receptor
- Tumor lysis syndrome
- Xanthine oxidase

REVIEW QUESTIONS

1. Features of retinoic acid syndrome include all the following **except**
   A. fever.
   B. altered mental status.
   C. respiratory failure.
   D. leukopenia.

2. Which of the following chemotherapeutic agents acts by blocking formation of the mitotic spindle?
   A. Hydroxyurea
   B. Cisplatin
   C. Vincristine
   D. Bleomycin

3. Oxidation of uric acid by rasburicase yields what product that is freely excreted in the urine, thus preventing uric acid nephropathy seen with chemotherapy-induced tumor lysis?
   A. Allantoin
   B. Hypoxanthine
   C. Urobilin
   D. Folic acid

Answers to Review Questions

CHAPTER 2

1. C
2. B
3. E
4. D

CHAPTER 3

1. C
2. B
3. E
4. C

CHAPTER 4

1. A
2. B
3. C
4. A

CHAPTER 5

1. A
2. D
3. C
4. B

CHAPTER 6

1. C
2. D
3. C
4. A

CHAPTER 7

1. C
2. B
3. C
4. D

CHAPTER 8

1. A
2. C
3. B
4. D

CHAPTER 9

1. B
2. B
3. D

CHAPTER 10

1. B
2. B
3. A
4. C
5. D

CHAPTER 11

1. B
2. C
3. A
4. A

CHAPTER 12

1. B
2. D
3. C
4. B

CHAPTER 13

1. B
2. D
3. C
4. A

CHAPTER 14

1. B
2. D
3. A
4. C
5. D

CHAPTER 15

1. D
2. B
3. C
4. A
5. D

CHAPTER 16

1. B
2. C
3. D
4. C

CHAPTER 17

1. B
2. B
3. C
4. A

CHAPTER 18

1. D
2. B
3. B
4. C

CHAPTER 19

1. D
2. C
3. A

Complete Blood Count

As judged by the frequency with which it is ordered, the complete blood count (CBC) is the most useful clinical laboratory test. The test is usually performed on (sodium citrate or sodium ethylenediaminetetraacetic acid [EDTA]) anticoagulated whole blood by automated determination of the red blood cell (RBC) count, hemoglobin concentration, hematocrit, mean corpuscular volume (MCV), mean corpuscular hemoglobin, mean corpuscular hemoglobin concentration, RBC distribution width, leukocyte (white blood cell) count, platelet count, mean platelet volume, and a five-part leukocyte differential that includes neutrophils, lymphocytes, monocytes, eosinophils, and basophils. Newer models of instruments also enumerate reticulocytes, nucleated RBCs, immature granulocytes, and reticulated (immature) platelets. Normal adult values and clinical significance of CBC results are presented in Tables Appendix B.1 and Appendix B.2.

After automated processing, Wright-stained blood smears may be prepared for morphologic review. RBC abnormalities that can be detected by blood smear microscopic examination include hypochromia, polychromasia, macrocytosis, microcytosis, anisocytosis (RBC size variation), poikilocytosis (RBC shape variation), cytoplasmic inclusions (hemoglobin C crystals, Howell-Jolly bodies, and so on), intracellular microorganisms (*Plasmodia* or *Babesia* spp.), nucleated RBC, rouleaux formation, and agglutination (Table Appendix B.3). Leukocyte abnormalities that can be detected on Wright-stained peripheral smears include abnormal segmentation (hyposegmented or hypersegmented neutrophils), abnormal cytoplasmic granulation ([toxic] hypergranulation, hypogranulation), cytoplasmic inclusions, intracellular microorganisms, and immature forms (Table Appendix B.4). **Pelger-Huët anomaly** is an autosomal dominant condition marked by hyposegmented (monolobated or bilobated) neutrophils that results from mutations in the ***Lamin B receptor* gene** on chromosome 1q42. The lamin B receptor plays a role in maintenance of the nuclear membrane. Homozygous disease is often accompanied by skeletal abnormalities. This anomaly is also seen as an acquired condition (acquired [or pseudo-] Pelger-Huët anomaly) in acute leukemia and myelodysplasia. In the mucopolysaccharidoses, leukocytes may contain large deep lilac-colored granular inclusions known as the **Alder-Reilly anomaly**. **Chediak-Higashi anomaly** is a

TABLE APPENDIX B.1 Complete Blood Count Normal Values in Adults

Parameter	Value	Unit of Measure
Red blood cell count	4 million–5 million	/μL
Hemoglobin concentration	12–17	mg/dL
Hematocrit	36–50	%
Mean corpuscular volume	80–98	fl
Mean corpuscular hemoglobin	27–34	pg
Mean corpuscular hemoglobin concentration	32–36	g/dL
Red blood cell distribution width	12–15	%
White blood cell count	4000–11,000	/μL
Platelet count	140,000–450,000	/μL
Mean platelet volume	9–12	fl
Neutrophil count	1500–7500	/μL
Lymphocyte count	1000–3500	/μL
Monocyte count	200–900	/μL
Eosinophil count	0–400	/μL
Basophil count	0–200	/μL
Reticulocyte count	0.4–1.8	%

TABLE APPENDIX B.2   Complete Blood Count Findings: Related Diseases

Parameter	Increased	Decreased
Red blood cell count	Polycythemia	Anemia
Hemoglobin	Polycythemia	Anemia
Hematocrit	Polycythemia	Anemia
Mean corpuscular volume	Macrocytic anemia	Iron deficiency, thalassemia
Mean corpuscular hemoglobin	Macrocytic anemia	Iron deficiency, thalassemia
Mean corpuscular hemoglobin concentration	Spherocytosis	Iron deficiency, thalassemia
Red blood cell distribution width	Anisocytosis (Fe-def > thalassemia trait)	No disease association
Platelet count	Inflammation, infection, myeloproliferative disorders	ITP, DIC, marrow failure
Neutrophil count	Infection, inflammation, leukemia	Increased risk of bacterial or fungal infection (<500/μL)
Lymphocyte count	Infectious mononucleosis, pertussis, CLL, ALL	Acute viral infection, sepsis, corticosteroid therapy, stress, congenital immunodeficiency
Monocyte count	Chronic inflammatory disease, chronic infection, CMML	Hodgkin lymphoma
Eosinophil count	Allergy, parasitic infection	Corticosteroids
Basophil count	Sinusitis, myeloproliferative disorder	Hyperthyroidism, pregnancy
Reticulocyte count	Hemolysis, blood loss	Marrow failure

ALL, Acute lymphoblastic leukemia; *CLL,* chronic lymphocytic leukemia; *CMML,* chronic myelomonocytic leukemia; *DIC,* disseminated intravascular coagulation; *ITP,* idiopathic thrombocytopenic purpura.

TABLE APPENDIX B.3   Common Red Blood Cell Morphologic Abnormalities

Abnormality	Disease Associations
Hypochromic microcytes	Iron deficiency, thalassemia
Macrocytes	Megaloblastic anemia, alcoholism, liver disease, myelodysplasia
Intracellular microorganisms	*Plasmodia* or *Babesia* spp. infection
Nucleated red blood cells	Asplenia, hemolytic anemia, sideroblastic anemia
Spherocytes	Hereditary spherocytosis, autoimmune hemolytic anemia
Dacrocytes (teardrops)	Myelofibrosis, thalassemia
Sickle cells	Sickle cell anemia
Hemoglobin C crystals	Hemoglobin C disease
Target cells	Thalassemia, hemoglobin C disease, iron deficiency, liver disease
Elliptocytes	Hereditary elliptocytosis, iron deficiency
Schistocytes	Microangiopathic hemolytic anemia, TTP
Acanthocytes	Liver disease, TTP
Reticulocytes (increased)	Hemolytic anemia, blood loss

TTP, Thrombotic thrombocytopenic purpura.

rare autosomal recessive disease characterized by albinism, increased risk of infection, and enlarged azurophilic granules in neutrophils. **Auer rods** are large needlelike azurophilic granules often seen in circulating myeloblasts in acute myelogenous leukemia. **Dohle bodies,** loose light blue cytoplasmic aggregates of rough endoplasmic reticulum in neutrophils, are often seen in the setting of acute infection. Dohle body–like RNA-rich inclusions are also characteristic of the **May-Hegglin anomaly,** an autosomal dominant condition marked by giant platelets, leukocyte inclusions, and variable thrombocytopenia.

TABLE APPENDIX B.4   Common Leukocyte Morphologic Abnormalities

Abnormality	Disease Associations
Hyposegmentation	Myelodysplasia, AML, Pelger-Huët anomaly
Hypersegmentation	Megaloblastic anemia
Toxic granulation	Acute inflammation or infection
Cytoplasmic inclusions	Parasites (*Ehrlichia* spp., *Anaplasma* spp.), abnormal granules (Chediak-Higashi, Alder-Reilly, Auer rods), RNA aggregates (Dohle bodies, May-Hegglin)
Immature myeloid cells (absent-rare blasts)	Infection, inflammation, CML
Immature and atypical monocytes	CMML
Atypical lymphocytes	Infectious mononucleosis
Myeloblasts, mono-blasts, promyelocytes	Acute myelogenous leukemia
Lymphoblasts	ALL

ALL, Acute lymphoblastic leukemia; *AML*, , acute myelogenous leukemia; *CML*, chronic myelogenous leukemia; *CMML*, chronic myelomonocytic leukemia.

Mean platelet volume is in most circumstances directly proportional to platelet age, with larger platelets being more immature. Mean platelet volume is decreased in conditions associated with decreased platelet production, as in aplastic anemia, and increased in conditions in which platelets are being destroyed peripherally, as in idiopathic thrombocytopenic purpura. Some inherited diseases are associated with abnormalities in platelet size. Small platelets are seen in **Wiskott-Aldrich syndrome**, an X-linked disorder marked by eczema, thrombocytopenia, and immune deficiency. Large platelets are seen in May-Hegglin anomaly and **Bernard-Soulier syndrome**, an autosomal recessive bleeding disorder caused by deficiency of the von Willebrand factor (VWF) receptor glycoprotein Ib.

An alternative and arguably more accurate measure of platelet age than mean platelet volume is reticulated platelets. Reticulated platelets are young (presumably large) platelets that retain a network of rough endoplasmic reticulum. Reticulated platelets can be detected in an automated cell counter after staining with the RNA-binding fluorescent dye thiazole orange.

AGE- AND PREGNANCY-RELATED HEMATOLOGIC CHANGES

Some hematologic parameters in healthy newborns, young children, pregnant women, and older adults differ from those in healthy young children and adults. Whereas hemoglobin concentration is increased in newborns (mostly hemoglobin F), it is decreased in pregnant women and older adults. To meet additional blood requirements for the placenta, maternal blood volume increases. The increase in plasma volume exceeds the increase in RBC mass, thus leading to **physiologic anemia of pregnancy**. In normal pregnancies, a mild increase in neutrophil count, sometimes accompanied by immature myeloid cells (bands, metamyelocytes, myelocytes, or a combination of these), is sometimes noted.

Because of increased RBC fragility and subsequent hemolysis, the RBC lifespan in newborns is only 60 to 80 days (compared with 120 days in adults), leading to a mild increase in reticulocytes compared with adults, and rare nucleated RBCs may be seen in the first few days of life. **Physiologic anemia of the newborn**, seen in the first few days of life, peaks about day 5, with steady improvement thereafter. Given the increased percentage of young RBCs in newborns, the MCV is increased. Infants and children up to the age of 4 years have an increased lymphocyte count compared with that of older children and adults.

The MCV may also be increased in older adults, perhaps related to mild deficiency of folic acid or vitamin B_{12}. Although the neutrophil count does not vary significantly with age, neutrophil function in older adults is impaired, with reduced phagocytic and oxidative ability. Functional lymphocyte defects are also noted in older adults. In particular, circulating T lymphocytes from older adults exhibit reduced ability to proliferate in response to antigen, a phenomenon sometimes referred to as *immune senescence*. Immune senescence has also been described in patients with chronic viral infection, human immunodeficiency virus infection in particular.

The bone marrow in newborns and young children is more cellular (80%) compared with that in adults (50%–60%). In contrast, marrow cellularity in older adults (older than 70 years) is normally reduced (20%–30%) compared with that in young adults. Although no significant age-related differences in the myeloid-to-erythroid ratio are seen, the number of small lymphocytes is increased in the marrow of young children compared with that of adults.

AGE- AND PREGNANCY-RELATED COAGULATION CHANGES

Because liver synthetic function in the newborn period is reduced in comparison with adults, levels of some coagulation factors (factors II, IX, X, XI, and XII) are reduced in newborns. In contrast, VWF levels are increased in newborns. During pregnancy, levels of coagulation factors II, VII, VIII, IX, and X and of VWF are increased, likely contributing to an increased thrombosis risk. Coagulation factors II, VII, and VIII and VWF

are also increased in older adults, possibly because of chronic inflammation.

KEY WORDS AND CONCEPTS

- Alder-Reilly anomaly
- Auer rods
- Bernard-Soulier syndrome
- Chediak-Higashi anomaly
- Dohle bodies
- *Lamin B receptor* gene
- May-Hegglin anomaly
- Pelger-Huët anomaly
- Physiologic anemia of pregnancy
- Physiologic anemia of the newborn
- Wiskott-Aldrich syndrome

Some Useful Immunophenotypic Markers for Hematologic Diagnosis

Name	Function	Normal Cell Expression	Useful Disease Associations
CD1a	MHC-like class I	Thymocytes, dendritic cells	T lymphoblastic malignancy, Langerhans cell histiocytosis
CD2	Adhesion molecule	T cells, NK cells	T/NK cell malignancy
CD3	Part of TCR complex	T cells	T-cell malignancy
CD4	MHC class II co-receptor	T-cell subset, monocytes	T-cell malignancy
CD5	Unknown	T cells, B-cell subset	CLL/SLL, mantle cell lymphoma
CD7	Unknown	Marrow stem cells, thymocytes, T cells	T-cell malignancy
CD8	MHC class I co-receptor	T-cell subset, NK cells	T/NK cell malignancy
CD10	Zinc metalloproteinase	B- and T-cell precursors	B lymphoblastic malignancy, follicular lymphoma, Burkitt lymphoma
CD13	Zinc metallopeptidase	Granulocytes, monocytes	Acute myeloid leukemia
CD14	LPS receptor	Monocytes, granulocytes	Acute (myelo)monocytic leukemia
CD15	Lewis^x trisaccharide	Granulocytes, monocytes	Hodgkin lymphoma
CD16	IgG Fc receptor	NK cells, macrophages, neutrophils	NK cell malignancy
CD19	Associated with BCR complex	B cells	B-cell lymphoma, B lymphoblastic malignancy
CD20	Calcium channel	B cells	B-cell lymphoma
CD21	C3d receptor	Mature B cells, follicular dendritic cells	Marginal zone lymphoma, FDC sarcoma
CD22	Sialoconjugate receptor	B cells	B-cell lymphoma
CD23	Low-affinity IgE receptor	B cells, monocytes, dendritic cells	CLL/SLL
CD25	IL-2 receptor alpha chain	Activated T and B cells, monocytes	ATLL, hairy cell leukemia
CD30	TNF-like receptor	Activated T, B, and NK cells; monocytes	Anaplastic large cell lymphoma, Hodgkin lymphoma
CD33	Carbohydrate lectin	Granulocytes, monocytes	Acute myeloid leukemia
CD34	Sialomucin	Hematopoietic stem cells, endothelial cells	Acute myeloid leukemia, lymphoblastic leukemia
CD38	Nicotinamide adenine dinucleotide glycohydrolase	B cells, activated T cells, plasma cells	Plasma cell myeloma, lymphoplasmacytic lymphoma
CD41	Platelet glycoprotein IIb	Platelets, megakaryocytes	Acute megakaryoblastic leukemia
CD42	von Willebrand receptor	Platelets, megakaryocytes	Acute megakaryoblastic leukemia
CD43	Leukosialin	All lymphocytes except resting B cells	CLL/SLL, mantle cell lymphoma, MALT lymphoma

Continued

Name	Function	Normal Cell Expression	Useful Disease Associations
CD45	Tyrosine phosphatase	All leukocytes and precursors	Hodgkin lymphoma (negative RS cells)
CD55	Complement inhibitor	All blood cells	PNH (decreased)
CD56	Neural cell adhesion molecule–like adhesion	NK cells, T-cell subset	T/NK cell malignancy
CD57	Oligosaccharide	NK cells, monocytes, T- and B-cell subsets	T/NK cell malignancy
CD59	Complement inhibitor	All blood cells	PNH (decreased)
CD61	Fibrinogen receptor	Platelets, megakaryocytes	Acute megakaryoblastic leukemia
CD68	Lysosomal protein	Monocytes, macrophages	Acute monocytic leukemia
CD71	Transferrin receptor	Erythroid cells	Erythroleukemia
CD79a	Part of BCR complex	B cells	B-cell lymphoma, plasma cell myeloma
CD103	Integrin	Lymphocyte subset	Hairy cell leukemia
CD117	SCF receptor	Immature hematopoietic cells, mast cells	Acute myeloid leukemia, mastocytosis
CD123	IL-3 receptor alpha	Stem cells, mast cells, plasmacytoid dendritic cells	Blastic plasmacytoid dendritic cell neoplasm
CD138	Heparan sulfate proteoglycan	B cells, plasma cells	Plasma cell myeloma
CD163	Hemoglobin scavenger receptor	Monocytes, macrophages	Histiocytic sarcoma
CD206	Mannose receptor	Monocytes, macrophages	Histiocyte-rich tumors
ALK	Tyrosine kinase receptor	Neural development	Anaplastic large cell lymphoma
BCL-2	Apoptosis inhibitor	Non-GC B cells, T cells	Follicular lymphoma (negative)
BCL-6	Transcriptional repressor	GC B cells	Follicular lymphoma, diffuse large B-cell lymphoma
Cyclin D1	G1-to-S cell cycle transition	Endothelial cells, histiocytes	Mantle cell lymphoma
Glycophorin A	MN blood group antigen	Erythroid cells	Erythroleukemia
Granzyme B	Cytotoxic enzyme	Cytotoxic T cells, NK cells	Cytotoxic T/NK cell lymphomas
MPO	Superoxide or hypochlorous acid formation	Myeloid cells	Acute myeloid leukemia
MUM-1	Transcription factor	Post-GC B cells, plasma cells	B-cell lymphoma, Hodgkin lymphoma, plasma cell myeloma
PAX-5	B-cell differentiation	B cells	B-cell lymphoma, Hodgkin lymphoma
Perforin	Induces cell lysis	Cytotoxic T cells, NK cells	Cytotoxic T/NK cell lymphomas
S-100	Multifunctional	Dendritic cells	Langerhans cell histiocytosis
SOX11	Nuclear transcription factor	Rare nonhematopoietic cells (cytoplasmic only)	Mantle cell lymphoma
TdT	Antigen receptor gene modification	Immature T and B cells	Lymphoblastic malignancy

ATLL, Adult T-cell leukemia/lymphoma; *BCR,* B cell receptor; *CLL,* chronic lymphocytic leukemia; *GC,* germinal center; *Ig,* immunoglobulin; *IL,* interleukin; *LPS,* lipopolysaccharide; *MALT,* mucosa-associated lymphoid tissue; *MHC,* major histocompatibility complex; *MPO,* myeloperoxidase; *NK,* natural killer; *PNH,* paroxysmal nocturnal hemoglobinuria; *RS,* Reed-Sternberg; *SCF,* stem cell factor; *SLL,* small lymphocytic lymphoma; *TCR,* T-cell receptor; *TdT,* terminal deoxynucleotidyl transferase; *TNF,* tumor necrosis factor.

Page numbers followed by "f" indicate figures, "t" indicate tables, and "b" indicate boxes.

A

ABH blood group antigens, 180–181
ABL tyrosine kinase inhibitor, 188
ABO-associated hemolytic disease of the newborn, 182
ABO blood group, 180–181
Acanthocytes, 194t
Acetylsalicylic acid, 165
Acid elution test, 38, 38f
Acid-fast bacilli, 173–174, 173f
Acid gel electrophoresis, 38–39
Acidosis, 30–31
Acquired hemophilia, 155
Acquired hemophilia A, 155
Acquired neutropenia, 66–67
Activated partial thromboplastin time, 155, 157, 160
Activated protein C resistance, 158
Activation-induced cytidine deaminase, 80–81
Acute erythroid leukemia, 112–113, 113f
Acute graft *versus* host disease, 184
Acute hemolytic transfusion reaction, 181
Acute intermittent porphyria, 26–28
Acute lymphoblastic leukemia, 107, 107t, 114f
  B cell, 114, 115f
  clinical presentation of, 114
  genetic defects in, 101
  intrathecal chemotherapy for, 109, 115–116
  key points about, 114–116
  T cell, 115
  treatment of, 115–116
Acute megakaryoblastic leukemia, 113–114, 113f
Acute monocytic leukemia, 109, 112, 113f
Acute myelogenous leukemia, 100t, 107
  functional groups of gene mutations in, 108t
  minimally differentiated (agranular) myeloblasts in, 111f
  myeloperoxidase-positive myeloid blasts in, 112f
Acute myeloid leukemia, 109
  blast cell characteristics, 111f
  features of, 107, 107t
  gene mutations associated with, 110–111
  genetic defects in, 101
  key points about, 109–114
  with maturation, 111
  with minimal differentiation, 111
  with multilineage dysplasia, 111
  mutations in, 111
  with 11q23 abnormalities, 110
  subtypes, 110
  without maturation, 111

Acute myelomonocytic leukemia, 109, 112, 112f
Acute promyelocytic leukemia, 109, 110, 110f
ADAMTS13, 152, 157
Adenoids, 89–92
Adenosine deaminase deficiency, 87
Adenosine deaminase inhibitor, 186–187
Adenosine diphosphate, 164
Adenylate cyclase, 165
Adult ITP, 167–168
Adult T cell leukemia/lymphoma, 143–144, 144f
Affinity maturation, 80–81
Agarose gel protein electrophoresis, 156
Albumin, 45
Alder-Reilly anomaly, 193–194
Alkaline gel electrophoresis, 38–39
Allantoin, 115–116
Allelic exclusion, 103
Allergic reaction, 68–69, 69f
Allergic transfusion reactions, 182
Alloantigens, 182
Allogeneic stem cell transplantation, 109, 183
  complications of, 184
Allopurinol, 115–116, 188
All-*trans* retinoic acid, 187
Alpha granules, 165
Alpha naphthyl acetate esterase (ANAE), 6
Alpha naphthyl acetate esterase-positive granulocytes, 13
Alpha naphthyl butyrate esterase, 6
Alpha naphthyl butyrate esterase-positive monocytes, 13, 14f
Alpha thalassemia, 35, 36t
Alternative pathway, complement, 82–83
Amegakaryocytic thrombocytopenia, 53
Aminolevulinic acid synthase, 26, 28f
Amyloidosis, 140, 140f
Amyloidosis A, 140
Anaphylactoid transfusion reaction, 182
Anaphylatoxins, 82
Anaplastic large cell lymphoma, 143, 143f
Anaplastic lymphoma kinase 1, 143
Anemia
  in adrenal insufficiency, 54
  aplastic. See Aplastic anemia
  causes of, 26, 26f, 27t
  of chronic disease, 30, 30f
  of chronic renal failure, 53–54
  classification of, 26, 27t
  congenital dyserythropoietic, 119
  of endocrine disease, 54
  hemolytic. See Hemolytic anemia
  in hypothyroidism, 54
  iron deficiency, 23–25

Anemia *(Continued)*
  of liver disease, 54
  megaloblastic, 56–59
  refractory, with excess blasts, 100–101
  sideroblastic, 120
Anergy, 79–80
Angioimmunoblastic T cell lymphoma, 142t, 144
Anisopoikilocytosis, 36–37
Antibody feedback mechanism, 81
Anticoagulation, 158–159
Antigen-binding fragment, 82
Antigens, blood group, 180–181
Anti-neutrophil antibodies, 53
Antiphospholipid antibody, 160–161
Antiphospholipid syndrome, 158
Antisense oligonucleotides, 188
Antithrombin III
  coagulation effects, 159
  deficiency of, 158
  description of, 153, 157
Anti-Xa test, 159
Aorto-gonado-mesonephros region, 4
AP-1, 83–84
Apaf-1, 99
Aplastic anemia, 52f
  Diamond-Blackfan anemia, 53
  drugs that cause, 51
  Fanconi anemia, 52
  hereditary, 52
  idiopathic, 51
  pure red cell aplasia, 52
Apoferritin, 22–23
Apoptosis, 98–99
  flippase inactivation in, 29–30
  mitochondrial-mediated, 99
  pathways of, 98–99, 98f
  triggers of, 98–99
Apoptosis inhibitor, 137–138
Apotransferrin, 30
Arachidonic acid, 165
L-Asparaginase, 186–187
Aspirin, 165
Asthma, 67–68
Atypical chronic myelogenous leukemia, 125
Auer rods, 111, 112f, 193–194
Autoantibody, 48
Autoimmune hemolytic anemia, 46–47
  cold, 47–48
  spherocytes in, 48f
  warm, 47–48
Autoimmune lymphoproliferative syndrome, 98–99
Autoimmune regulator, 78
Autologous stem cell transplantation, 183